CANCER
THERAPIES

MARGARET BARTON-BURKE, PhD, RN
Assistant Professor
University of Massachusetts
Amherst, Massachusetts

GAIL M. WILKES, MSN, RNC
Oncology Nurse Practitioner and Clinical Instructor
Boston Medical Center
Boston, Massachusetts

JONES AND BARTLETT PUBLISHERS
Sudbury, Massachusetts
BOSTON   TORONTO   LONDON   SINGAPORE

World Headquarters

Jones and Bartlett Publishers
40 Tall Pine Drive
Sudbury, MA 01776
978-443-5000
info@jbpub.com
www.jbpub.com

Jones and Bartlett Publishers
Canada
6339 Ormindale Way
Mississauga, Ontario L5V 1J2
CANADA

Jones and Bartlett Publishers
International
Barb House, Barb Mews
London W6 7PA
UK

Jones and Bartlett's books and products are available through most bookstores and online booksellers. To contact Jones and Bartlett Publishers directly, call 800-832-0034, fax 978-443-8000, or visit our website at www.jbpub.com.

Substantial discounts on bulk quantities of Jones and Bartlett's publications are available to corporations, professional associations, and other qualified organizations. For details and specific discount information, contact the special sales department at Jones and Bartlett via the above contact information or send an email to specialsales@jbpub.com.

Library of Congress Cataloging-in-Publication Data
Barton-Burke, Margaret.
    Cancer therapies / Margaret Barton-Burke, Gail Wilkes.
       p. ; cm.
    Includes bibliographical references and index.
    ISBN 0-7637-2682-6 (pbk.)
    1. Cancer—Treatment.   I. Wilkes, Gail M. II. Title.
    [DNLM: 1. Neoplasms—therapy. QZ 266 B293c 2006]
    RC270.8.B37 2006
    616.99'406—dc22
                                                2005023403

6048

Production Credits
Executive Publisher: Christopher Davis
Associate Editor: Kathy Richardson
Production Director: Amy Rose
Production Editor: Renée Sekerak
Marketing Manager: Emily Ekle
Manufacturing Buyer: Amy Bacus
Composition: GGS Book Services
Cover and Text Design: Anne Spencer
Printing and Binding: Malloy, Inc.
Cover Printing: Malloy, Inc.

Printed in the United States of America
10 09 08 07 06   10 9 8 7 6 5 4 3 2 1

CONTENTS

Chapter 4 Biologic Therapy for Cancer Treatment 117

Paula M. Muehlbauer, R.N., M.S.N., O.C.N.®

Chapter 5 Molecular Targeted Therapy 181

Gail M. Wilkes, M.S.N., R.N.C.

Chapter 6 Hematopoietic Stem-Cell Transplantation 215

Janice P. Maienza, R.N., M.S.N., A.O.C.N.

Chapter 7 Cancer Therapy in Malignant and Nonmalignant Conditions: Safety and Administration Issues 255

Ann Marie B. Peterson, R.N., M.S., C.N.S., and Margaret Barton-Burke, Ph.D, R.N.

Chapter 8 Drug Interactions with Antineoplastic Medications 289

Michael Steinberg, Pharm. D., B.C.O.P

Appendix I Standardized Nursing Care Plans 311

Index 351

Margaret Barton-Burke, PhD, RN
  Assistant Professor of Nursing
  University of Massachusetts
  Amherst, MA

Janice P. Maienza, RN, MSN, AOCN
  Clinical Nurse Specialist
  Tufts New England Medical Center
  Boston, MA

Paula M. Muehlbauer, MSN, RN, OCN
  Oncology Clinical Nurse Specialist
  National Institute of Health Clinical Center
  Nursing Department
  Bethesda, MD

Ann Marie B. Peterson, RN, MS, CNS
  National Institutes of Health Clinical Center
  Bethesda, MD

Michael Steinberg, PharmD, BCOP
  Assistant Professor of Pharmacy Practice
  Massachusetts College of Pharmacy and
  Health Sciences
  Worcester, MA

Gail M. Wilkes, MSN, RNC
  Oncology Nurse Educator/Nurse Practitioner
  Boston Medical Center
  Boston, MA

Linda Workman, PhD, RN, FAAN
  Nursing Specialist
  Case Western Reserve
  Cleveland, OH

DURING THE PAST DECADE, numerous developments in science, technology, and knowledge related to cancer have changed the way cancers are treated in clinical settings. These changes have affected all members of the healthcare team. This book is a reflection of these changes and presents this new knowledge in such a way that it can be used most effectively by nurses and other healthcare providers. It is also the result of a partnership that began almost 20 years ago, when Gail M. Wilkes and I first conceived of writing a book about cancer chemotherapy for nurses. At that time, few textbooks covered this subject. Over the years, however, this area of nursing knowledge has grown along with the scientific and the technologic advances.

While this book covers cancer chemotherapy principles and many of the most commonly used chemotherapeutic agents, it also seeks to expand nurses' knowledge of both the cellular origins and the genetic causes for cancer. This insight into the disease at the cell and gene levels contributes to even greater understanding of these newer treatments. Specific chapters cover topics such as monoclonal antibodies, growth factors, recombinant technology, targeted therapies, and cancer vaccines. Another chapter deals with the safe administration and handling of "hazardous drugs," the term currently used by the National Institute for Occupational Safety and Health (NIOSH) to describe many of the agents used to treat cancer. As more cancer therapies emerge as treatments for both malignant and nonmalignant conditions, this topic will become an even more critical issue for members of the healthcare team. Finally, as many caregivers realize, interactions between these newer therapies and other medications have the potential to cause patients undue harm. The last chapter of the book deals with what is known regarding emerging therapies and their interactions with other drugs.

Clearly, this book aims to present a great deal of new knowledge about caring for the person with cancer. It synthesizes information about what we know from research and, more importantly, translates this knowledge into a practical clinical guide for nurses. To that end, an appendix to this edition provides the expanded care plans from our previous books. As we are all aware, care planning sometimes seems to be an aspect of care from another era. Nevertheless, these care plans have endured—a testimony to their ongoing relevance—and can be used either totally or in part when caring for the person with cancer. More importantly, the care plans are comprehensive enough that they can serve as a template for care of the person with cancer, regardless of that individual's particular treatment regimen.

A book is never the work of one person. Even a single-authored text requires manuscript preparation, editing, and marketing, to mention only a few aspects of the complex world of publishing. Gail and I must say "thank you" to so many people who have been involved at various points in the development of this book.

First, a "thank you" to Jones and Bartlett Publishers, which has been publishing our cancer chemotherapy books for 15 years. The next "thank you" goes to Dr. Penny Glynn, formerly an editor at Jones and Bartlett Publishers, who suggested we write this book. She encouraged us to rethink our book, *Cancer Chemotherapy: A Nursing Process Approach*, and to update oncology nurses' knowledge base by writing a book about cancer therapies that aligned with the twenty-first-century science taking shape in the field of oncology and cancer care. Additional staff within Jones and Bartlett have worked tirelessly to produce a book that we can be proud of, including Tracey Chapman, Renée Sekerak, Kathy Richardson, Chris Davis, and many other people who we never get to meet but who work behind the scenes.

Authors from previous editions of our books have also contributed to our thinking and writing in one way or another. One never knows how one's thinking and writing will change by being part of something as important as publishing a book. We thank the many people with whom we have been fortunate enough to write over the past 15 years.

To my husband, Thom, my best friend and toughest critic, you continue to be the wind beneath my wings.

Finally, Gail and I would like to thank our patients. It has been a privilege to be allowed into their lives. They have taught us—and continue to teach us every day—what it is like to live with cancer.

Margaret Barton-Burke, Ph.D., R.N.
Gail M. Wilkes, M.S.N., R.N.C.

All of our previous books have contained disclaimers, and this book is no different. The drug information presented in *Cancer Therapies* is an amalgam of information from many sources, including manufacturer's current prescribing guidelines, package inserts, standard reference sources, and current published research on cancer therapies including, but not limited to, chemotherapeutic drugs, targeted therapies, monoclonal antibodies, and cancer vaccines. As such, the information contained in this book has not been tested or verified by the authors or the publisher. The authors, editors, and publisher have made every effort to ensure that dosages and regimens set forth in the text are accurate and in accord with current labeling at the time of publication. However, in view of the constant flow of information resulting from ongoing research, clinical practice, and government regulations, readers are urged to check the manufacturer's product information sheet for the most up-to-date recommendations on dosages, precautions, and contraindications, and to consult with a pharmacist for each drug they administer to be certain that no changes have occurred since this book's publication. This search for the most current information is particularly important when a drug is new, is infrequently ordered, or is seldom administered to a patient. The drugs in this book were chosen on the basis of their frequency of use and as examples of newer cancer therapies. The authors and the publisher take no responsibility for the use of the products described herein.

The Biological Basis of Cancer

Linda Workman, Ph.D., R.N., F.A.A.N.

Introduction

Cancer is a common health problem worldwide, although cancer types vary considerably between affluent and less affluent countries. All cancer is genetic in that cancer arises from normal cells that have experienced alterations (mutations) at the gene level. The most significant genetic alterations leading to transformation of normal cells to cancer cells occur in those genes that regulate cell proliferation. As a result, the strict processes controlling normal cellular growth, function, and cell death have been lost. Although these alterations can occur in any cell type and result in cancer, they occur most commonly among cell types that have retained the ability to divide.

The relationship between genetic changes and cancer development are becoming better understood. Cancer cells have features, responses, and growth advantages that are different from those of normal cells as a result of genetic changes. All forms of cancer chemotherapy, including traditional cytotoxic chemotherapy, hormonal manipulation, targeted therapies, and some biologic response modifier therapies, attempt to take advantage of these genetically induced differences. Thus, knowledge of basic genetics, normal cell biology, and cancer cell biology are key to understanding how different chemotherapeutic agents exert both their therapeutic effects and their side effects.

Basic Genetics

The nucleus of a cell contains the DNA (deoxyribonucleic acid) that contains the codes or patterns for construction of every protein made by every cell within the body (Figure 1.1). All hormones, growth factors, enzymes, and other substances synthesized by the human body are composed of protein. Examples of these protein substances include insulin, interferon, thyroxin, and interleukin-2, to name only a few. The controlling factors for development and anything the cell can ever do are the genes. A gene is a specific segment of DNA that codes for the pattern or plan for a specific gene product (a protein).

All cells make substances that are used for the normal housekeeping duties of the cell. In addition, some cells make at least one specific substance that leaves the cell and is either used by other cells or controls the activity of other cells. All of these substances are proteins, and the process involved in making these proteins is termed protein synthesis. Protein synthesis can only occur if the specific segment of DNA (the gene) that contains the coding pattern for a protein is present to direct the actual synthesis of the protein.

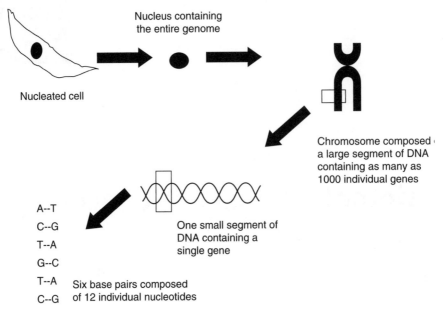

FIGURE 1.1 Different forms of cellular (nuclear) DNA.

DNA Structure

DNA is composed of two very long chains (strands) of interlocking nucleotides. Each nucleotide is composed of a molecule of any one of the following four bases: adenine (A), guanine (G), thymine (T), and cytosine (C) (Figure 1.2). These bases are attached to a five-carbon sugar called a pentose sugar (deoxyribose), which is connected to a phosphate group. The phosphate groups link the bases so that long strands are formed. When each base is attached to the sugar molecule and linked to a phosphate group, it is then a nucleotide (Figure 1.2).

Human cellular DNA is double stranded in an antiparallel arrangement. The two strands are not

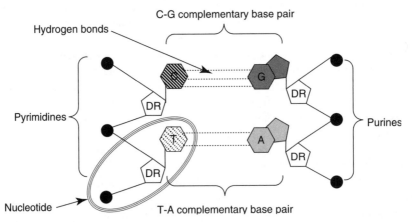

FIGURE 1.2 Four nucleotides arranged as complementary base pairs. C = cytosine; G = guanine; A = adenine; T = thymine; DR = deoxyribose; ● = phosphorous.

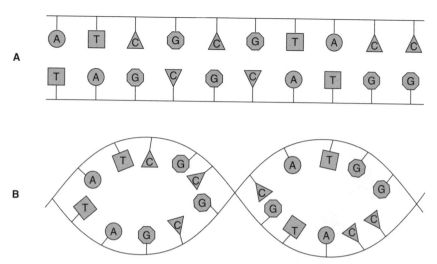

FIGURE 1.3 Double-stranded DNA. (A) Linear and straight complementary strands. (B) Same strands arranged in a soft helix. T = thymine; C = cytosine; A = adenine; G = guanine.

directly physically connected together; relatively weak hydrogen bonds hold the strands close. These ionic forces are different for the two groups of bases, and thus, adenine always pairs with thymine (and vice versa), and guanine always pairs with cytosine. The two strands of DNA are lined up together and composed of interacting bases that form base pairs. Because the base pairs are specific in their attractions, the two strands of DNA are complementary to each other in terms of their nucleotide sequence. Therefore, it is possible, if the sequence of one DNA strand is known, to be able to predict with accuracy the sequence of the complementary DNA strand (Figure 1.3).

Except when cells are in the act of dividing, the double-stranded DNA has a loosely coiled helical arrangement within the nucleus. This double helix is not just one very long piece of DNA. It is divided into 46 separate chunks that pack together tightly during the last part of cell division to form the dense structures of chromosomes (Figure 1.4). Therefore, chromosomes are actually temporary arrangements of large sections of DNA. Each chromosome contains many genes. The location of some genes is known. For example,

the gene for blood type is on chromosome 9, the BRCA1 gene is on chromosome 17, and the gene for the beta chain of hemoglobin is on chromosome 11.

The two long structures making up the two longitudinal halves of the chromosome present during metaphase of cell division are called chromatids. Chromatids on the same chromosome are called *sister* chromatids. The point at which the two sister chromatids are joined together is called the centromere. Many chromosome features are described in relation to the centromere. The distal ends of the chromosome are the telomeres. These special pieces of DNA literally cap the chromosome and keep the DNA of each chromosome together throughout the life of the cell. The DNA in the telomeres gets shorter with every round of cell division, and its presence is related to cell aging. The rate at which a person ages is related to the rate of telomeric DNA loss. Faster cellular aging occurs with faster rates of telomere loss. Slower cellular aging occurs with slower rates of telomere loss. Telomeres have a role in the normal cellular process of apoptosis (discussed later under the biology of normal cells).

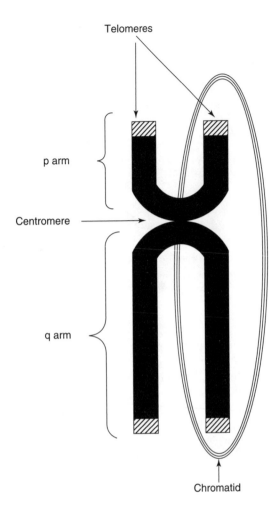

FIGURE 1.4 DNA in chromosome form.

Labels on figure: Telomeres, p arm, Centromere, q arm, Chromatid

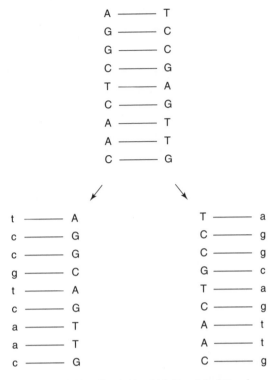

A	T
G	C
G	C
C	G
T	A
C	G
A	T
A	T
C	G

t	A	T	a
c	G	C	g
c	G	C	g
g	C	G	c
t	A	T	a
c	G	C	g
a	T	A	t
a	T	A	t
c	G	C	g

FIGURE 1.5 DNA replication in which the original strands separate and each original strand serves as a template for the synthesis of a new complementary strand. The result is two complete sets of DNA, each containing one original strand and one newly replicated strand. Capital letters indicate the original strand. Lowercase letters indicate the newly replicated strand.

DNA Replication

The genes within the DNA regulate every aspect of individual cell function. Thus, it is important that each cell have the correct amount of DNA with all the genes in its nucleus. When one cell divides to form two new daughter cells, each new daughter cell must have the same DNA and gene content as the original parent cell. For each new cell to have the correct DNA and gene content, the parent cell must first make an exact copy of its DNA. The making of an exact copy of DNA is

termed DNA replication and occurs during the DNA synthesis phase of the cell cycle.

DNA is replicated by using the original strands of DNA as models or templates. The two original strands of DNA loosen up from the tight helical arrangement. The loosened strands separate into two single strands so that each single strand can be used as a template for the new DNA (Figure 1.5). A series of enzymes is required for this process (Table 1.1). The steps in this process involve having the DNA relax, unwind from the helix, and straighten out. An additional enzyme enters the straightened out area and separates the two DNA strands. Another enzyme enters and prevents the two strands from rejoining. A different enzyme

TABLE 1.1 Enzymes Involved in DNA Replication

Enzyme	Action
DNA polymerases	DNA chain elongation (building the strands)
Exonucleases	DNA editing and repair
DNA ligases	Connect short, newly synthesized DNA segments together
DNA helicases	Unwind DNA and separate the two strands
DNA topoisomerases	Create a transient "nick" to disrupt DNA supercoils before transcription can begin
Single-stranded DNA binding proteins (SSB proteins)	Keep separated DNA strands apart long enough to allow transcription to take place

attaches itself to one strand, travels down the strand (from the 5' to 3' direction), and reads (transcribes) the base sequence of this strand. Another enzyme, a polymerase, builds a new strand of DNA complementary to the one being read by lining up individual nucleotides and connecting them together in the sequence dictated by the original DNA strand.

This process occurs in thousands of sites within the DNA so that all of the DNA is correctly replicated in a relatively short period of time. The process is somewhat like turning a 250-mile two-lane highway into a four-lane highway by having 10 separate work crews each build a 25-mile segment of the new highway. Each segment is built independently of the other segments, but the segments must be connected together as the final step. For DNA replication, special enzymes ensure that the independently generated segments of DNA are linked together correctly when DNA synthesis is complete.

The result of DNA replication during the S phase of the cell cycle is the presence of two complete sets of double-stranded DNA being present in the nucleus. Each set is composed of one old strand of DNA (that served as the template) and one new complementary strand of DNA. Thus, at this phase of cell division, the original cell now has twice as much DNA in its nucleus than it did when cell division began. One of these two compete sets will be placed into one new daughter cell, and the second complete set will be placed into the other new daughter cell when cell division is complete.

Implications for Chemotherapy

Some cancer therapy drugs target the DNA or the process of DNA replication in an attempt to kill cancer cells or at least slow their growth. For the more traditional cytotoxic chemotherapeutic agents, the mechanisms of action are not limited to cancer cells but also affect normal cells, accounting for some of the common acute side effects of chemotherapy. The following sections discuss the general mechanisms of action for several different categories of chemotherapeutic agents that target DNA processes.

Alkylating Agents

The alkylating agents work by inducing the formation of tight bonds (covalent bonds) between the double strands of DNA. This action prevents the two strands of DNA from separating and inhibits DNA replication. Without DNA replication, cell division does not occur.

Antimetabolites

Antimetabolites are similar to normal metabolites needed to make the four bases that are converted into nucleotides for DNA synthesis. Antimetabolite drugs result in the making of counterfeit nucleotides that closely resemble the normal nucleotides in size and shape. However, when these counterfeit nucleotides are placed into the growing DNA strands during DNA replication, they result in nonfunctional DNA and impaired cell division. It is much the same effect as using a Canadian quarter, which is the same size and weight as an American quarter, in a vending machine. The vending machine does not respond appropriately by dispensing the desired product and, in fact, may become jammed so that it doesn't work at all.

Antitumor Antibiotics

Antitumor antibiotics often bind to the cell's DNA and interrupt DNA synthesis and/or protein synthesis. Different drugs bind to different areas of the DNA at different times during cell division. Exactly how the interruptions occur varies with each agent.

Topoisomerase Inhibitors

Topoisomerase is an enzyme needed for DNA replication (Table 1.1). It nicks and straightens the DNA helix, allowing the DNA to be copied, and then reattaches the DNA together. Topoisomerase inhibitors prevent these processes, causing DNA breakage and cell death.

Gene Function

Gene Expression

Genes are relatively small segments of DNA that are the instructions for the making of all the different proteins our bodies need. Specific genes direct each cell regarding what protein to make, how to make it, when to make it, and how much to make. Think of each gene as a unique recipe for making a certain protein. The specific protein coded by any one gene is known as that gene's product. All human cells with a nucleus contain the entire set of human genes. This complete set of genes is called the genome. The human genome contains about 35,000 individual genes.

All cells with a nucleus contain all the genes even though not every cell uses all these genes. For example, the beta chain of hemoglobin (beta-globin) is produced only by red blood cells even though every cell type has the gene for beta-globin. So, in all other body cells, the gene for beta-globin is unexpressed (turned off). Only in red blood cells is the gene for beta-globin selectively expressed (turned on) when hemoglobin production is needed.

Consider all of the DNA in any cell's nucleus to be a giant recipe book containing all the recipes needed to make all the proteins, hormones, enzymes, and other substances needed by the body.

The chromosome pairs are analogous to the different book chapters, and the genes are the individual recipes contained within the chapters.

The purpose of a gene is to code for the making of a specific protein used by a cell, tissue, or organ within a person. For example, the beta chain of hemoglobin is a protein. When a person is anemic and needs to make more hemoglobin, immature red blood cells rapidly make all parts of hemoglobin, including the beta chain, to correct the anemia. During the synthesis of the beta chain of hemoglobin, the beta-globin gene is expressed.

Protein Synthesis

Protein synthesis is the process by which genes are expressed to make the proteins needed for physiologic function. Actual proteins are composed of individual amino acids connected together in a specific order. There are 22 different amino acids. Every protein has a specific amount of the amino acids and a specific order in which they are put together. If even one amino acid is out of order or completely deleted from the sequence, the protein will be incorrect and may be unable to perform its normal function or unable to perform it as efficiently.

For example, the beta chain of hemoglobin contains 146 amino acids in a specific sequence. If any of the amino acids are missing or are in the wrong position, the protein made would be different from normal beta-globin and would not function properly. Thus, the actual order of the amino acids is critical for the final function of any protein.

Within the DNA, there is a code for each amino acid. Each amino acid code is 3 bases (nucleotides) long. A gene is the recipe for making a specific protein. It contains all the amino acid codes in exactly the right order for that specific protein. For example, the beta chain of hemoglobin has 146 amino acids. Thus, the minimum number of bases needed in the gene for beta-globin would be 438 (3 bases per amino acid × 146 amino acids).

When a specific protein needs to be synthesized, the chromosome with the specific gene opens around the area of the gene, and the right gene is found. The code sequence of the gene is copied (transcribed) into ribonucleic acid (messenger RNA, sometimes just called the *message*). The message then leaves the nucleus and moves to the area of the cell where all the amino acids are waiting to be assembled into a specific protein. This area is the endoplasmic reticulum. Once in the endoplasmic reticulum, the message is read by enzymes, and a team of structures assembles the amino acids together in the exact order specified by the gene.

RNA itself is similar to DNA with a few differences. First, the sugar attached to the base is a ribose sugar (hence the name ribonucleic acid). In addition, thymine does not exist in RNA. Instead the base uracil, which is structurally similar to thymine, is placed in RNA instead of thymine. There is a specific three-base RNA code in messenger RNA (called a codon) for each amino acid (Table 1.2). These RNA codes are complementary to the DNA amino acid codes, with uracil in place of thymine. In addition to the amino acid codes, RNA contains some stop codes that tell the process when the protein is finished.

The total number of amino acids in a specific protein and the exact order in which they are connected together determine the nature and activity of the protein. The making of protein, or protein synthesis, is very similar to some of the steps in DNA synthesis, using similar enzymes but carried out on a smaller level (Figure 1.6).

When a specific protein, such as beta-globin, is needed, the DNA area that contains the amino acid code sequence (gene) for beta-globin loosens and unwinds slightly, using similar enzymes to those used in transcription for DNA replication. Once the appropriate area of DNA is opened, the two strands in the area are separated, and an RNA enzyme determines which strand contains the actual gene for beta-globin (the sense strand) and which strand contains a DNA sequence complementary to the gene (the antisense strand). The enzyme then binds to the gene area of the sense strand of DNA and reads it, synthesizing a strand of messenger RNA complementary to the beta-globin gene. This completed message is translated to put together the 146 amino acids in exactly the right order for normal beta-globin. After beta-globin is made, it connects to the other proteins (alpha-globin and heme) needed to complete hemoglobin production.

Mutations

Mutations are DNA changes that are passed from one cell generation to another. When mutations occur in general body cells (somatic cells), they are known as somatic mutations. Because these mutations occur in a person's cells after conception, the person cannot pass a somatic mutation on to his or her children. One possible consequence of somatic mutations is the increased risk for cancer in the cells that have undergone such mutations. Germline mutations occur in sex cells and can be passed on to one's children.

DNA bases can be altered or mutated accidentally. Sometimes, the wrong base is put into a certain position during DNA replication (point mutation). A mutation can also arise from a base being deleted during DNA replication or an extra base (or several bases) being added during DNA replication (frameshift mutations). Usually, the editing work of enzymes during DNA replication prevents or corrects these changes. When mutations occur in a gene, the resulting change can alter the expression of that gene, and the gene product may be incorrect or not synthesized at all.

TABLE 1.2 Sample DNA Codes (Triplets) and RNA Codons for Selected Amino Acids

Amino acid	DNA code(s)	RNA codons
Leucine	AAT, AAC	UUA, UUG
Methionine	TAC	AUG
Phenylalanine	AAA, AAC	UUU, UUG
Serine	AGA, AGG, AGT, AGC	UCU, UCC, UCA, UCG
Valine	CAA, CAG, CAT, CAC	GUU, GUC, GUA, GUG
Start		AUG
Stop		UAA, UAG, UGA

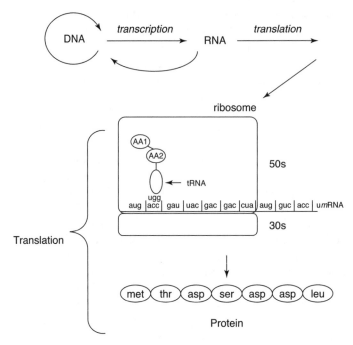

FIGURE 1.6 The process of protein synthesis. mRNA = messenger RNA; aug, acc, gua, uac, gac, cuc, aug, guc, acc = individual RNA codons for specific amino acids; met = methionine; thr = threonine; asp = aspartic acid; leu = leucine; AA = amino acid.

Point Mutation

Point mutations are the substitution of one base for another. A change has been made at a single point of DNA, and the type of change is a base substitution, not a deletion or an addition. As a result, a three-base amino acid code may be incorrect and result in an amino acid position change in the final gene product during protein synthesis.

The following sentences are an analogy to a point mutation. The top sentence represents the correct reading sequence of amino acid codes for a specific gene.

THE FAT DOG HIT HIS TOE
THE FAT DOG BIT HIS TOE

A point mutation, as seen in the bottom sentence, has changed the H in HIT to a B. The coded message is similar but not exactly the same.

Sometimes a point mutation can change the protein (gene product) a little, but it may still function, although not very efficiently. For example, the normal beta chain of hemoglobin (beta-globin) has a glycine as the number 6 amino acid in the chain of 146 amino acids. A point mutation in the 18th base in the gene for beta-globin results in valine being the 6th amino acid instead of glycine (Figure 1.7). This mutation is the basis for sickle cell disease. A person who has inherited a pair of mutated beta-globin genes produces red blood cells that contain mostly hemoglobin S instead of normal hemoglobin A. The hemoglobin S does function to carry oxygen but not very efficiently, and it folds incorrectly when low tissue oxygen levels exist, causing the red blood cell to assume a sickle shape. Some point mutations result in protein synthesis being stopped too early, and the resulting new protein is both incomplete and nonfunctional.

Frameshift Mutation

A frameshift mutation occurs when a DNA base is added or deleted. Such a mutation always disrupts the DNA reading frame and causes all amino

HbA	1	2	3	4	5	6	
DNA	CAC	GTG	GAC	TGA	GGA	CTC	A
RNA	GUG	CAC	CUG	ACU	CCU	GAG	
AAs	val	his	leu	thr	pro	glu	

HbS	1	2	3	4	5	6	
DNA	CAC	GTG	GAC	TGA	GGA	CAC	B
RNA	GUG	CAC	CUG	ACU	CCU	GUG	
AAs	val	his	leu	thr	pro	val	

FIGURE 1.7 An example of the consequences of a point mutation. (A) Normal adult hemoglobin with glutamine in the sixth amino acid position. (B) Point mutation in hemoglobin with valine in the sixth amino acid position, resulting in sickle cell disease. DNA = deoxyribonucleic acid; RNA = ribonucleic acid; AAs = amino acids; HbA = normal adult hemoglobin; HbS = sickle cell hemoglobin.

acid codes from the site of the mutation on down to be in the wrong position. As a result, either a nonfunctional garbage protein is made or no protein is made at all from that gene. Usually, a frameshift mutation is serious because the person who has such a mutation is not able to synthesize a needed and important protein.

The following sentences are an analogy to a frameshift mutation. The top sentence represents the correct reading sequence for a specific gene.

THE FAT DOG HIT HIS TOE

THF ATD OGH ITH IST OE

THE PFA TDO GHI THI STO E

A base deletion mutation, as seen in the middle sentence, has removed the E in THE, shifting the rest of the bases to the left (for the three-base codes) and disrupting the reading frame. A base addition mutation, as seen in the bottom sentence, has added a P to FAT, shifting the three-base reading codes to the right and disrupting the reading frame. The coded message has been lost completely.

Biology of Normal Cells

Normal human function is dependent on cells in all tissues and organs operating efficiently and correctly. In addition to ensuring proper cell work, an important aspect of normal function is the tight regulation of when cells divide, when they die, and how or if they are replaced. Some human cells no longer grow by mitosis (cell duplication division) after maturation of the tissue or organ is complete. Such cells include cardiac muscle cells and neurons. A disadvantage of the lack of mitotic cell division is that, when these nondividing tissues experience cell damage or death, the tissue is replaced by scar tissue rather than by the same type of tissue that was lost. For example, if a person has a myocardial infarction and loses 20% of his or her ventricular myocardial cells as a result of ischemia and necrosis, the dead cells die and slough. These cells are replaced with scar tissue composed of collagen and fibrous connective tissue. The replacement cells are not myocardial tissue and will not contract rhythmically to assist in cardiac output. Thus, when normal cells are replaced with scar tissue, some of the function of that tissue or organ is lost. The degree of loss is proportional to the amount of scar tissue replacing normal tissue.

Many human cells continue to grow by mitotic cell division throughout the life span long after tissue maturation is complete, although the rate of mitosis diminishes with age. Such cells are located in tissues where constant damage or wear is likely and continued cell growth is needed to replace dead tissues. Tissues that retain mitotic ability have the advantage of replacing dead, aged, or damaged cells with new cells. Cells of the skin, hair, mucous membranes, bone marrow, and linings of organs, such as the lungs, stomach, intestines, bladder, uterus, and other organs, retain the ability to divide throughout a person's life span. The growth of these cells is well controlled, ensuring that only the right number of functionally active cells is always present in any tissue or organ.

Any new or continued cell growth not needed for normal development or replacement of dead and damaged tissues is called *neoplasia*. This cell growth is always abnormal even if it is not malignant and causes no harm. Whether the new cells are benign or malignant, neoplastic cells develop from normal cells (parent cells). Cancer cells were once normal cells but changed to no longer look, grow, or function normally. To understand how cancer cells grow, it is important to first understand the function and growth regulation of normal cells.

Features of Normal Cells

Appearance
Each normal cell type has a distinct and recognizable appearance, size, and shape. The size of the normal cell nucleus is small compared with the size of the rest of the cell, including the cytoplasm. Thus, normal cells have a small nuclear-to-cytoplasmic ratio.

Function
Every normal cell has a minimum of one specific, differentiated function that it performs to contribute to whole-body homeostasis. For example, pancreatic beta cells secrete insulin, ovaries secrete estrogen, cardiac muscle cells contract, nerve cells generate action potentials, and erythrocytes synthesize hemoglobin.

Tight Tissue Adherence
Normal cells make proteins that protrude from the cell surface and interact with each other to bind cells closely and tightly together. These proteins form a large family known as cell adhesion molecules (CAMs). One CAM is fibronectin, which keeps normal cells within one tissue or organ bound tightly to each other. As a result of CAMs, normal cells are not migratory and do not leave their parent organ or tissue. Cells that are expected to move about the body as part of their function, such as erythrocytes and leukocytes, do not produce fibronectin and do not usually adhere together.

Ploidy
Most normal cells have the normal diploid number of human chromosomes of 23 pairs (or 46 individual chromosomes). Human cells containing just the right number of chromosomes are termed euploid. Mature erythrocytes have extruded the

nucleus and do not contain any chromosomes. The mature sex cells (oocytes or eggs, and spermatocytes or sperm) are haploid, containing only half of each pair of chromosomes, or a total of 23 chromosomes. For mature sex cells, this is the euploid condition.

Contact Inhibition
Normal cells capable of mitosis will only undergo cell division as long as some membrane surface remains untouched by the membrane of another cell. Once a normal cell is in direct contact on all surface areas with other cells, it no longer undergoes mitosis. Thus, normal cell division is contact inhibited or displays density-dependent inhibition of cell growth. This feature prevents overgrowth of a tissue or organ. For example, if a tissue, such as skin cells, was not contact inhibited, skin growth in an area of injury could continue beyond normal wound closure and result in excess skin flaps or folds in that area.

Orderly and Well-Controlled Growth
Normal cells do not divide unless there is a need for more cells and sufficient resources are present. Cell division or mitosis occurs in a well-recognized pattern described by the cell cycle. The phases and normal regulation of the cell cycle are described in detail in the next section, Mitosis.

Normal cells are restricted from entering the cell cycle unless new cells are absolutely needed either for normal growth and development or to replace damaged and dead cells. These restrictions are controlled by specific gene products, and normal cells respond appropriately to the presence of these products. Normal cell populations are regulated by a balance between gene products that promote entering and completing the cell cycle and gene products that restrict or inhibit entering and moving through the cell cycle.

Mitosis

Cells not actively reproducing are outside of the cell cycle in a state known as G_0. These cells are termed *quiescent*, which is not really appropriate for these cells because the definition means quiet or sleeping. In reality, cells in G_0 are functionally very active, just not reproducing. They are busy performing all their usual differentiated functions needed for whole-body homeostasis. Most cells spend the vast majority of their functional lives in this state. Cells that are not capable of mitosis only leave this state to die. Cells that retain the ability to divide must exit the G_0 state to enter the cell cycle for reproduction.

Even among normal cells capable of mitosis, the step of leaving G_0 and entering the first phase of the cell cycle (G_1) is severely restricted. Once a cell enters the cell cycle, it does not respond to external changes. After entry into the cycle, the cell cannot go backwards; it either must progress through the cycle or is arrested at some point in the cycle. If the cell arrests rather than completes the cell cycle, it is nonfunctional and usually dies. New targeted agents inhibit the proteins and enzymes that promote progression through the cell cycle.

Mitotic cell division makes one cell divide into two daughter cells. These two cells are identical to each other and to the original cell that started the mitotic cell division (Figure 1.8). The steps of entering and completing the cell cycle are tightly controlled. Much of this control is regulated by proteins produced by suppressor genes.

Some of the checks, known as restriction point controls, placed on a cell before it can enter the cell cycle include:

- need for cell division in the specific tissue where the cell resides
  Are more cells needed in this tissue as a result of previous cell damage or loss?
  Are more cells needed in this tissue because the tissue needs to increase in size (as in normal development)?
- presence of adequate nutrition (especially protein, glucose, and oxygen) to support the cells that already exist as well as new cells
- adequate production of energy
- adequate supplies of substances needed in the synthesis of more membranes, more DNA, intracellular proteins, and organelles

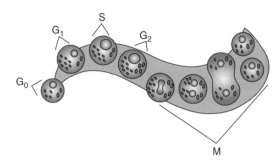

FIGURE 1.8 The steps of mitotic *cell division*. *Source*: Modified with permission from: Ignatavicius, D., and Workman, M.L. 2002. *Medical-surgical nursing: Critical thinking for clinical care*. Philadelphia: W.B. Saunders.

G_1 Phase of the Cell Cycle

Once the cell responds to tissue mitotic signals indicating that it is time to divide and that all systems are ready for this reproductive event, the cell exits G_0 and enters the first phase of the cell cycle, G_1. Once the cell has entered G_1, whether or not it can progress to the next phase is determined by the presence of cyclins.

Cyclins are members of a family of proteins that, when present in an active form, drive the cell forward in the cell cycle, allowing progression through all phases and resulting in cell division where one cell forms two daughter cells. Most of these cyclin proteins are activated when a phosphorous molecule is added to its chemical structure, which is a process known as phosphorylation. Removal of a phosphorous molecule, or dephosphorylation, usually results in deactivating or inhibiting the protein. Enzymes that phosphorylate molecules are known as kinases. The kinases that activate cyclins are known as cyclin-dependent kinases (CDKs). CDKs combine with cyclins to form a complex that sets into motion all the cellular machinery needed to make the cell reproduce. Normally, cyclins and CDKs are carefully regulated in amount and activation so that cell division only occurs when it is needed.

The amount of cyclin and the type of cyclins present in the cell during cell division varies by the phase of the cycle. These differences in types

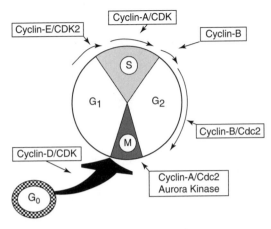

FIGURE 1.9 Cyclin activity in the cell cycle.

of cyclins determine when or if a cell moves from one phase of the cycle to the next. Twenty different families of cyclins have been identified (A through T). The type of cyclins that have been best characterized at this time are the A, B, and D families of cyclins. The most common signal for entering and starting the cell cycle at G_1 is the combining of a cyclin-D with the appropriate CDK, forming a complex (cyclin-D/CDK) (Figure 1.9).

Each of these proteins, cyclin-D and CDK, are made in the cell in response to turning on the right genes. Some of the new chemotherapy agents, the cell cycle inhibitors, target either cyclin-D (preventing its production) or CDK (inhibiting its ability to combine with cyclin-D and form a complex or preventing its production). Drugs that prevent activation of the cyclin-D/CDK complex are cell cycle–inhibiting proteins that work in opposition to the complex. This family of drugs is known as cyclin-dependent kinase inhibitors (CDKIs). Because there are many different CDKs and not all drugs inhibit all types of CDKs, the drugs are labeled by which specific CDK they inhibit. For example, INK4 is a CDKI that specifically inhibits the activity of CDK4. Another group of CDK inhibitors are the KIPs (kinase inhibitor proteins) that selectively inhibit other cyclin/CDK complexes. Therefore, there are many specific

cyclins and specific CDKs that form complexes to promote movement through the cell cycle. The development of different and specific inhibitor proteins as drugs may negatively regulate cancer cell growth by inhibiting progression through the cell cycle at different times in the cell cycle.

Late in the G_1 phase of the cell cycle, movement of the cell from G_1 into the S phase of the cell cycle is regulated by the combining of certain proteins with transcription factors that promote DNA transcription and synthesis. Progression into S phase requires that regulator proteins be phosphorylated to work with the transcription factors. The synthesis of the transcription factors and the regulator proteins is another process that is governed by specific gene products. For example, the Tp53 gene product restricts the progression of cells from G_1 into S phase. Anything that damages the Tp53 gene can result in less restriction at this point in the cell cycle.

S Phase of the Cell Cycle

The major activity of S phase is the replication of DNA, resulting in the synthesis of two complete sets of DNA. The process of DNA replication is described earlier in the chapter under the heading of Basic Genetics. The cyclin activity important for ensuring DNA synthesis is cyclin-E combining with CDK2 to form cyclin-E/CDK2. This complex works with the retinoblastoma gene product to produce transcription factors to allow expression of the cyclin-E gene. Cyclin-E combines with CDK2 to activate some of the enzymes needed to produce nucleotides. Another cyclin, cyclin-A, is activated by combining with CDK. This cyclin-A/CDK complex then permits the synthesis of all substances needed for DNA replication.

Late in S phase, cyclin-B makes an appearance. This substance is responsible for activating other kinases that control the ability of the cell to complete S phase and progress into the G_2 phase of the cell cycle.

G_2 Phase of the Cell Cycle

The main activity of the cell during the G_2 phase of the cell cycle is intense protein synthesis. Not only are the normal housekeeping proteins of the cell made, but also those proteins with a role in mitosis must be synthesized. This activity is regulated by the cyclin-B/Cdc2 complex. At the end of G_2, this complex moves into the cell's nucleus, reducing the intracellular concentration of cyclin-B/Cdc2 complexes and initiating processes that help the cell progress toward the M phase of mitosis. In the nucleus, the cyclin-B/Cdc2 complex induces the production of anaphase-promoting complexes and proteins that stimulate the production of centrioles and spindle fibers and promote the survival of the cell during the dangerous M phase.

Chemotherapy agents that prevent or disrupt protein synthesis, such as the antitumor antibiotics, have the greatest effect in this phase of the cell cycle. Under the influence of these drugs, the proper proteins needed to complete cell division are not made.

M Phase of the Cell Cycle

The part of the cell cycle in which two new cells are formed from the original cell is called mitosis and is the only time in which the DNA is organized into chromosomes. This phase is further divided into the subphases of prophase, prometaphase, metaphase, anaphase, and telophase (Figure 1.10). During M phase, each chromosome forms and moves to the center of the cell that is about to divide. String-like fibers called microtubular spindle fibers form from the centrioles located on each side of the cell. One end of the spindle fiber is attached to one centriole, and the other end is attached to one chromatid of a chromosome. The other chromatid of the chromosome has a spindle fiber attached to the opposite centriole. Just before the cell splits into two cells (cytokinesis), each chromosome is pulled apart so that half of each chromosome goes into one new cell and the other half goes into the other new cell. The process of pulling the chromosomes apart is called nucleokinesis.

Centriole development, maturation, and movement to opposite sides of the cell before mitosis is directed by some of the cyclins and an activat-ing enzyme called aurora kinase. This substance and the protein survivin direct spindle fiber formation and attachment.

Antimitotic chemotherapy agents exert their effects in this phase of the cell cycle. Some of these drugs prevent spindle fiber formation. This action prevents nucleokinesis and cytokinesis. Other antimitotic agents (especially the taxanes) allow the spindle fibers to form but prevent them from degrading at the proper time. When the fibers remain, they interfere with all other aspects of cell function.

Apoptosis

Not only do cells have to live and sometimes reproduce for normal human function, some cells also have to die for optimum function of the human body. For tissues composed of cells that can undergo mitosis, like the liver, cells perform their physiologic functions, age, and eventually die. For example, optimum liver function requires that most of the cells in the liver, at any one time, be at their peak performance level. As a cell ages, as measured by the number of cell divisions it can undergo, it begins to perform at less than optimum levels. If a cell is damaged, this reduced performance can occur at earlier cell ages, even when the cell has undergone fewer cell divisions than expected for the cell type. Damaged cells and older cells take themselves out of the organ workforce through a process known as apoptosis (programmed cell death).

With each round of cell division, the telomeric DNA at the tips of the cell's chromosomes shortens. When the cell has achieved its preprogrammed number of cell divisions, the telomeric DNA that capped the chromosomes is completely gone. The DNA then unravels and fragments, triggering a variety of genetic and intracellular signals for self-destruction. The cell shrinks as enzymes (endonucleases) degrade the DNA. The mitochondria in the cell release a substance called cytochrome c. This substance activates a protein known as apoptotic protease activation factor (Apaf-1).

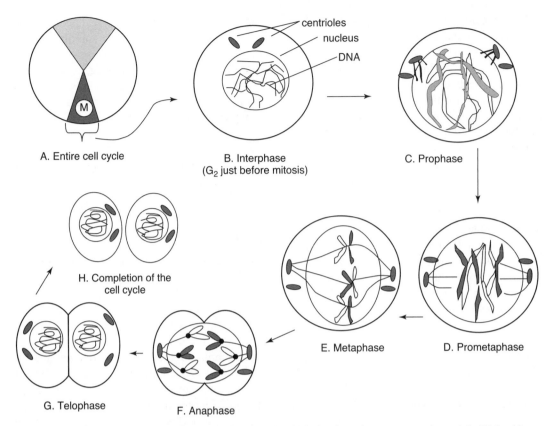

FIGURE 1.10 The activities occurring during M phase of the cell cycle (using three chromosomes as the model). (A) Graphic model of the entire cell cycle. (B) Interphase cell. Cell is still in late phase of G_2 and is about to enter M phase. DNA is beginning to coil more tightly. Centrioles are about to replicate. (C) Prophase section of M phase. DNA is becoming more dense. Loose chromosome structures are appearing. Two centrioles are beginning to synthesize spindle fibers. (D) Prometaphase section of M phase. Chromosomes becoming more dense. Spindle fibers forming and elongating from the two centrioles, which are now at the opposite poles of the cell. (E) Metaphase section of M phase. Chromosomes are highly contracted and very dense. They have lined up on the equatorial plate down the center of the cell. Each half of the chromosome is connected to a separate spindle fiber. (F) Anaphase section of M phase. The spindle fibers have pulled each chromosome into two halves. One half is pulled toward the right pole, and the other half is pulled toward the left pole. Eventually, each half will go into one of the two new daughter cells. (G) Telophase section of M phase. The chromosomes have completely separated, with each half in one side of the cell. Nucleokinesis is complete, as there are two nuclei in this cell. The chromosome structures are losing density within each nucleus as the DNA uncoils into a relaxed helical state. Cytokinesis (separation of this one large cell containing two nuclei) is beginning. (H) Completion of the cell cycle. Cytokinesis is complete. Two new separate daughter cells now exist, each with one nucleus and a pair of centrioles. The nucleus of each new cell contains the total genome. Each cell can now remain in the state of G_0 or is capable (under the right conditions) of entering the cell cycle to undergo cell division.

Apaf-1 then, in turn, activates the enzyme caspase 9. In a manner similar to the blood clotting cascade, in which small events set into motion a large rapid response, when caspase 9 is activated, a rapid activation of the whole family of caspases occurs, resulting in the degradation of most of the cell's internal structures. The membrane bubbles up, forming blebs, and the cell breaks into progressively smaller fragments called apoptotic bodies. Eventually, the white blood cells, particularly the neutrophils and macrophages, engulf these apoptotic bodies and eliminate them from the body.

The process of apoptosis ensures that only healthy and maximally functional cells compose body tissues. It is an active, energy-requiring process under strict genetic control so that healthy functional cells do not self-destruct faster than they can be replaced and that older or damaged cells unable to perform vital functions do not become immortal and reduce overall organ efficiency. Thus, maintenance of healthy tissues and organs is dependent upon the proper balance of cell division with apoptosis.

Apoptosis is regulated by different gene products. One of the most well-characterized proteins that directs cells to undergo apoptosis at the proper time is the product coded by the tumor suppressor gene, Tp53. When cells reach a certain age or experience DNA damage, the Tp53 gene is turned on (expressed). When the Tp53 gene functions well and the correct gene product is made, older and damaged cells are either stimulated to undergo apoptosis or prohibited from mitosis by arresting the cell cycle at either the G_1 or G_2 phase. This master regulating gene turns on other genes that make proteins important in signaling the mitochondria to release cytochrome c. In addition, expression of the Tp53 gene triggers the making of another protein, p21. The p21 protein prevents various anti-apoptotic substances from leaving the cell nucleus.

Biology of Cancer Cells

Body cells are exposed to personal and environmental conditions that can mutate the genes and alter how the cells grow or function. At times, these gene alterations change a cell that used to express normal features and functions into a cell that expresses malignant features and functions. This change is known as carcinogenesis or malignant transformation. Once transformed, cancer cells are always abnormal, serve no useful purpose, and harm normal body tissues and organs.

Features of Cancer Cells

Appearance
Cancer cells gradually lose the specific differentiated appearance of their parent cells, becoming anaplastic over time. The shape changes and becomes smaller and rounded. As cells become more malignant and do not retain any parental cell features, it may be difficult to determine from what normal tissue the cancer arose.

The nucleus of a cancer cell is much larger than that of a normal cell, reflecting the increased synthesis of DNA and the possible presence of abnormal amounts of DNA. The cancer cell itself is small, with the nucleus occupying much of the space within the cancer cell. Thus, cancer cells have a large nuclear-to-cytoplasmic ratio compared with normal body cells.

Function
Cancer cells gradually lose some or all differentiated functions that the parent cells performed. Cancer cells serve no useful purpose. As they progress in degree of malignancy, cancer cells become less and less differentiated in both appearance and function.

Poor Adherence
Most cancer cells lose the ability to synthesize cell adhesion molecules (CAMs), such as fibronectin. As a result, they adhere poorly to each other, easily break off from the main tumor, and extend into surrounding tissues and migrate to distant sites. This ability to metastasize and invade other body tissues is a key feature of cancer cells and a major cause of death among people with cancer.

Ploidy
As cancer cells become more malignant, they lose or gain chromosomes. Other changes at the chromosome level include breakage and rearrangement of chromosomes as well as chromosome fragmentation. This abnormal chromosome number and/or structure is called aneuploidy. Usually, the more malignant a cancer cell becomes, the greater the degree of aneuploidy its chromosomes have.

Cancer cells do not experience reduction of telomeric DNA with cell division. Some cancer cells have unusually long telomeres, whereas others have normal-length telomeres that do not lose DNA, and the chromosomes do not unravel. The enzyme telomerase is responsible for maintaining telomeric DNA. Cancer cells produce large amounts of telomerase and do not respond to apoptotic signals.

Loss of Contact Inhibition

Cancer cells continue to divide even when their membranes are in direct contact with other cells. This loss of contact inhibition allows persistence of cancer cell division regardless of how many cancer cells are occupying a given space.

Poorly Regulated Growth

Cancer cells do not respond to growth-restricting signals or apoptotic signals. Many cancer cells do not necessarily go through the cell cycle faster than normal cells; they just keep reentering the cell cycle and spend very little time in the reproductive resting state of G_0. In this respect, cancer cells more closely resemble early embryonic cells than normal cells. The basic defect in cancer cell division is an imbalance between those factors and gene products that restrict mitotic cell division and those factors and gene products that promote mitotic cell division.

Malignant Transformation (Carcinogenesis)

The process of changing a group of normal cells into cancer cells is called malignant transformation. Other terms for this process are carcinogenesis and oncogenesis. The process first begins with a change in the genes that either turns on the factors and proteins that promote cell growth or turns off the factors and proteins that restrict cell growth. Carcinogenesis occurs through four main steps and is a continually evolving process on a continuum that extends from totally normal to as highly malignant as possible (Figure 1.11). Thus, cancer cells are able to become even more malignant over time. The cells evolve in such a way that, when the cell first becomes malignant, it still retains some features of the parent cell from which it arose. After many cell divisions and continuing gene changes, cancer cells lose all normal features and express only malignant features. This process occurs through the steps of *initiation*,

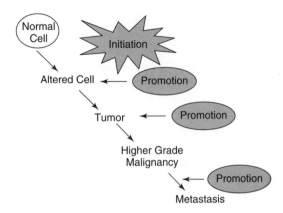

FIGURE 1.11 Continuum of malignant transformation.

promotion, progression, and *metastasis.* Gene changes continue to occur at each step.

Role of Oncogenes and Suppressor Genes in Cancer Development

Genetic control of normal cell function and growth changes with maturation of tissues and organs. In early embryonic development, just after conception, the fertilized egg divides rapidly, and the cells have neither a specific differentiated appearance nor a specific differentiated function. Early embryonic genes directed these cells to exit and reenter the cell cycle as fast as possible to generate a large population of undifferentiated stem cells. The stem cells in early embryonic development each have the potential to become any body cell under the right conditions and are thus considered multipotent or totipotent. Developmental biologists suggest that the behavior of these early embryonic stem cells is directed by the gene products that promote cell division and movement through the cell cycle, the cyclins. Furthermore, the genes for restricting or controlling growth, such as the Tp53 gene, are either not expressed at all at this time or are only minimally expressed. At 8 days after conception, the embryonic stem cells commit to differentiate, and their growth becomes more controlled. The genetic processes regulating this change involve either shutting down the action of the cyclin and cyclin-activating genes or, at least, greatly suppressing their activity. At the same time, the genes that restrict cell division become much more active.

The early embryonic genes promoting cell division are the oncogenes. After commitment, these genes and their gene products are severely restricted. When these oncogenes are restricted in their activity, they are known as proto-oncogenes. Exposure to carcinogens can damage DNA and result in removing the restrictions on proto-oncogenes, allowing them to be inappropriately active and their gene products to be heavily expressed. When these proto-oncogenes are fully expressed at any time after commitment has occurred, they revert back to being oncogenes. Oncogene expression forces cells to lose their normal features and take on the features of cancer cells, especially the features surrounding uncontrolled growth. Thus, damaging a proto-oncogene and converting it to an oncogene makes it more functionally active. Many oncogenes have been identified, and their activation leads to development of specific cancers. Table 1.3 lists

some known oncogenes and the cancers most associated with their overexpression.

The genes that became more active and heavily expressed at embryonic commitment are suppressor genes. Suppressor gene products keep all cell growth under rigid control, and their high level of expression is needed throughout the individual's lifetime. Exposure to carcinogens can damage DNA and result in knocking out suppressor gene function. Loss of suppressor gene function allows removal of growth restriction and increases the risk for cancer in the tissues that have experienced this gene damage. Table 1.4 lists

TABLE 1.3 Selected Malignancies Associated with Altered Oncogene Activity

Oncogene	Malignancies
ABL1	Chronic myelogenous leukemia, other leukemias
BRAF	Gastric
ERBB-1	Glioblastomas, squamous cell carcinoma
ERBB-2 (HER-2/neu)	Breast, salivary gland, ovarian carcinomas
HRAS	Breast, melanoma, lung, kidney, bladder, colon
Ki-RAS	Colorectal
MYC	Burkitt's lymphoma, T-cell and B-cell neoplasms, breast, gastric, lung
MYCL	Lung
MYCN	Small-cell lung cancer, neuroblastoma
NRAS	Ovarian, thyroid, melanoma, leukemia
PRAD-1	Breast, squamous cell cancers
RET	Thyroid, multiple endocrine neoplasias
TRK	Colorectal, thyroid

TABLE 1.4 Selected Malignancies Associated with Altered Suppressor Gene Activity

Suppressor gene	Malignancies
APC	Colorectal, stomach and pancreatic
ATM	Leukemia, lymphoma, breast, ovarian
BRCA1	Breast, ovarian, colorectal
BRCA2	Breast, ovarian
CDK4	Melanoma
CDKN1C	Wilms' tumor, rhabdomyosarcoma
CDKN2A	Mesotheliomoa, melanoma
DCC	Colorectal
DPC4	Pancreatic, colon
Ink4a	Melanoma
MEN1	Parathyroid, pituitary, adrenal, carcinoid, pancreatic islet cell
MLH1	Colorectal
MSH2	Colorectal
MTS1	Melanoma, brain tumors, leukemia, sarcomas, breast, bladder, ovarian, lung, kidney
NF1	Neurofibroma, colon, astrocytoma
NF2	Neurofibroma, meningioma, schwannoma
PTEN	Breast, prostate, endometrial
RB1	Retinoblastoma, sarcomas, bladder, esophageal, small-cell lung
TP53	Breast, bladder, colorectal, esophageal, liver, lung, ovarian, brain tumors, sarcomas, leukemia, lymphoma
VHL	Renal cell carcinoma, pheochromocytoma, hemangioblastoma
WT1	Wilms' tumor (nephroblastoma)

some known suppressor genes and the cancers most associated with their loss of function.

For all genes, there are two alleles, one on each chromosome pair. For example, the BRCA1 gene is a suppressor gene located on chromosome 17. There is one BRCA1 gene allele on one chromosome 17 and another BRCA1 gene allele on the other chromosome 17. When both of these gene alleles are functioning well, cell growth in most tissues is well controlled and follows the rules for restriction point control. When one of the pair of BRCA1 alleles is damaged, its function is lost. Thus, in cells whose growth rates are controlled by BRCA1, there is less control available because only one gene allele is functioning. This is the case in people who have inherited a specific mutation in one BRCA1 gene allele. Their risk for cancer is higher even though there is a remaining active normal BRCA1 gene allele because, from birth, they are relying on maintaining the function of just the one normal allele. If at some point during their lifetime the remaining healthy BRCA1 gene allele is damaged by a carcinogen, some cells in the exposed tissue are no longer growth regulated, and the risk for cancer development is high.

Stepwise Process of Malignant Transformation

Initiation

The first step in carcinogenesis is initiation. Normal cells can become cancer cells if their proto-oncogenes are turned back on at any time after early embryonic life. Anything that can penetrate a cell, get into the nucleus, and damage the DNA can damage the genes. This damage can turn on genes that should remain suppressed (proto-oncogenes) and turn off normal genes (suppressor genes). Substances that change the activity of a cell's genes so that the cell becomes a cancer cell are carcinogens. Carcinogens may be chemicals, physical agents, or viruses. In addition, some gene damage can occur through spontaneous DNA replication error taking place in cells still capable of mitosis. When this error is unrepaired and remains fixed in the DNA, it can result in the activation of proto-oncogenes into oncogenes or cause suppressor genes to lose their functions.

Pure carcinogens initially mutate a cell's genes and are thus called *initiators*. Initiation is an irreversible event that can lead to cancer development if it does not interfere with the cell's ability to divide.

Once a cell has been initiated, it can become a cancer cell if the cellular changes that occurred during initiation are enhanced by promotion. A cancer cell can only form a tumor if it can divide. If the initiated cancer cell can divide, it can lead to the development of widespread metastatic disease.

Promotion

After a normal cell is initiated by a carcinogen and becomes a cancer cell, growth enhancement can lead to tumor development. Usually, there is a lag time between when cells are initiated and when an overt tumor develops. This lag time is the latency period and can range from months to years.

Promoters are growth-enhancing substances that promote mitosis of the initiated cancer cell and shorten the latency period. Promoters may be hormones, drugs, or a wide variety of chemicals.

Progression

After cancer cells have developed into an overt tumor, other events must occur for this tumor to become more widespread and impinge on the function of normal tissues and organs. When the tumor is small, it receives nutrition from surrounding fluids by diffusion alone. After the tumor reaches a centimeter in diameter, diffusion alone is not adequate to supply needed nutrients, and the tumor must develop its own blood supply. At this stage, the tumor activates genes responsible for synthesis of tumor angiogenesis factor (TAF). This protein stimulates blood vessels into the tumor, thus connecting the tumor to the body's general circulation.

As tumor cells continue to divide, some of the new cells change features from the original, initiated cancer cell. Subpopulations of cancer cells appear within the tumor. These cancer cell subpopulations usually differ from the original cancer cell, expressing selection advantages that allow them to survive and grow even when body conditions are poor. Some of the selection advantages include the loss of contact inhibition and the ability to take up all types of nutrients more efficiently than surrounding normal cells. These advantages literally allow the cancer cells to "wax fat" while normal cells starve. Changes that occur during this progressive or progression stage cause tumor cells to become more and more malignant and express fewer normal cell features.

Some of the features gained by cancer cells during progression are either not present at all in normal cells or only slightly present. These different features allow specific sites or processes of cancer cells to be targeted. Targeted therapies combine biologic therapy and gene therapy, such as antibodies that target a cellular element of the cancer cell or antisense drugs that work at the gene level. For example, the drug imatinib mesylate (Gleevec) binds to the energy site of tyrosine kinase and prevents its activation. This drug is most useful in cancers that overexpress the ABL1 oncogene, such as Philadelphia chromosome–positive chronic myeloid leukemia. Another targeted therapy involves blocking specific receptors for substances that enhance the growth of cancer cells. For example, in some colorectal cancers, epidermal growth factor binds to the epidermal growth factor receptor (EGFR) site and activates it, leading to the generation of signals that increase the growth potential of the cancer cell. Blocking EGFR reduces this potential. Anti-EGFR antibodies target the EGFR receptor and prevent it from binding to epidermal growth factor.

Metastasis

In metastasis, cancer cells move from the primary site by direct extension and invasion of nearby tissues and by breaking off from the original tumor, entering the bloodstream, arresting at distant sites, and establishing remote colonies. Although metastasis is a common occurrence and often leads to death of the person with cancer, it is a relatively slow process. Cancer cells need to

TABLE 1.5 Usual Sites of Metastasis for Common Tumors

Malignancy	Sites of metastasis
Breast cancer	Bone, brain, lung, liver
Colorectal cancer	Adjacent lymph nodes, liver
Leukemia	Visceral organs, central nervous system
Lung cancer	Lymph nodes, brain, bone, liver, pancreas
Prostate cancer	Bone, adjacent lymph nodes, lung

overcome many hostile and protective elements to achieve metastasis. Thus, cancer cells that do metastasize are those that have the greatest selection advantages and represent the most malignant populations. Table 1.5 lists the usual sites of metastasis for common malignancies.

Summary

The following concepts and facts about cancer development and progression are used as a basis to develop effective cancer treatments that induce less harm on normal cells.

- Normal cell division, function, and cell death are controlled by gene activity.
- All cancer is genetic in that all cancers involve changes at the gene level.
- All cancers arise from parent cells that were once normal.
- A single cancer cell, under the right growth conditions, can lead to widespread metastatic disease.
- Gene changes can be induced by carcinogens or may occur as a result of spontaneous DNA replication error that is not repaired appropriately. People vary in their ability to recognize and correct DNA damage.
- Gene changes that occur in somatic cells can cause cancers in those cells but cannot be passed on to one's children.
- Gene changes that occur in germline cells (sex cells) can be passed on to one's children,

increasing the risk for cancer in anyone who inherits these mutations.

- Currently, gene mutations cannot be corrected as a result of medical or surgical intervention.
- The gene changes that have occurred in cancer cells allow the potential for therapies to be specifically targeted to cancer cells and have fewer effects on healthy cells.
- Anything that interfere's with a cancer cell's ability to divide at least slows its growth and may result in its death.
- Proto-oncogenes are a normal part of cellular DNA whose main function is in early embryonic development and are strictly controlled after that time.
- Gene damage can activate a controlled proto-oncogene into a functional oncogene that promotes cell division and growth.
- Gene damage can destroy the activity of the suppressor genes that function as guardians of the cell cycle.
- Cytotoxic chemotherapies, including the alkylating agents, antimetabolites, and antitumor antibiotics, prevent DNA replication and arrest cell division.
- Hormonal manipulation can deprive a cancer cell of hormones needed for growth. This therapy is not cytotoxic but does assist in controlling the growth of cancer cells.
- Antimitotic agents either prevent or interfere with chromosome separation and cytokinesis.
- Agents that inhibit the activation of cyclins can restore growth control to cancer cells.

References

American Cancer Society. 2004. *Cancer facts and figures 2004*. Atlanta: American Cancer Society.

American Cancer Society. 2003. *Cancer prevention and early detection: Facts and figures 2003*. Atlanta: American Cancer Society.

Bargonetti, J., and Manfredi, J. 2002. Multiple roles of the tumor suppressor p53. *Current Opinion in Oncology* 14(1):86–91.

Ford, H., and Pardee, A. 1999. Cancer and the cell cycle. *Journal of Cellular Biochemistry* 75(Suppl 32/33): 166–172.

Hanahan, D., and Weinberg, R. 2000. The hallmarks of cancer. *Cell* 100(1):57–70.

Hawkins, R. 2001. Mastering the intricate maze of metastasis. *Oncology Nursing Forum* 28(6):959–965.

Johnson, D., and Walker, C. 1999. Cyclins and cell cycle checkpoints. *Annual Review of Pharmacology and Toxicology* 39(1):295–312.

Levine, A. 1997. p53: The cellular gatekeeper for growth and division. *Cell* 88(3):323–331.

Loescher, L. 2003. The biology of cancer. In A. Tranin, A. Masny, and J. Jenkins (Eds): *Genetics in oncology practice: Cancer risk assessment*. Pittsburgh: Oncology Nursing Society.

Macleod, K. 2000. Tumor suppressor genes. *Current Opinion in Genetics and Development* 10(1):81–93.

Malumbres, M., and Barbacid, M. 2001. To cycle or not to cycle: A critical decision in cancer. *Nature Reviews: Cancer* 1(3):222–231.

Nussbaum, R., McInnes, R., and Willard, H. 2001. *Thompson & Thompson: Genetics in medicine* (ed 6). Philadelphia: W.B. Saunders.

Paulovich, A., Toczyski, D., and Hartwell, L. 1997. When checkpoints fail. *Cell* 88(3):315–321.

Peltomaki, P. 2003. Role of DNA mismatch repair defects in the pathogenesis of human cancer. *Journal of Clinical Oncology* 21(6):1174–1179.

Peters, J., Loud, J., Dimond, E., and Jenkins, J. 2001. Cancer genetics fundamentals. *Cancer Nursing* 24(6):446–461.

Reed, J. 1999. Dysregulation of apoptosis in cancer. *Journal of Clinical Oncology* 17(9):2941–2953.

Shah, M., and Schwartz, G. 2003. Cell cycle modulation: An emerging target for cancer treatment. *Horizons in Cancer Therapeutics* 4(3):3–21.

Tranin, A., Masny, A., and Jenkins, J. 2003. *Genetics in oncology practice: Cancer risk assessment*. Pittsburgh: Oncology Nursing Society.

Volker, D. 2001. Carcinogenesis: Application to clinical practice. *Clinical Journal of Oncology Nursing* 5(5): 225–226, 229.

Zimmerman, V. 2002. Gene mutations and cancer. *American Journal of Nursing* 102(8):28–37.

Cancer Chemotherapy and Cell Cycle Kinetics

Margaret Barton-Burke, Ph.D., R.N.

Gail M. Wilkes, M.S.N., R.N.C.

History of Cancer Therapy

The disease of cancer dates back as far as prehistoric times. There is evidence that cancer affected animals long before humans were on earth. The studies of the remains of a Cretaceous dinosaur and a Pleistocene cave bear indicate the existence of tumors of the vertebrae (Brothwell 1967). Evidence of malignant neoplasms was documented in Egyptian mummies some 5000 years ago (Wells 1963). The number of cases of these prehistoric and ancient tumors are small, but they support the assumption that cancer is a very old disease, afflicting animals and man long before written history.

As cancer dates back to antiquity, so too is there evidence in the earliest Egyptian writing of medical treatment for benign tumors (such as lipomas and polyps) and for malignant cancers of the stomach and uterus (Breasted 1930). Early treatment of these tumors by Egyptians consisted of surgical removal of benign lipomas and polyps with a knife or red-hot iron. Cancer of the stomach was treated with boiled barley mixed with nuts, and cancer of the uterus was treated with a mix of fresh dates and pig's brain, which was then introduced into the vagina (Ebbell 1937).

As early as the Greco-Roman period (500 BC–AD 500), cancer was recognized and given a grave prognosis. Evidence of cancer was documented in the writings of Hippocrates (the "father of medicine") and other medical authorities of the period, such as Celsus, Artaesus, and Galen (Shimkin 1977). Shimkin's book describes the predominant theory regarding cancer during this period. At this time in history, the body of man was defined by the four Humors: blood, phlegm, yellow bile, and black bile. When in proper proportions in regard to mixture, quantity, and force, man remained healthy. If any Humor was out of proportion (diminished or increased), man became ill. The four Humors were the biologic counterparts for air, fire, water, and earth, which, in certain proportions, produced heat, cold, wet, and dry. Cancer was believed to be the result of an excess of black bile (also called *melanchole* or *atrabilis*). Cancer was and still is, in many respects, a melancholy disease.

The Medieval period (AD 500–1000) saw little progress in science and medicine. These years were dominated by political and religious struggles. Cancer was still believed to be caused by an excess of black bile. Superficial tumors and ulcers were treated by wide excision and cauterization. Caution was used if tumors could not be treated by excision. The more extensive tumors and ulcers were treated with caustic pastes, and treatment included a combination of phlebotomy, herbal potions, diet, powder of crab, and other symbolic charms. Medicine during this time remained a combination of astrology, herbal potions, caustic pastes, excisions and cauterizations, and bloodletting. None of the pastes, potions, or symbolic charms had any benefit systematically, but some did have escharotic effects on local tumors. In particular, arsenic paste might have had an antitumor effect. The use of arsenic compositions continued throughout the centuries up to 1865, when marked improvements were observed by Lissauer after a solution of potassium (Fowler's Solution) was given to a patient with chronic leukemia. A few years later, Billroth demonstrated a dramatic response of lymphosarcoma to Fowler's Solution (Haddow 1970). Today, this solution has made a comeback and is being used once again to treat cancer.

Shimkin (1977) describes the evolution of cancer treatments through the centuries. The 17th century saw a change in the theory of cancer. Cancer was no longer thought to be a result of an excess of black bile but was now seen as a result of stasis and abnormalities of lymph. Surgery continued to be used for local tumors. In breast tumors, the technique of mastectomy was used. Without anesthesia or antiseptic techniques, the breast was removed by a total slice removal followed by cauterization. The opinion that cancer was contagious began to develop during this century.

Up until this time in history, cancer chemotherapy remained a treatment using caustic pastes and potions, which showed little concrete value. An important development occurred in the 1600s that would later encourage the investigation and use of chemotherapy for cancer. The success of cancer chemotherapy is linked directly to the successful discovery of the use of chemotherapy for infections. Beginning in 1630, the first real chemotherapeutic *drug* (chemical used to treat disease) was used by the Jesuits who used a tea made from the bark of a chinchona tree to treat malaria. Dysentery was treated using a drug from the bark of a tree in Brazil. From these crude and simple extracts came quinine and emetine (ipecac), which are established treatments for malaria and amoebic dysentery, respectively (Burchenal 1977). These drugs can be considered the first successful curative chemotherapeutic agents. They were used without knowledge of the etiology of disease, the identity of chemicals, or the action of the drugs (DeVita 2001). These successes provided support that drugs could cure diseases. Further advances in chemotherapies of infectious diseases and cancer would have to wait until the early 20th century, when the important discoveries of Paul Ehrlich, the "father of chemotherapy," affected the treatment of infectious diseases and cancer.

During the 18th century, surgery remained the primary means for treating localized tumors. The theory that cancer was originally a localized, respectable disease caused by inflammation developed during this time. Attention was given to the disease known as cancer, and the first hospitals specifically for cancer opened in France (1740) and England (1792). Treatment of cancer emerged but was in an embryonic state. Toward the end of the century, it was discovered that environmental carcinogens could be epidemiologically linked to cancer. The use of snuff and the exposure to chimney soot was related causally to nasal cancers and scrotal cancers, respectively.

The 19th century was an age of inventions. Oncology was ushered into a new era. Better understanding of tumor histology resulted from the invention of the achromatic microscope. The use of anesthesia and the introduction of antisepsis permitted surgical removal of deeper cancers in internal organs. The first chemical agent to be used against malignant disease was arsenic in the form of potassium arsenite. Another mixture, the first biologic therapy, was used in 1893 by Coley. A mixture of streptococci and bacilli (Coley's toxins) demonstrated objective response in sarcoma. This treatment was dangerous, with results that were unpredictable. Still, a few people were cured of cancer in the 19th century.

Discoveries occurring at the turn of the 20th century had an impact on the treatment of cancer.

The development of the radical "en bloc" mastectomy by Halsted, where the primary tumor and the draining lymph nodes were removed surgically, and the discovery of x-rays by Roentgen offered a new modalities. Tumors could now be visualized, and radiation was introduced as therapy. The use of radiation therapy in the treatment of cancer first occurred in 1896; by 1905, the first patient with carcinoma of the uterus was treated with radium. The 21st century appears to be bringing revolutionary changes to cancer treatment. Targeted therapy, molecular therapy, gene therapy, and cancer vaccines are being developed and studied for various cancers. This century offers a new hope to patients with cancer.

Advent of Cancer Chemotherapy

The idea that drugs could be used for treatment of malignant disease was supported by the successes seen with synthetic chemicals and natural products used to cure parasitic and common bacterial infections and tuberculosis in rodent models and humans. Paul Ehrlich tested drugs on rodent models, the model most likely to predict the effectiveness of drugs in humans. It was the theory of using rodent models that led George Clowes of Roswell Park Memorial Institute in the early 1900s to develop inbred rodent lines that could carry transplanted rodent tumors. These rodent models were the testing ground for early cancer chemotherapeutic agents (DeVita 2001). Potential cancer chemotherapeutic drugs were investigated and tested for their effect against tumors in humans.

The modern era of chemotherapy was initiated by the discovery of the effective use of estrogens in prostate and breast cancer (Shimkin 1977). The alkylating agents were discovered by looking at the toxic effects of poison gases. In an accident in Naples Harbor, sailors were exposed to poisonous mustard gas. As a result, many developed marrow and lymphoid hypoplasia. Looking at this effect, it was thought that a derivative of this gas could be useful in treating cancers. Given a code designation of HN2 (and subsequently known as *nitrogen mustard*), this agent was used to treat lymphomas. It was given to patients with Hodgkin's disease at Yale University in 1943. Patients' tumors responded to the treatment (i.e., tumors became smaller) (DeVita 2001). The clinical effect of nitrogen mustard interested researchers who were treating cancers, but the tumor response was short lived, and all the patients relapsed. From these studies came other chemotherapeutic agents, such as busulfan and melphalan (Burchenal 1977).

In 1947, Dr. Sydney Farber discovered a treatment for childhood acute leukemia (Farber *et al.* 1948). He demonstrated the activity of the antifols as effective cancer agents. A related drug, methotrexate, would later be developed as an effective agent for treating choriocarcinomas (DeVita 2001), leading to more than 50% of patients being cured of their disease. In 1956, the first patient with Wilms' tumor was cured using chemotherapy, and the first bone marrow transplant was performed. As a result of these important discoveries, the development of cancer chemotherapeutic agents began in earnest.

The appropriation of funds for the development of the Cancer Drug Development Program initiated more reliable testing and development for cancer chemotherapeutic agents. Over the years, changes have occurred in treatment regimens that have brought dramatic results in the treatment of certain cancers. Single-agent drug therapy was the accepted treatment regimen in the earlier days of chemotherapy development. Today, combination chemotherapy has resulted in long-term remissions, more effective prevention of resistance, and tolerable side effects with maximal dose. A cure is possible now in patients with gestational choriocarcinoma, advanced Hodgkin's disease, non-Hodgkin's lymphomas, Burkitt's lymphoma, childhood leukemias, and testicular cancers. Increased survival has been reported in many other lymphomas and leukemias (Stonehill 1978).

High-dose chemotherapy with stem-cell rescue (autologous) and transplant of bone marrow from a compatible door (allogeneic) have led to cures for some patients with acute myelocytic leukemia and chronic myelocytic leukemia. New strategies to harness the immune system show promise in increasing cure rates.

Another approach that has shown evidence of increased survival rates and longer disease-free intervals is the use of adjuvant chemotherapy. It is known that, despite surgery and radiation, many cancers recur. This recurrence is believed to be a result of undetectable micrometastases. The modern use of chemotherapy primarily evolved from a need to treat metastatic, disseminated disease. Adjuvant chemotherapy has proved effective in Wilms' tumor, osteosarcoma, Ewing's sarcoma, embryonal rhabdomyosarcomas in children, non-seminomatous testicular cancer, and both pre-menopausal and postmenopausal breast cancer.

Forty years ago, it was believed that chemotherapy was ineffective against cancer. Fifteen years ago, only hematologic and embryonic tumors were thought to be treatable by cancer chemotherapy. Today combination chemotherapy and adjuvant chemotherapy have achieved great success in the treatment of malignant disease. Fortunately, however, our understanding of the molecular processes of malignant metastasis have led to the development of molecular targeted agents. The goal is to optimize the activity of chemotherapy in combination with molecular targeted agents to prevent cell division, slow cell division, encourage apoptosis (programmed cell death), and prevent the development of blood vessels (angiogenesis) that permit metastases. With the success of the Human Genome Project, the doors of molecular oncology have opened, ushering in new hope and promise.

The Cell Cycle and Its Importance

The cell cycle has been described in detail previously in Chapter 1. The cell cycle describes a sequence of steps through which both normal and neoplastic cells grow and replicate. This process of cell growth and replication involves five steps,

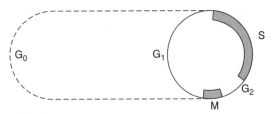

FIGURE 2.1 Stages in the Cell Replication Cycle. S = DNA synthesis; G_2 = the gap between DNA synthesis and mitosis; M = mitosis; and G_1 = the gap between the end of mitosis and the start of DNA synthesis (G_0 = resting phase, no replication).

Source: Tortorice, P.V. 2000. Cancer Nursing: Principles and Practice. Sudbury, MA: Jones & Bartlett publishers. Reprinted with permission.

or phases, which are designated by the letters and subscript numbers G_0, G_1, S, G_2, and M. The phases of the cell cycle are shown in Figure 2.1.

The letter G denotes gap phases, which are time periods in which cells are either preparing for the more active phases of DNA (deoxyribonucleic acid) synthesis and mitosis or resting. G_1 is referred to as the *first gap* or *first growth phase*. During this phase, the cell prepares for DNA synthesis by producing RNA (ribonucleic acid) and protein. G_1 includes a *resting phase* called G_0. Cells in G_0 are considered to be out of the cell cycle; that is, cellular activity does not include replication when the cell is in G_0. Cells can remain in G_0 for varying lengths of time and can be recruited back into G_1 according to the organism's needs. In this way, cells in G_0 are in a cellular reservoir; resting cells can be drawn from G_0 to add to the supply of dividing cells in the cell cycle (Ford and Pardee 1999).

The *synthesis* of DNA is the major event occurring during the S phase. DNA is the genetic code of information necessary for the growth, repair, and reproduction of the cell. Normal and neoplastic cells differ in the amount of time they spend in the S phase. Many antineoplastic drugs work by causing irreparable disruption in the organization of the DNA code during DNA synthesis. The disruption ultimately results in cell death. The S phase lasts between 10 and 30 hours (Tortorice 2000).

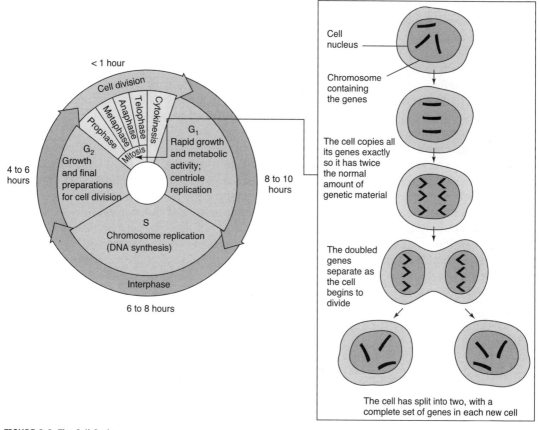

FIGURE 2.2 The Cell Cycle.

G_2 is the *second growth period* or *second gap*. The synthesis of RNA and proteins continues as the cell prepares itself for mitosis. The production of the mitotic spindle apparatus (where chromosomes are condensed in preparation for division) also occurs during this phase. G_2 lasts between 1 and 12 hours.

Actual cell division, or *mitosis*, occurs during the M phase. The mitotic process consists of four phases: prophase, metaphase, anaphase, and telophase. The major events occurring during the M phase are shown in Figure 2.2.

During the M phase, the cell divides into two daughter cells, each one containing the same number and kind of chromosomes as the parent cell. At the completion of the M phase, the cells either reenter the cell cycle at G_1 to undergo further maturation and replication or await activation by resting in G_0. Normally, cells spend about an hour in M phase.

The amount of time required to complete the cell cycle (called the *generation time*) varies depending on the type of cell. Although the time from the beginning of S phase to the end of M phase seems to be fairly constant, the time the cell spends in G_1 phase can vary greatly (from 12 to 48 hours). The temporal length of G_1 phase determines the rate of cell proliferation (Baserga 1981).

Research into cyclins tells us more about the growth and regulation of the cell. Cyclins are proteins that cause the cell to enter mitosis and begin division (Johnson and Walker 1999). Cyclin research elucidates cell cycle activity for malignant cells. Malignant cells from a variety of tumors bear abnormalities in a four-protein molecular structure responsible for cell cycle control (Figure 2.3). Cyclin is one of the four proteins. Chapter 1 discusses the specific molecular and cellular processes that are active in normal and cancerous cells, including the concept of apoptosis.

Apoptosis occurs when proteins in the nucleus of the cell fragment the cell's nuclear DNA, resulting in cell death. The absence of growth factors or hormones in some malignant cells can lead to apoptosis, whereas various other genetic events have been found to lead to a resistance to apoptosis. Treatment with some chemotherapeutic agents, monoclonal antibiotics, oncolytic viruses, and other agents results in a breakdown of resistance

to apoptosis in some cancer cells. Elucidation of the molecular mechanisms underlying apoptosis will shed light on the question of why some tumor cells survive chemotherapy and others do not.

Antineoplastic drugs affect both normal and malignant cells by altering cellular activity during one or more phases of the cell cycle. Although both types of cells die as a result of irreparable damage caused by chemotherapy, normal cells have a greater ability to repair minor damage and to continue living than neoplastic cells. The increased vulnerability of malignant cells is exploited to achieve the therapeutic effects seen with the administration of antineoplastic drugs.

Most antineoplastic agents are classified according to their structure or cell cycle activity. Two major classes of chemotherapeutic agents

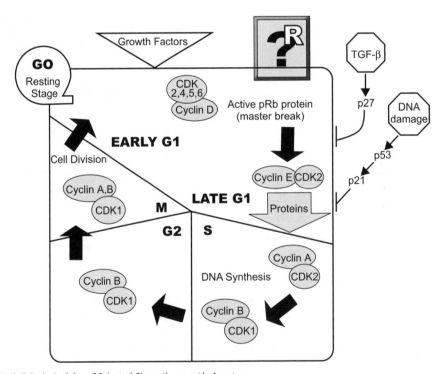

FIGURE 2.3 Cell Cycle Activity of Selected Chemotherapeutic Agents.

Source: Yarbro, C. 2006. *Cancer Nursing Principles and Practice.* 6th ed. Sudbury, MA: Jones and Bartlett. Reprinted with permission.

have been established: cell cycle phase–specific and cell cycle phase–nonspecific agents.

Cell Cycle Phase–Specific Agents

Cell cycle phase–specific agents kill proliferating cells only in a specific phase of the cell cycle (phases G_1 though M) (Tortorice 2000). For example, the vinca alkaloids, vincristine and vinblastine, are lethal only to cells in the M phase, where as hydroxyurea and cytosine arabinoside (cytarabine) inhibit DNA synthesis and, therefore, are specific to the S phase. Because phase-specific agents depend on cells being in a specific phase to work, they are most effective against cells that are rapidly cycling. Rapid cycling ensures that the cell passes through the phase in which it is vulnerable to the effects of the drugs. The antimetabolites and bleomycin are examples of phase-specific agents.

Some authors (Fischer *et al.* 2003) classify phase-specific agents under a broad class of agents called *cell cycle–specific agents*. These drugs damage both proliferating and resting cells, although they tend to be more effective against actively dividing cells than cells in G_0 (Fischer *et al.* 2003). Therefore, cells that spend most of their time in G_0 are not affected significantly by cycle-specific agents. For purposes of simplicity and clarity and because the distinctions between the classes of antineoplastic drugs are often relative, the drugs are classified as either cell cycle–specific or cell cycle phase–nonspecific drugs.

Cell Cycle Phase–Nonspecific Agents

Cell cycle phase–nonspecific agents do not depend on the phase of the cell cycle to be active. Rather, these agents affect cells in all phases of the cell cycle; resting cells are as vulnerable as dividing cells to the cytotoxic effects of these agents. Consequently, phase-nonspecific agents have been found to be some of the most effective drugs against slow-growing tumors (Fischer *et al.* 2003).

However, because DNA is the target site for these drugs, maximum cell kill is not possible when cells are in the S phase at the time of drug administration. Nitrogen mustard, dacarbazine, and mitomycin are some examples of phase-nonspecific agents.

Chemotherapy and Cell Kinetics

A basic understanding of tumor cell kinetics is helpful in comprehending the rationales behind various chemotherapy schedules and regimens.

Tumor Growth

Tumors grow by a progressive, steady expansion. According to Tortorice (2000), three characteristics of cells should be considered when assessing tumor growth: cell cycle time, growth fraction, and rate of cell loss. *Cell cycle time* is defined as the amount of time needed for the cell to complete an entire cycle from mitosis to mitosis. Cycle times for cancer cells vary from 24 to 120 hours, with most ranging from 48 to 72 hours. It is interesting to note that some of the more rapidly dividing normal cells (e.g., colon and rectum crypt cells at 39–48 hours and bone marrow precursor cells at 19–40 hours) have similar, if not faster, cell cycle times than cancer cells. It originally was thought that cancer cells cycled and grew faster than normal cells (Tortorice 2000). It is easily understandable, then, how toxicities to normal cells occur because chemotherapy acts on *all* rapidly dividing cells and not just those that are malignant. The *growth fraction* is the fraction of cells in the tumor that are cycling at a given time. In the early stages of tumor development (i.e., when tumor volume is low), the growth fraction is high, and the tumor doubles its volume relatively rapidly. As the tumor grows, however, space becomes restricted, and it outgrows the blood and nutrient supply so that the *tumor doubling time* decreases. Common tumor doubling times range from 5 days to 2 years.

The last factor influencing net tumor growth is the *rate of cell loss*, which is the fraction of cells that die or leave the tumor mass. Tumor growth is the net effect of the three factors of cell cycle time, growth fraction, and rate of cell loss and follows a *Gompertzian growth curve* (Figure 2.4).

The growth curve is a visual depiction of the idea that, as the tumor mass increases in size, tumor doubling time slows. The earliest point at which a solid tumor can be detected clinically is when it contains 5×10^8 cells (at this point, it measures 1 cm in diameter) (Gussack *et al.* 1984).

Tumor growth characteristics at least partially determine the choice of chemotherapeutic agents used against a tumor. For example, when tumor volume is low, a relatively large percentage of cells are dividing and thus are vulnerable to chemotherapeutic agents that affect dividing cells (cell cycle phase–specific agents). Likewise, when tumor volume is high, fewer cells divide, and cell cycle phase–specific agents are used and found to be effective regardless of cell division.

Cell Kill Hypothesis

The *cell kill hypothesis* is the theoretical ability of chemotherapeutic agents to kill cancer cells. According to the hypothesis, which was first described in studies by Skipper and colleagues (Skipper *et al.* 1964; Skipper *et al.* 1965; Skipper 1968), drugs kill cancer cells on the basis of *first-order kinetics*; a certain drug dosage kills a constant percentage of cells rather than a constant number of cells. Thus, repeated doses of therapy are needed to reduce the total number of cells, and the number of cells left after therapy depends on the results of previous therapy, the time between repeated doses, and the doubling time of the tumor. For example, if a therapy has a 90% cell kill rate against a given tumor and the tumor is composed of a million cells, 100,000 cells are left living after the first treatment. Repeated treatments eventually should reduce the tumor to a small enough number of cells so that the immune system can kill any remaining cells (Tortorice 2000).

Unfortunately, cells can mutate over time and become resistant to chemotherapy. Patients with similar tumors can respond to treatment differently, sometimes making therapeutic decisions difficult. Consequently, the cell kill hypothesis cannot serve as the only predictor of a host's response to chemotherapy.

Relevance of Cytostatic Versus Cytotoxic Agents in Designing Chemotherapy Regimens

One way in which chemotherapeutic regimens are planned uses the principles of synchronization and recruitment. *Synchronization* refers to the process of increasing the percentage of tumor cells that are in a specific phase of the cell cycle (Hill 1978). This can be done by administering *cytostatic* agents (agents that block or retard cell development in a specific phase of the cell cycle) or by administering *cytotoxic* agents (agents that kill cells in a specific sensitive phase and lead to a relative increased percentage of cells in the insensitive phases). Low doses of antineoplastic agents tend to cause cells to arrest or block in certain phases, whereas high doses tend to cause cell death, particularly in certain phases (Gussack *et al.* 1984; Ingwersen 2001). According to Hill (1978), the chemotherapeutic purpose of synchronization is to gather cells in a specific phase

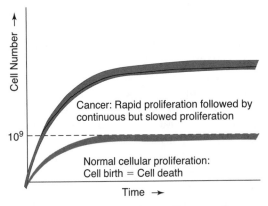

FIGURE 2.4 Gompertzian Growth Curve. Tumor growth differs from normal growth. Chemotherapy is effective when cell division is rapid.

of the cell cycle so that they are rendered vulnerable to agents that are cytotoxically specific for that phase. For example, cytosine arabinoside's cytostatic properties cause cells to arrest at the boundary of phases G_1 and S (the G_1/S boundary) (Hill 1978). In causing this G_1/S arrest, an increased percentage of cells are caught in late G_1–early S, rendering them vulnerable to agents specific for the S phase.

Recruitment is another theoretical construct used to design chemotherapeutic regimens. The term refers to the transformation of resting cells to dividing (or cycling) cells. It can occur as an indirect consequence of cell killing, when cell population depletion leads to the recruitment of resting cells back into the cell cycle. Cells that are recruited in this way are more vulnerable to the effects of drugs that work when cells are dividing (i.e., cycle phase–specific drugs) (Gussack *et al.* 1984; Ingwersen 2001).

Classification of Antineoplastic Agents

Antineoplastic agents are drugs that are specifically for the purpose of killing cancer cells. The terms *cancer chemotherapeutic drugs* and *cytotoxic compounds* are interchangeable. Cancer chemotherapeutic drugs generally are grouped into seven major classes: alkylating agents, antimetabolites, antibiotics, plant alkaloids or mitotic inhibitors, hormones, miscellaneous agents, and investigational agents.

Alkylating Agents

Alkylating agents are highly reactive compounds that work by interacting chemically with the cellular DNA to prevent replication of the cell. More specifically, by substituting an alkyl group for the hydrogen atoms in cellular molecules, alkylating agents cause single- and double-strand breaks in DNA to cross link and bond covalently (Ratain 2001). The DNA strands are thus unable to separate, which is an action necessary for the replication of cellular genetic material. Alkylating agents prevent replication by causing a misreading of the DNA code and by inhibiting RNA, DNA, and protein synthesis in rapidly dividing tissues. The nucleic acid base most often involved in the process is guanine, but adenine and cytosine have undergone alkylation as a result of drug administration. A schematic diagram showing sites and mechanisms of action of all the major chemotherapeutic agents is shown in Figure 2.5.

Alkylating agents are considered cycle nonspecific. They exert their lethal effects on cells throughout the cell cycle but tend to be more effective against rapidly dividing cells. One author postulates that this may be because rapidly dividing cells have less time to repair damaged caused in G_1 before they enter the sensitive S phase of the cycle (Ratain 2001). Because alkylating agents are active against cells in G_0, they can be used to debulk (reduce the size of) tumors, causing resting cells to be recruited into active division. At this point, those cells are vulnerable to the cell cycle–specific agents.

Alkylating agents have been proven to be cytotoxically active against lymphomas, Hodgkin's disease, breast cancer, and multiple myeloma. Unfortunately, patients exposed to high doses of alkylating agents are at a higher risk of developing second primary sites of cancer (secondary malignancies), such as bladder cancer (after exposure to cyclophosphamide) and leukemias (after melphalan). Some of the alkylating agents (most notably, cyclophosphamide and diaziquone) have a pronounced effect on bone marrow stem cells, producing cumulative myelosuppression after repeated administrations of the drug. The nitrosoureas (carmustine, lomustine, and methyl-lomustine) are associated with a delayed myelosuppression, with a nadir at 3–5 weeks after administration, which may continue for several more weeks. Changes in gonadal function also have occurred after treatment with alkylating agents. Oligospermia and azospermia, most often associated with the agents cyclophosphamide and chlorambucil, may be reversible after discontinuation of treatment.

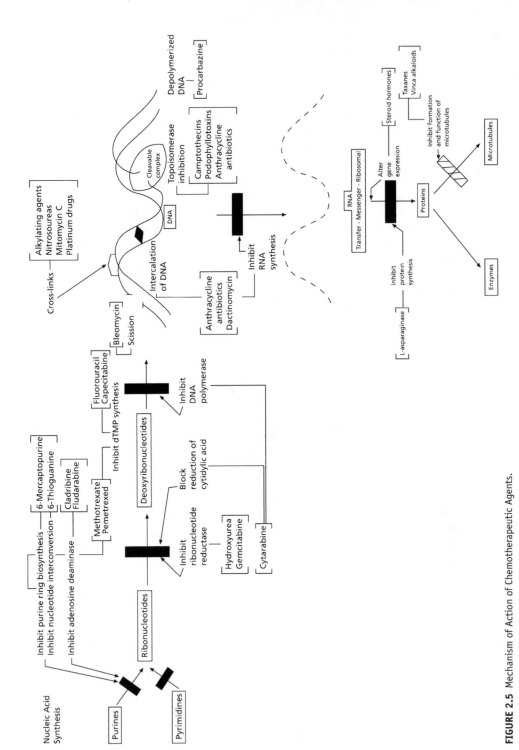

FIGURE 2.5 Mechanism of Action of Chemotherapeutic Agents.

Source: Yarbro, C. 2006. *Cancer Nursing Principles and Practice.* 6th ed. Sudbury, MA: Jones and Bartlett. Reprinted with permission.

Amenorrhea is a common occurrence, but it too may be reversible in some patients.

Common Alkylating Agents

busulfan (Myleran)

carboplatin (Paraplatin)

carmustine (BiCNU, BCNU)

chlorambucil (Leukeran)

cisplatin (*Cis*-Platinum, CDDP, Platinum, Platinol)

cyclophosphamide (Cytoxan, Endoxan, Neosar)

dacarbazine (DTIC-Dome, imidazole carboxamide)

estramustine phosphate (Estracyte, Emcyt)

ifosfamide (Ifex, IFX, Isophosphamide)

lomustine (CCNU, CeeNU)

mechlorethamine (nitrogen mustard, Mustargen, HN_2)

melphalan (Alkeran, L-PAM, Phenylalanine Mustard, L-Sarcolysin)

streptozocin (Streptozotocin, Zanosar)

thiotepa (triethylene thiophosphoramide, TSPA, TESPA)

Antimetabolites

Cells depend on various nutrient products of normal cell metabolism, *metabolites*, for the biologic synthesis of RNA and DNA. The *antimetabolites* are a group of agents that interfere with DNA and RNA synthesis by mimicking the chemical structure of essential metabolites. They prohibit cell replication in one of two ways: antimetabolites deceive cells into incorporating them along certain metabolic pathways essential for the synthesis of RNA or DNA so that a false genetic message is transmitted; or antimetabolites block the enzymes necessary for the synthesis of essential compounds. The end result is that DNA synthesis is prevented.

Most antimetabolite cytotoxic activity occurs during the synthetic phase (S) of the cell cycle. It logically follows, then, that these agents would be most effective when used against rapidly cycling cell populations. This explains why antimetabolites are more effective against fast-growing tumors than slow-growing tumors.

The most common toxicities to normal cells occur as a result of the agent's attack on rapidly dividing cell populations. For example, oral mucosal cells, bone marrow stem cells, and cells lining the gastrointestinal (GI) tract are affected by antimetabolite administration. Toxicities that follow such cytotoxic activity include stomatitis, bone marrow depression (myelosuppression), and diarrhea (and other GI sequelae resulting from death of normal cells and tissue sloughing). Commonly used antimetabolites include folate antagonists (methotrexate, trimetrexate), purine antagonists (6-mercaptopurine and 6-thioguanine), fluoropyrimidines (5-fluorouracil and floxuridine), and cytosine arabinoside (ARA-C, cytarabine).

Common Antimetabolites

capecitabine (Xeloda)

cytarabine (ARA-C, Cytosar-U, cytosine arabinoside)

floxuridine (FUDR, 5-FUDR, 5-fluoro-2'-deoxyuridine)

5-fluorouracil (fluorouracil, Adrucil, 5-FU)

gemcitabine (Gemzar)

hydroxyurea (Hydrea)

6-mercaptopurine (purinethol, 6-MP)

methotrexate (Amethopterin, Mexate, Folex)

6-thioguanine (thioguanine)

Antibiotics

The antitumor antibiotics are agents that are isolated from micro-organisms. They have both antimicrobal and cytotoxic activity, although the latter predominates. As a class, the antibiotics are cell cycle nonspecific and appear to have several different mechanisms by which they produce their cytotoxic effects. For example, bleomycin's primary action is to produce single- and double-strand breaks in DNA. The anthracyclines (daunomycin and doxorubicin) intercalate DNA (forming a bond so that DNA is prevented from functioning as a template for RNA and DNA synthesis), cause oxidation-reduction reactions, and react directly with cell membranes at low concentrations to change membrane function. As our understanding of molecular functioning advances, so too does our understanding of mechanisms of drug action. For example, doxorubicin acts as a topoisomerase II inhibitor as well.

Mitomycin produces cellular reactions similar to those of the anthracyclines but also functions as an alkylator. Mithramycin inhibits DNA-directed RNA synthesis, whereas actinomycin-D's primary action is the intercalation of DNA (Ratain 2001). To summarize, in general, antibiotics function by binding or reacting with DNA, by inhibiting the synthesis of RNA, or both.

Major dose-limiting toxicities associated with the antibiotics are myelosuppression (all but bleomycin); skin and GI toxicity (actinomycin-D); pneumonitis leading to fibrosis (bleomycin); cardiotoxicity and mucositis (doxorubicin and daunorubicin); and hepatic, renal, and blood clotting dysfunctions (mithramycin) (Ratain 2001).

Common Antibiotics

bleomycin (Blenoxane)
dactinomycin (actinomycin-D, Cosmegan)
daunorubicin (daunomycin, rubidomycin, Cerubidine)
doxorubicin (Adriamycin)
idarubicin (Idamycin)
mithramycin (Mithracin, plicamycin)
mitomycin (Mutamycin)
mitoxantrone (Novantrone)

Plant Alkaloids (Mitotic Inhibitors)

The search for new cytotoxic compounds led to the screening of many plant extracts. Compounds of note (vincristine, vinblastine, and etoposide) have survived clinical trials to become recognized as worthwhile antineoplastic agents. Vincristine and vinblastine are called vinca alkaloids and are derived from the shrub *Vinca rosea*. Etoposide is derived from products of the mandrake plant.

The vinca alkaloids work by crystallizing the microtubular mitotic spindle proteins during metaphase, which arrests mitosis and causes cell death. At high concentrations of the drug, inhibition of nucleic acid synthesis and protein synthesis has also been noted. The action of plant alkaloids is considered cell cycle phase specific, occurring during the M phase. Etoposide is premitotic in its cytotoxic activity, exerting most effect in G_2 (Fischer *et al.* 2003), but also acts as a topoisomerase II inhibitor. Major dose-limiting toxicities of plant alkaloids include myelosuppression (with vinblastine and etoposide) and neurotoxicity (with vincristine and, to a lesser extent, vinblastine).

Common Plant Alkaloids

etoposide (VP 16-213, Vepesid, epipodophyllotoxin)
vinblastine (Velban, vinblastine sulfate)
vincristine (Oncovin, vincristine sulfate)
vinorelbine (Navelbine)

Hormones

The growth and development of certain tumors depend to some extent on their existing in a specific hormonal environment. When that environment is changed, tumor growth is impaired or arrested. Breast, thyroid, prostate, and uterine cancers are examples of solid tumors that are sensitive to hormonal manipulation. With these diseases, the action of hormones or hormone antagonists depends on the presence of hormone receptors in the tumors themselves (i.e., estrogen receptors in breast cancers). Normally, proteins in the cytoplasm of a cell act as receptors that bind to hormones and transfer them to the nucleus of the cell. Once there, the hormone receptors facilitate the binding of chromatin to the nucleus—a process necessary for the synthesis of messenger RNA, which transmits the genetic information necessary for the synthesis of new proteins.

The blocking of this process occurs when hormones or their antagonists are administered. Commonly used gonadal or sex hormones are estrogens (diethylstilbestrol [DES], ethinyl estradiol [Estinyl]), progestins (medroxyprogesterone acetate [Provera], megestrol acetate [Megace]), antiestrogens (tamoxifen citrate [Nolvadex]), androgens (fluoxymesterone [Halotestin, Utadren], testosterone propionate [Oreton]), and antitestosterones (leuprolide acetate [Luporon], bicalutamide [Casodex], flutamide [Eulexin]).

Corticosteroids, such as prednisone and prednisolone, are another class of agents useful in the treatment of certain neoplasms. The discovery of their lympholytic action led to their use against lymphatic leukemias, myeloma, and malignant lymphoma. Some evidence exists to suggest that corticosteroids also can recruit malignant cells out of the G_0 phase of cell cycle–specific chemotherapeutic agents (Bingham 1978).

Side effects from hormonal therapy occur as a result of the administering of higher than physiologic doses of a drug to achieve the desired antineoplastic effects (Tortorice 2000). For the sex hormones, side effects include changes in secondary sexual characteristics (e.g., deepening of voice and hirsutism), changes in libido, and fluid retention. For the corticosteroids, side effects include hypertension, fluid retention, hyperglycemia, ulcers, osteoporosis, emotional instability, muscle wasting, increased appetite, Cushingoid features, increased susceptibility to infection, and masking of fevers.

Common Hormonal Agents

Adrenocorticoid Agents
  cortisone
  dexamethasone
  hydrocortisone
  methylprednisone
  methylprednisolone
  prednisone
  prednisolene
Androgens
  fluoxymesterone (Halotestin, Ora-Testryl)
  testolactone (Teslac)
  testosterone propionate (Neo-hombreol, Oreton)
Estrogens
  conjugated equine estrogen (Premarin)
  diethylstilbestrol (DES)
  diethylstilbestrol diphosphate (Stilphostrol, Stilbestrol Diphosphate)
  ethinyl estradiol (Estinyl)
Antiestrogens
  tamoxifen citrate (Nolvadex)

Antitestosterones
  bicalatamide (Casodex)
  flutamide (Eulexin)
  leuprolide (Lupron)
Progesterones
  medroxyprogesterone acetate (Provera, Depo-Provera)
  megestrol acetate (Megace, Pallace)

Miscellaneous Agents

Miscellaneous agents are those agents whose mechanisms of action differ from the major classes just mentioned. One of the most commonly used miscellaneous agents is L-asparaginase.

Asparagine is a nonessential amino acid required by some tumor cells for normal growth and development. The enzymes needed to synthesize asparagine are present in many normal tissues but are lacking in certain tumors, especially tumors arising from T lymphocytes (Ratain 2001). Cells that lack these enzymes derive asparagine from circulating pools of amino acids. L-asparaginase depletes these pools rapidly and completely. Because normal tissues can synthesize their own asparagine, L-asparaginase has very little toxicity to normal tissues. However, it is a foreign protein and can cause serious anaphylactic reactions.

Common Miscellaneous Agents

L-asparaginase (Elspar)
mitotane (Lysodren)
mitoxantrone (Novantrone)
procarbazine (Matulane)

Camptothecins

The camptothecins are drugs that inhibit the enzyme topoisomerase I. Topoisomerase I is one of the enzymes responsible for relaxing the tension in the DNA helix by causing single-strand breaks in the helix and eventually reattaching them in the religation step of the process. Topotecan and irinotecan work by binding to topoisomerase I, thereby arresting the cell in the G_2 phase. Dose-limiting toxicities include diarrhea (with irinotecan) and myelosuppression (with both irinotecan and topotecan).

Common Camptothecins

irinotecan (Camptosar, camptothecan-11, CPT-11)

topotecan (Hycamptin)

Taxanes

Like the plant alkaloids, paclitaxel (Taxol) and docetaxel (Taxotere) are plant derivatives, originally from the needles of the Pacific yew tree. The taxanes promote microtubule assembly and stability, thereby blocking the cell cycle in mitosis. Docetaxel is more potent in enhancing microtubule assembly and induces apoptosis.

Common Taxanes

docetaxel (Taxotere)

paclitaxel (Taxol)

Investigational Chemotherapeutic Agents

Investigational agents are those agents that currently are undergoing clinical trials and thus are not yet approved by the U.S. Food and Drug Administration (FDA). Such agents include not only new drugs but also approved drugs that are being administered in a manner different from that for which approval was obtained previously.

In clinical trials, drugs are procured directly from the National Cancer Institute (NCI) or indirectly through cooperative group protocols (the Cancer and Leukemia Group B, the Pediatric Oncology Group, etc.) and cancer centers. Although patients generally need to be treated on an NCI-approved protocol to receive investigational drugs, such agents may be obtained from the pharmaceutical company for "compassionate use." This term refers to the use of an investigational agent off protocol in a patient for whom no other clinically established treatment options exist.

Rationale of Single-Agent Therapy Versus Combination Therapy

Single-agent therapy was often used in the early history of cancer chemotherapy. Starting in the 1960s, however, combinations of chemothera-

peutic agents were found to produce superior clinical responses with less overall toxicity than single-agent therapy (Fischer *et al.* 2003). With a few exceptions, combination chemotherapy has replaced single-agent therapy in the medical management of cancer.

The major disadvantages of single-agent therapy led to clinical trials with combinations of drugs. Some of these disadvantages are as follows: single agents are unsuccessful at achieving long-term remissions; they produce cell lines that are resistant to further drug therapy; and they produce severe or lethal toxicities when given in doses adequate to eradicate the tumor (Fischer *et al.* 2003). The most significant of these disadvantages is tumor drug resistance because this is found to be the most common reason for treatment failure.

The improved therapeutic effects of combination chemotherapy resulted from both the additive and synergistic effects of the drugs used. According to Carter and Livingston (1982), three conceptual approaches have been used in designing drug combinations. The *biochemical approach* asserts that by using drugs that individually produce different biochemical damage, one can attack different sites in the biosynthetic pathways or inhibit processes that are necessary for the normal function of essential macromolecules. The goal of the biochemical approach is to decrease the production and the availability of the end products needed by the tumor for normal growth and development.

The *cytokinetic approach* is based on principles of cell cycle kinetics. This approach suggests that drugs should produce changes in cells that render them more vulnerable to cycle-specific agents. For example, it is known that debulking a tumor by surgery or chemotherapy causes an increase in the growth fraction (the number of cells undergoing active division) of the remaining cells. Activating cells in this way would make them vulnerable to cycle-specific agents.

The third approach is the empirical approach. Numerous effective combinations of agents have evolved through the use of individual agents that

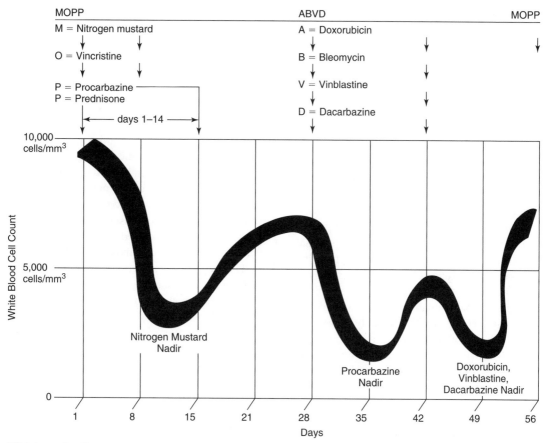

FIGURE 2.6 The Effect of MOPP Combined with ABVD on the White Blood Cell Count.

Source: Goodman, M.S. 1987. *Cancer: Chemotherapy and Care*. Bristol-Myers Oncology Division. Reprinted with permission.

alone have demonstrated antineoplastic activity against a particular tumor. When combined, the mechanisms of action of the different drugs often complement each other to produce maximal cell kill. A distinct advantage of combination chemotherapy is that the toxicities of the individual drugs often differ, allowing the administration of nearly full tolerated doses without severe toxicity. One example of an empirically derived drug combination is MOPP (mechlorethamine, vincristine, prednisone, and procarbazine) for the treatment of Hodgkin's disease. The effect on the bone marrow of the drug combination MOPP plus ABVD (doxorubicin, bleomycin, vinblastine, and dacarbazine) used against Hodgkin's disease is shown in Figure 2.6.

A closer look at this drug combination illustrates some of the principles used in the empirical approach.

Principle: *Each drug in the combination should be active against the tumor when used alone.* Mechlorethamine, vincristine, procarbazine, prednisone, doxorubicin, bleomycin, vinblastine, and dacarbazine have all been shown to be active against Hodgkin's disease.

Principle: *The mechanisms of action of the different drugs should complement each other to produce maximal cell kill.* The drugs listed for the first principle are both cell cycle phase specific and cell cycle phase nonspecific. For example, dacarbazine and mechlorethamine are alkylating agents and are cell cycle phase nonspecific, whereas vincristine and vinblastine are both specific for the S and M phases. Using these drugs in combination theoretically ensures that cells will be affected regardless of their cycling characteristics at the time of drug administration.

Principle: *Drugs that produce toxicities in different organ systems should be combined so that maximal doses of each can be administered without excessive morbidity.* In the MOPP combination, mechlorethamine is a potent myelosuppressant, whereas vincristine's dose-limiting toxicity is often neurotoxicity. Prednisone does not affect bone marrow but sometimes causes imbalances in glucose metabolism and protein breakdown (Fischer *et al.* 2003). Procarbazine's dose-limiting toxicities are nausea and vomiting and myelosuppression, although the myelosuppression occurs much later than that of mechlorethamine (Goodman 1992).

Principle: *Drugs should be combined that have toxicities occurring at different times.* As mentioned, mechlorethamine's myelosuppressive nadir occurs at 10–14 days, whereas procarbazine's nadir is 2–3 weeks after cessation of therapy (Fischer *et al.* 2003).

Some of the advantages of combination chemotherapy are that it allows for maximal cell kill within the range of toxicity tolerated by the patient for each drug; it provides for a broader range of coverage of new resistant tumor cell lines (this seems to be the major reason for the success of combination chemotherapy over single-agent therapy); and it prevents or slows the development of new resistant cell lines (DeVita 2001). An important advance made with the institution of combination chemotherapy was the use of intermittent treatment schedules, which permit the recovery of normal tissues between treatment cycles.

In summary, combination chemotherapy has replaced single-agent chemotherapy in the medical management of most tumors because of its improved clinical responses and decreased toxicity compared with single-agent therapy.

Mechanisms of Drug Resistance

One of the factors preventing the development of curative chemotherapy is the development of tumor resistance to the drug. Laboratory evidence has shown that exposure of a cancer cell to a *single* antineoplastic agent can lead to resistance to multiple agents, and many of the drugs causing this multidrug resistance are natural products, such as vinblastine and doxorubicin (Beck and Dalton 2001).

The presence of a large cell-surface glycoprotein, called p-glycoprotein, on cancer cells appears to be one of the most important causes of multidrug resistance. Cancer cells with multidrug resistance have a very high number of these cell-surface glycoproteins, whereas cells sensitive to chemotherapy agents have very few cell-surface glycoproteins, if any.

The p-glycoprotein molecule works like a pump so that chemotherapeutic drugs enter the cell but then are pumped quickly back out of the cancer cells, leaving cells undamaged by the chemotherapy. Certain normal body cells have p-glycoprotein molecules on their surface, possibly as an evolutionary protective mechanism to remove ingested toxins. As might be expected, these normal cells are found in organs frequently resistant to chemotherapy, such as the kidneys, adrenal glands, liver, and parts of the GI tract, whereas cells that are extremely chemosensitive, such as blood cells, have almost no p-glycoprotein.

Genetically, the cells that contain p-glycoprotein and demonstrate multidrug resistance (MRD) usually have gene amplification of MDR, or PGY1. According to Goldstein *et al.* (1989), this amplified gene is transcribed into the RNA that produces the p-glycoprotein molecule. The investigators also found that the highest levels of the gene (cells having the most amplified genes) were found in chemoresistant cancers of the colon, kidney (renal cells), liver, adrenal cortex, and lung (non–small-cell with neuroendocrine properties) and in pheochromocytoma, islet tumor of the pancreas, carcinoid tumor, and chronic myelogenous leukemia in blast crisis (Beck and Dalton 2001).

Reasons for drug resistance include:

- Defective transport of the drug into the cell with increased drug excretion, so there are decreased intracellular concentrations of the drug
- Defective drug metabolism
- Increased drug inactivation
- Altered DNA repair with increased cell efficiency to excise or repair DNA damage caused by the drug
- Altered drug target, so drug cannot recognize intracellular target (i.e., enzyme, nucleotide)

Current research efforts include the following:

- Identifying agents that inactivate the p-glycoprotein molecule in cells
- Screening agents that overcome resistance to known drugs
- Identifying drugs that affect cellular pathways leading toward cell division or apoptosis
- Identifying chemomodifiers that may be combined with chemotherapy agents to increase their effectiveness, such as the calcium channel agents
- Finding drugs that interact with unique chromosomal abnormalities of tumors

As more is learned about the mechanisms of drug resistance, models can be developed and tested that target these mechanisms and attempt to make the cancer cells sensitive to chemotherapeutic agents.

Conclusion

Drug therapy, supportive therapy, bone marrow transplantation, biologic response modifiers, and molecular targeted agents are in the forefront of cancer treatment methodology. All of these therapies are used in combination to enhance drug effectiveness. New drugs are being tested and developed in a variety of programs through the National Cancer Institute, as well as in programs in pharmaceutical companies. The development of new drugs has been the cornerstone of cancer chemotherapy. Newer theories of chemotherapy administration, such as neoadjuvant or induction chemotherapy, confer a definite survival advantage in several sarcomas and rectal cancers and improve surgical results in other solid tumors. Chemoprevention has been shown to prevent the development of second primary cancers in patients with head and neck cancers, and it is also being explored in other tumors. Newer strategies related to a more effective use of chemotherapy, hormones, and biologic agents are underway.

Both allogeneic (matched donor) and autologous (self-donor) bone marrow transplantations have shown success in a variety of cancers. This area holds a great deal of promise. Also, the use of growth factors to hasten bone marrow recovery permits more consistent and higher drug dosing.

The field of cancer treatments has grown over the years. More than 40 chemotherapeutic agents have proven useful in treating malignant diseases. Cancer chemotherapy, hormones, and biotherapy are here to stay. The science is constantly changing in an attempt to improve the survival of persons with cancer as well as their quality of life. The new millennium will see continuing changes in therapeutics, such as the technology of bone marrow transplantation, genetic reengineering, and drug development; oncology nursing will be in the forefront of these scientific and practice advancements.

References

Baserga, R. 1981. The cell cycle. *New England Journal of Medicine* 304(8):453–459.

Beck, W.T., and Dalton, W.S. 2001. Mechanisms of drug resistance: Chapter 11. In V.T. DeVita, S. Hellman, and S.A. Rosenberg (Eds): *Cancer: Principles and practice of oncology* (ed 6). Philadelphia: Lippincott Williams & Wilkins.

Bingham, C.A. 1978. The cell cycle and cancer chemotherapy. *American Journal of Nursing* 78(7):1201–1205.

Breasted, J.H. 1930. *The Edwin Smith Surgical Papyrus*. Chicago: University of Chicago Press.

Brothwell, D. 1967. The evidence of neoplasms. In D. Brothwell and A.T. Sanderson (Eds): *Disease of antiquity*. Springfield, IL: C.C. Thomas, pp 320–345.

Burchenal, J.H. (1977). The historical development of cancer chemotherapy. *Seminars in Oncology* 4(2):135–146.

Carter, S., and Livingston, R. 1982. Principles of cancer chemotherapy. In S. Carter, E. Glatstein, and R. Livingston (Eds): *Principles of cancer treatment*. New York: McGraw-Hill, pp 95–110.

DeVita, V.T., Jr. 2001. Principles of cancer management: Chemotherapy. In V.T. DeVita, Jr., S. Hellman, and S.A. Rosenberg (Eds): *Cancer: Principles and Practice of Oncology* (ed 6). Philadelphia: Lippincott Williams & Wilkins.

Ebbell, B. 1937. *The Papyrus Ebers: The greatest Egyptian medical document*. Copenhagen: Levin and Munksgaard.

Farber, S., Diamond, L., Mercer, R., *et al.* 1948. Temporary remissions in acute leukemia in children produced by folic acid antagonists, 4-aminopteroyglutamic acid (aminopterin). *New England Journal of Medicine* 238:787–793.

Fischer, D.S., Knobf, M.T., Durvage, H., Beaulieu, N. 2003. *The cancer chemotherapy handbook* (ed 6). St. Louis: Elsevier Press.

Ford, H., and Pardee, A. 1999. Cancer and the cell cycle. *Journal of Cellular Biochemistry* 75(Suppl 32/33):166–172.

Goldstein, L.J., Glaski, A., Fojo, M., Willingham, M., Lai, S.L., Gazdar, A., and Pirker, R. 1989. Expression of a multidrug resistance gene in human cancers. *Journal of the National Cancer Institute* 81(2):116–124.

Goodman, M.S. 1992. *Cancer: Chemotherapy and care* (ed 3). New York: Bristol-Myers Oncology Division.

Gussack, G.S., Brantley, B.A., and Farmer, J.C. 1984. Biology of tumors and head and neck cancer chemotherapy. *Laryngoscope* 94(9):1181–1187.

Haddow, A. 1970. David A. Karnofsky Memorial Lecture: Thoughts on chemical therapy. *Cancer* 26(4):737–754.

Hill, B.T. 1978. Cancer chemotherapy: The relevance of certain concepts of cell cycle kinetics. *Biochemica and Biophysica Acta* 516:389–417.

Ingwersen, K.C. 2001. Cell cycle kinetics and antineoplastic agents: Chapter 2. In M. Barton-Burke, and G.M. Wilks (Eds): *Cancer chemotherapy: A nursing process approach*. Boston: Jones and Bartlett, pp 23–44.

Johnson, D., and Walker, C. 1999. Cyclins and cell cycle checkpoints. *Annual Review of Pharmacology and Toxicology* 39(1):295–312.

Ratain, M.J., 2001. Pharmacokinetics and pharmacodynamics: Chapter 19. In V.T. DeVita, Jr., S. Hellman, and S.A. Rosenberg (Eds): *Cancer: Principles and practice of oncology* (ed 6). Philadelphia: Lippincott Williams & Wilkins, pp 335–340.

Shimkin, M.S. 1977. *Contrary to nature*. Washington, DC: U.S. Department of Health, Education, and Welfare, Public Health Service, Publication 76–720.

Skipper, H.E. 1968. 21st Annual Symposium on Fundamental Cancer Research at M.D. Anderson Hospital and Tumor Institute, Houston, Texas. In *The proliferation and spread of neoplastic cells*. Baltimore: Williams and Wilkins, pp 213–233.

Skipper, H.E., Schabel, F.M., Jr., and Wilcox, W.S. 1964. *Cancer Chemotherapy Reports* 35:1–111.

Skipper, H.E., Schabel, F.M., Jr., and Wilcox, W.S. 1965. Experimental evaluation of potential anticancer agents. XIV. Further Study of certain basic concepts underlying chemotherapy of leukemia. *Cancer Chemotherapy Reports* 45:5–28.

Stonehill, E.H. 1978. Impact of cancer therapy on survival. *Cancer* 42:1008–14.

Tortorice, P.V. 2000. Chemotherapy: Principles of therapy: Chapter 18. In C.H. Yarbro, M.H. Frogge, M. Goodman, and S.L. Groenwald (Eds): *Cancer nursing: Principles and practice*. Boston: Jones and Bartlett, pp 352–385.

Wells, C. 1963. Ancient Egyptian pathology. *Journal of Laryngology and Otology* 77:261–265.

Chemotherapy Drugs

Margaret Barton-Burke, Ph.D., R.N.

Gail M. Wilkes, M.S.N., R.N.C.

Drug Name: Acridinyl anisidide (AMSA, M-AMSA)

A

Class:	Investigational
Mechanism of Action:	Cell cycle phase specific; S phase. The primary mechanism of action is not yet clearly understood. It is believed that AMSA binds with DNA by intercalating between base pairs and thus prohibiting RNA synthesis.
Indications:	Per protocol
Dosing:	Drug is undergoing clinical trials. Consult individual protocol for specific dosages.
Administration:	Intravenous (IV). Dilute the AMSA solution further in 5% dextrose in water (D_5W) and infuse over 1 hour unless contraindicated.

AMSA is available as two sterile liquids: one ampule with an orange-red solution of AMSA and a second with the dilutant L-lactic acid. The solution, once mixed, is chemically stable for 48 hours. It should be discarded after 8 hours because of lack of bacteriostatic preservatives. AMSA is not stable in sodium chloride–containing solutions. Precipitates form. Only 5% dextrose solutions should be used.

Drug is a vesicant. Drug is investigational. No anaphylaxis reported. Do not dilute AMSA with chloride-containing solutions. Impaired liver function may require dose modifications. Drug is orange-red when reconstituted.

Side Effect Profile:	Common:

Neutropenia

Cardiotoxicity

Less Common:

Anemia

Thrombocytopenia

Nausea and vomiting

Skin discoloration

Drug is a vesicant

Phlebitis and vein irritation

Rare:

Neurotoxicity

Nursing Implications: Assess ANC, WBC, Hgb/Hct, and platelet count prior to drug administration. Administer antiemetic prior to chemotherapy, and review patient prescription for antiemetic administration at home. Transfuse with red blood cells as ordered. Patient teaching/nurse assessment: (1) self-assessment of infection, bleeding, fatigue; notify MD or RN T > 100.5°F, signs/symptoms of infection, bleeding; energy-conserving activities, self-care strategies to manage fatigue; (2) try to increase fluid intake and call RN or MD if nausea/vomiting severe or if unresolved in 24 hours or if unable to take oral fluids.

A **Drug Name: Adrenocorticoids (cortisone, hydrocortisone, dexamethasone, methylprednisone, methylprednisolone, prednisone, prednisolone)**

Class: Hormones

Mechanism of Action: Cause lysis of lymphoid cells, which led to their use against lymphatic leukemia, myeloma, and malignant lymphoma. May also recruit malignant cells out of G_0 phase, making them vulnerable to damage caused by cell cycle phase–specific agents.

Indications: These drugs are used as single agents or in combination with other cancer therapies, including antiemetic therapies. Chronic steroid use is associated with numerous side effects. Intermittent therapy is safer and, in some conditions, just as effective as daily therapy.

Dosing: Varies according to which preparation is used. Dexamethasone is 25 times the potency of hydrocortisone.

Sample doses:

Cortisone	25 mg
Hydrocortisone	20 mg
Prednisone, prednisolone	5 mg
Methylprednisolone	4 mg
Dexamethasone	0.75 mg

Administration: Oral preparation

Side Effect Profile: Common:

Gastric irritation

Hyperglycemia

Sodium and water retention

Fluid and electrolyte imbalance

Immunosuppression

Less Common:

Cushing's syndrome

Osteoporosis

Decreased bone mineral density

Bone fractures

Steroid-induced psychosis: ranging from emotional lability, insomnia, mood swings, and euphoria to psychosis

Rare:

Cataracts or glaucoma

Nursing Implications: Observe patients for these side effects and taper doses; do not withdraw steroids rapidly. Teach patient that these side effects may occur and to report them. Assess patient coping with mood changes and provide emotional support; discontinue drug if psychoses occurs.

Drug Name: Altretamine (Hexalen, Hexamethylmelamine)

Class: Alkylating agent

Mechanism of Action: The exact mechanism of action is unknown. May inhibit incorporation of thymidine and uridine into DNA and RNA, respectively.

Hexamethylmelamine is felt not to act as an alkylating agent in vitro, but it may be activated to an alkylating agent in the body in vivo. Also may act as an antimetabolite, with activity in the S phase.

Indications: Treatment of refractory ovarian cancer

Dosing: 4–12 mg/kg/day (divided in 3 or 4 doses) for 21–90 days *or* 240 mg/m^2 (6 mg/kg)–320 mg/m^2 (8 mg/kg) daily for 21 days, repeated every 6 weeks

Administration: Oral preparation

Side Effect Profile: Common:

Neutropenia

Less Common:

Anemia

Thrombocytopenia

Peripheral neuropathy

Nausea and vomiting

Diarrhea and anorexia

Skin rash

Nursing Implications: Assess ANC, WBC, Hgb/Hct, and platelet count prior to drug administration. Nadir 3–4 weeks after treatment. Administer antiemetic prior to chemotherapy, and review patient prescription for antiemetic administration at home. Nausea and vomiting can be minimized if patient takes dose 2 hours after meal and at bedtime. Vitamin B$_6$ may be administered concurrently to decrease neurologic complications. Patient teaching/nurse assessment: (1) self-assessment of infection, bleeding, fatigue; notify MD or RN T > 100.5°F, signs/symptoms of infection, bleeding; energy-conserving activities, self-care strategies to manage fatigue; (2) try to increase fluid intake and call RN or MD if nausea/vomiting severe or unresolved in 24 hours or if unable to take oral fluids.

Drug Name: Amifostine for injection (Ethyol, WR-2721)

Class: Free radical scavenger, metabolized to a free thiol that can neutralize cisplatin in normal cells

Mechanism of Action: Drug is phosphorylated by alkaline phosphatase bound in tissue membranes, producing free thiol. Inside the cell, free thiol binds to and detoxifies reactive metabolites of cisplatin and other chemotherapeutic agents, thus neutralizing the chemotherapeutic drug in normal tissues so that cellular DNA and RNA are not damaged. Normal cells are protected because of differences in cell physiology (higher alkaline phosphate concentrations and tissue pH, as well as more effective vascularity in normal cells compared with malignant cells) and transport that promote the preferential uptake of free thiol into normal tissues. Free thiol may also scavenge free radical reactive oxygen molecules resulting from chemotherapy or radiotherapy and may upregulate p53 expression, so that cells accumulate in the G_1-S cell cycle phase, enabling DNA repair.

Indications: Chemoprotectant in protecting multiple organ systems, including cisplatin-induced nephrotoxicity in patients with advanced ovarian cancer and NSCLC; radioprotectant in patients with head and neck cancer whose radiation covers parotid glands. Is being studied in the treatment of myelodysplastic syndrome and reversal of neurotoxicity (Wilkes and Barton-Burke 2005).

Dosing: IV: Renal Protectant: 910 mg/m² administered IV 30 minutes prior to beginning cisplatin-based therapy, but some investigators suggest initial dose of 740 mg/m². If patient is unable to receive the full dose because infusion was stopped for hypotension and not resumed, the next dose and subsequent doses should be reduced to 740 mg/m². IV: Radioprotectant: 200 mg/m² IV over 3 minutes 15–30 minutes before radiation therapy (RT) daily.

Subcutaneous: 500 mg in two divided subcutaneous (SC) doses 30 minutes prior to RT daily (Law *et al.* 2004).

Administration: Hypertension medicines should be stopped 24 hours prior to drug administration. Place patient in sitting or supine position. Administer antiemetics prior to IV and SC doses and antihistamine prior to SC dose. Infuse amifostine IV over 15 minutes, beginning 30 minutes prior to cisplatin.

Side Effect Profile: Common (appear to be dose dependent):

Nausea and Vomiting

Hypotension

Allergic reactions

Nursing Implications: Asses BP before, during, and after administration of drug. Premedicate with antihistamines and antiemetics. Teach patient about the side effects that may occur; important that the patient take oral premedications as prescribed, and notify MD or RN if any of the side effects occur.

Drug Name: 9-Aminocamptothecin (9-AC) investigational

Class: Topoisomerase inhibitor

Mechanism of Action: Cell cycle phase specific. Induces protein-linked DNA single-strand breaks and blocks DNA and RNA synthesis in dividing cells, preventing cells from entering mitosis.

Indications: Being studied in solid tumors

Dosing: 35 $\mu g/m^2/h$ every 2 weeks or 45 $\mu g/m^2/h$ every 3 weeks (phase II trials) as 72-hour infusion. Prolonged infusion studies under way.

Administration: IV infusion over 72 hours

Side Effect Profile: Neutropenia is dose-limiting toxicity

Common:

Nausea, vomiting, and diarrhea

Alopecia

Anemia and fatigue

Nursing Implications: Assess ANC, WBC, Hgb/Hct, and platelet count prior to drug administration; administer antiemetic prior to chemotherapy, and review patient prescription for antiemetic administration at home. Transfuse with red blood cells as ordered. Patient teaching/nurse assessment: (1) self-assessment of infection, bleeding, fatigue; notify MD or RN T > 100.5°F, signs/symptoms of infection, bleeding; energy-conserving activities, self-care strategies to manage fatigue; (2) increase fluid intake and call RN or MD if nausea/vomiting severe or unresolved in 24 hours or if unable to take oral fluids.

Drug Name: Aminoglutethimide (Cytadren, Elipten)

Class: Adrenal steroid inhibitor

Mechanism of Action: Causes chemical adrenalectomy. Blocks adrenal production of steroids, reducing levels of glucocorticoids, mineralocorticoids, and estrogens. Also inhibits peripheral aromatization of androgens to estrogens.

Indications: Treatment of metastatic breast cancer but, because of toxicity, is rarely used today

Dosing: 750–2000 mg orally (PO) daily in divided doses

40 mg hydrocortisone daily given to replace glucocorticoid deficiencies

Administration: Oral preparation

Side Effect Profile: Common:

Adrenal insufficiency

Drug rash accompanied by low-grade fever

Transient neurologic symptoms, lethargy, somnolence, blurred vision, vertigo, ataxia, nystagmus

Less Common:

Hypotension

Nausea and vomiting

Anorexia

Nursing Implications: Monitor VS. Skin rash may develop within 5–7 days, lasting 8 days, often with malaise and fever (100–102°F; 37.5–39°C). If not resolved in 7–14 days, drug should be discontinued. Teach patient that these side effects may occur and to report them. Premedicate with antihistamine to prevent scratching of the skin and with antiemetics per MD order. Adjuvant corticosteroids need to be administered.

A | Drug Name: Anastrozole (Arimidex)

Class: Nonsteroidal aromatase inhibitor

Mechanism of Action: Inhibits the enzyme aromatase. Aromatase is one of the P-450 enzymes and is involved in estrogen biosynthesis. Circulating estrogen in postmenopausal women (mainly estradiol) arises from the aromatase-mediated conversion of androstenedione (made by the adrenals) to estrone and then estrone to estradiol in the peripheral tissues, such as adipose tissue. Anastrozole is highly selective for this enzyme and does not affect steroid synthesis, so that estradiol synthesis is potently suppressed (to undetectable levels), whereas cortisol and aldosterone levels are unchanged.

Indications: Indicated for the adjuvant treatment of postmenopausal women with hormone receptor–positive early breast cancer. Second-line therapy for postmenopausal women with advanced breast cancer.

Dosing: 1 mg PO qd. No dosage adjustment required for mild to moderate hepatic impairment.

Administration: Oral preparation. Take with or without food at approximately the same time daily. Well tolerated with low toxicity profile. Coadministration of corticosteroids is not necessary. Absolutely contraindicated during pregnancy.

Side Effect Profile: Common:

Hot flashes

Asthenia or loss of energy

Headache

Vaginal dryness may occur

Mild nausea

Mild diarrhea

Thrombophlebitis

Nursing Implications: Explore with patient and partner their patterns of sexuality and impact of therapy. Teach patient that vaginal dryness may be from menopause, not the drug, and estrogen creams SHOULD NOT be used. Teach use of lubricants. Teach patients to report/come to emergency room for pain, redness, swelling in arms or legs, or if SOB or dizziness occur. Teach patient to treat headache with nonprescription analgesics and report headaches if unrelieved. Encourage rest as needed. Discuss strategies to minimize nausea, including diet and dosing time. Teach patient that diarrhea is usually relieved by non-prescription medications, such as loperamide HCl and kaopectate and report unrelieved diarrhea.

Drug Name: Androgens: testosterone propionate (Neohombreol, Oreton), fluoxymesterone (Halotestin, Ora-Testryl), testolactone (Teslac)

Class: Hormones

Mechanism of Action: Has stimulatory effect on red blood cells that results in an increased Hct. Other mechanism of action unknown.

Indications: These drugs are used as single agents or in combination with other cancer therapies. Chronic steroid use is associated with numerous side effects.

Dosing: Testosterone propionate 50–100 mg intramuscular (IM) 3 times weekly

Fluoxymesterone 10–30 mg PO daily (3–4 divided doses)

Testolactone 100 mg IM 3 times weekly or 250 mg PO 4 times daily

Drug comes in ready-to-use vials or tablets.

Administration: Oral preparation; before IM administration, shake vial vigorously and give injection immediately to avoid solution settling.

Side Effect Profile: Common:

Sodium and water retention

Fluid and electrolyte imbalance

Nausea

Less Common:

Hypercalcemia

Obstructive jaundice

Nursing Implications: Observe patients for the side effects of hormone therapy. Teach patient that these side effects may occur and to report them. Fluoxymesterone may increase sensitivity to oral anticoagulants. Should be administered in divided doses because of its short action. Call RN or MD if nausea is unresolved in 24 hours or if unable to take oral fluids.

Drug Name: Arsenic trioxide (Trisenox)

Class: Miscellaneous antineoplastic agent

Mechanism of Action: Not completely understood, but drug appears to cause changes in DNA with fragmentation typical of apoptosis or programmed cell death. Drug also damages and causes degradation of the fusion protein PML-RARα, characteristic of acute promyelocytic leukemia. The gene responsible for the fusion protein is corrected in many cases (cytogenetic complete response) so that immature malignant myelocytic cells mature into normal white blood cells.

Indications: Drug is indicated for induction of remission and consolidation in patients with acute promyelocytic leukemia (APL) who are refractory to, or have relapsed from, retinoid and anthracycline chemotherapy and whose APL is characterized by the presence of the t(15;17) translocation or PML/RARα gene expression.

Dosing: Induction dose of 0.15 mg/kg/day IV until bone marrow remission, not to exceed 60 doses. Consolidation begins 3–6 weeks after induction therapy is completed, at a dose of 0.15 mg/kg/day IV for 25 doses over a period of up to 5 weeks.

Administration: Administer immediately after reconstitution. The prescribed dose is mixed in 100–250 ml 5% dextrose injection, USP, or 0.9% sodium chloride injection, USP.

Administer IV over 1–2 hours or for up to 4 hours if acute vasomotor reactions occur (does not require a central line).

Drug is chemically and physically stable for 24 hours at room temperature and 48 hours when refrigerated.

Drug does not contain any preservatives, discard unused portions.

Do not mix with any other medications.

Overdose: if symptoms of acute arsenic toxicity appear (seizures, muscle weakness, confusion) discontinue drug immediately and consider chelation therapy (dimercaprol 3 mg/kg IM q 4 hours until immediate life-threatening toxicity has subsided, then give penicillamine 250 mg PO up to qid [≤ 1 g/day]).

Avoid drugs that prolong the QT interval (e.g., certain antiarrhythmics or orthioridazine) or lead to electrolyte abnormalities (e.g., diuretics or amphotericin B). Monitoring and correction of abnormalities (e.g., hyperkalemia, hypokalemia, hypomagnesemia, hyperglycemia, hypoglycemia, hypocalcemia) is critical.

Side Effect Profile: Common:

Leukocytosis

Nausea

Vomiting

Diarrhea

Abdominal pain

Fatigue

Edema

Hyperglycemia

Dyspnea

Cough

Rash

Itching

Headaches

Dizziness

Nursing Implications: Prior to treatment, a baseline 12-lead EKG, serum electrolytes, and renal function tests. Electrolyte abnormalities should be corrected. Any drugs that prolong the QT interval, such as serotonin antagonist antiemetics, should be discontinued

Serum potassium should be kept > 4.0 mEq/dl and serum magnesium > 1.8 mg/dl. Monitor for syncope and rapid or irregular heart rate. Assess temperature and VS, oxygen saturation, cardiopulmonary status at baseline and at each visit. Assess weight daily and teach patient to report any SOB, fever, or weight gain immediately. Monitor cardiac signs or pulmonary symptoms (breath sounds and changes in oxygen saturation) at baseline and monitor daily during treatment. Notify physician and discuss obtaining CXR, cardiac echo, and focused exam if changes occur.

APL differentiation syndrome characterized by fever, dyspnea, weight gain, pulmonary infiltrates, and pleural or pericardial effusions, with or without leukocytosis. Steroids should be instituted (dexamethasone 10 mg IV bid) for at least 3 days or longer until signs and symptoms abate.

Drug is a human carcinogen; pregnant or breast-feeding women should avoid handling drug, patient waste, or waste products.

Assess GI, nutritional status, presence of function at baseline and with each visit. Administer antiemetics and teach patient self-administration. Assess presence of pain, and discuss pharmacologic and nonpharmacologic analgesic plan with physician.

Assess baseline energy, activity level, and level of comfort. Assess need for assistance with ADLs. Teach patient self-care strategies to minimize exertion, such as clustering activity during shopping, alternating rest and activity periods, diet, gentle exercise.

Assess baseline mental and neuro status and monitor during therapy. Assess sensory function and teach patient to report numbness, tingling, dizziness, tremor, seizure, decreases in alertness, and changes in sleep. Assess for paresthesias and motor and sensory function prior to treatment. Teach self-care strategies, including maintaining safety when walking, getting up, taking a bath, or washing dishes if unable to feel temperature changes. Teach self-care measures to manage sleep problems, and discuss possible need for sleeping medication.

Assess baseline skin integrity, and monitor at each visit. Teach patient to report any skin changes or itching. Teach patient symptomatic local measures to manage dermatitis, itch, or other changes.

Drug Name: Asparaginase (Elspar)

Class: Miscellaneous/enzyme

Mechanism of Action: Hydrolysis of serum asparagine occurs, which deprives leukemia cells of the required amino acid. Normal cells are spared because they generally have the ability to synthesize their own asparagine. Cell cycle specific for G_1 post-mitotic phase. Some leukemic cells are unable to synthesize asparagine. These cells must obtain asparagine from an exogenous source—the patient's serum. Administration of the enzyme L-asparaginase causes hydrolysis of asparagine to aspartate, resulting in rapid depletion of the asparagine concentration in the patient's serum.

Indications: Indicated in the therapy of patients with acute lymphocytic leukemia

Dosing: IM or IV

Administration: Use in a hospital setting. Make preparations to treat anaphylaxis at each administration of the drug.

Side Effect Profile: Common:

Neutropenia

Cardiotoxicity

Less Common:

Anemia

Thrombocytopenia

Nausea and vomiting

Skin discoloration

Drug is a vesicant

Phlebitis and vein irritation

Rare:

Neurotoxicity

Nursing Implications: Potential reduction in antineoplastic effect of methotrexate when given in combination. Anaphylaxis is associated with the administration of this drug. Intravenous administration of L-asparaginase concurrently with or immediately before prednisone and vincristine administration may be associated with increased toxicity.

Assess ANC, WBC, Hgb/Hct, and platelet count prior to drug administration; administer antiemetic prior to chemotherapy, and review patient prescription for antiemetic administration at home. Transfuse with red blood cells as ordered. Patient teaching/nurse assessment: (1) self-assessment of infection, bleeding, fatigue; notify MD or RN T > 100.5°F, signs/symptoms of infection, bleeding; energy-conserving activities, self-care strategies to manage fatigue; (2) try to increase fluid intake and call RN or MD if nausea/vomiting severe or unresolved in 24 hours or if unable to take oral fluids.

Drug Name: 5-Azacytidine (azacytidine, 5AZ) IV formulation

Class: Investigational

Mechanism of Action: Interferes with nucleic acid metabolism by acting as a false metabolite when incorporated into DNA and RNA; cell cycle phase specific for S phase.

Indications: Per protocol

Dosing: 100–400 mg/m^2 daily, weekly, biweekly, or continuous infusion schedule. Consult individual clinical trial protocol for specific dose.

Administration: This drug is supplied by the National Cancer Institute. The powder is reconstituted with sterile water for injection. **Do not reconstitute with 5% dextrose.**

SC administration may be painful and result in discoloration at the injection site.

IV bolus or continuous infusion. This drug is rapidly metabolized, and once reconstituted, it decomposes quickly. The infusion bottles need to be changed every 3–4 hours because of drug decomposition. Stable in lactated Ringer's solution for 4 hours.

Side Effect Profile: Common:

Neutropenia

Thrombocytopenia

Anemia

Nausea and vomiting

Diarrhea

Stomatitis

Hepatotoxicity

Less Common:

Nephrotoxicity

Neurotoxicity: syndrome of lethargy, myalgia, muscle pain and weakness, and coma (rare)

Rash

Fever and hypotension

Nursing Implications: Assess ANC, WBC, Hgb/Hct, and platelet count prior to drug administration; administer antiemetic prior to chemotherapy, and review patient prescription for antiemetic administration at home. Transfuse with red blood cells as ordered. Patient teaching/nurse assessment: (1) self-assessment of infection, bleeding, fatigue; notify MD or RN T > 100.5°F, signs/symptoms of infection, bleeding; energy-conserving activities, self-care strategies to manage fatigue; (2) try to increase fluid intake and call RN or MD if nausea/vomiting severe or unresolved in 24 hours or if unable to take oral fluids. Monitor LFTs and renal function. Assess baseline neurologic status. Teach patient about all side effects and how and when to contact the staff to discuss. Thromboembolic phenomena may occur.

A

Drug Name: Bicalutamide (Casodex)

Class: Nonsteroidal antiandrogen

Mechanism of Action: Binds to androgen receptors in the prostate; affinity is 4 times greater than that of flutamide.

Indications: Use in combination therapy with a luteinizing hormone–releasing hormone analog (LHRH-A) for the treatment of stage D2 metastatic carcinoma of the prostate.

Dosing: 50 mg PO qd

Administration: Oral preparation

Side Effect Profile: Less Common:

Gynecomastia and hot flashes

Nausea

Constipation

Nursing Implications: Observe patients for the side effects of hormone therapy. Teach patient that these side effects may occur and to report them. Use cautiously in patients with moderate to severe hepatic dysfunction. Observe closely for toxicity because dosage adjustment may be required. No dose modification needed for renal dysfunction. In a study comparing castration to bicalutamide 50 mg/day, there was no difference in time to disease progression or subjective tolerance, but overall health of group receiving castration was better (McLeod 1997).

Drug Name: Bleomycin sulfate (Blenoxane)

Class: Antitumor antibiotic—isolated from fungus *Streptomyces verticullus*. Possesses both antitumor and antimicrobial actions.

Mechanism of Action: Cross links DNA strands so DNA cannot be copied and cell dies. Primary action of bleomycin is to induce single-strand and double-strand breaks in DNA. DNA synthesis is inhibited. The action of drug is not exerted against RNA.

Indications: Treatment of testicular and head and neck cancers, choriocarcinoma, teratocarcinoma, and lymphoma; treatment of recurrent pleural effusions as a sclerosing agent.

Dosing: 5–20 U/m^2 once a week

10–20 U/m^2 twice a week (frequency and schedule may vary according to protocol and age)

Administration: Dilute powder in normal saline or sterile water

IV, IM, or SC doses may be administered. Some clinical trials may use 24-hour infusions. There is a risk for anaphylaxis and hypotension with some diseases and with higher doses of drug. It may be recommended that a test dose be given before the first dose to detect hypersensitivity.

Side Effect Profile: Common:

Nausea and vomiting

Anorexia and weight loss

B

Stomatitis

Fever and chills and pain at tumor site

Skin changes including alopecia, discoloration, rash, hyperpigmentation, skin peeling of fingertips, and hyperkeratosis

Rare:

Interstitial pneumonitis

Anaphylaxis

Nursing Implications: Monitor and obtain PFTs and CXR before each course or as outlined by protocol to track pulmonary toxicities. Maximum cumulative lifetime dose: 400 U. Incidence of anaphylaxis increases over the age of 70. Watch for signs/symptoms of hypotension and anaphylaxis. Test dose may be needed. Administer premedications, such as acetaminophen, antihistamines, and, in some cases, steroids, because drug may cause chemical fevers up to 103–105°F or 39.5–40.5°C (60%).

May cause irritation at site of injection (is considered an irritant, not a vesicant). Patient teaching: (1) self-assessment of temperature and symptomatic treatment; notify MD or RN T > 100.5°F; (2) try to increase fluid intake and call RN or MD if nausea/vomiting severe or unresolved in 24 hours or if unable to take oral fluids.

Drug Name: Busulfan (Myleran)

Class: Alkylating agent

Mechanism of Action: Forms carbonium ions through the release of a methane sulfonate group. This results in the alkylating of DNA. Acts primarily on granulocyte precursors in the bone marrow and is cell cycle phase nonspecific.

Indications: Chronic myelogenous leukemia

Dosing: Oral preparation:

4–8 mg/day PO for 2–3 weeks initially, then maintenance dose of 1–3 mg/m^2 PO qd or 0.05 mg/kg PO qd. Dose titrated to WBC count.

Administration: Available in 2-mg scored tablets given PO

Side Effect Profile: Common:

Neutropenia

Anemia

Thrombocytopenia

Less Common:

Pulmonary fibrosis

Drug is teratogenic and is a reproductive hazard

Nursing Implications: If WBC is high, patient is at risk for hyperuricemia. Allopurinol and hydration may be indicated. Follow weekly CBC and platelet count initially, then monthly. Dose is decreased to maintenance when leukocyte count falls below 50,000 mm^3. Hyperpigmentation of skin creases may occur due to increased melanin production. If given according to accepted guidelines, patient should have minimal side effects. Assess ANC, WBC, Hgb/Hct, and platelet count prior to drug administration; administer antiemetic prior to chemotherapy, and review patient prescription for antiemetic administration at home. Transfuse with red blood cells as ordered. Patient teaching/nurse assessment: (1) self-assessment of infection, bleeding, fatigue; notify MD or RN T > 100.5°F, signs/symptoms of infection, bleeding; energy-conserving activities, self-care strategies to manage fatigue.

Drug Name: Busulfan injection (Busulfex)

Class: Alkylating agent

Mechanism of Action: Forms carbonium ions through the release of a methane sulfonate group. This results in the alkylating of DNA. Acts primarily on granulocyte precursors in the bone marrow and is cell cycle phase nonspecific.

Indications: Drug is currently indicated ONLY for patients who are getting conditioning regimen for hematopoietic progenitor-cell transplantation.

Dosing: IV preparation:

0.8 mg/kg of ideal body weight (IBW) or actual body weight (whichever is lower) q 6 hours as a 2-hour infusion for a total of 16 doses, followed by cyclophosphamide tablets

Administration: Administer using an IV pump over 2 hours. When mixed in NS, drug is stable (refrigerated) for 12 hours. In D_5W, drug is stable at room temperature for 8 hours. Infusion must be completed within these two time frames.

Side Effect Profile: Common:

Neutropenia

Anemia

Thrombocytopenia

Nausea and vomiting

Anorexia

Stomatitis

Diarrhea

Hepatotoxicity including veno-occlusive disease and graft-versus-host disease

Less Common:

Pulmonary fibrosis

Cardiac including tachycardia, thrombosis, hypertension, and vasodilation

Fluid and electrolyte imbalance

Drug is teratogenic and is a reproductive hazard

Nursing Implications: Profound myelosuppression occurs in all patients. Follow weekly CBC and platelet count closely. Assess ANC, WBC, Hgb/Hct, and platelet count prior to drug administration. Administer antiemetic prior to chemotherapy.

B

Transfuse with red blood cells as ordered. Patient teaching/nurse assessment: (1) self-assessment of infection, bleeding, fatigue; notify MD or RN T > 100.5°F; signs/symptoms of infection, bleeding; energy-conserving activities, self-care strategies to manage fatigue. Premedicate with phenytoin before administration because drug crosses the blood-brain barrier. Probable increased risk of hepatic veno-occlusive disease with patients who have history of RT, greater than three cycles of chemotherapy, or prior progenitor-cell transplantation. Elevated LFTs are common. Hyperpigmentation of skin creases may occur because of increased melanin production.

Drug Name: Capecitabine (Xeloda, N4-pentoxycarbonyl-5-deoxy-5-fluorocytidine)

Class: Fluoropyrimidine carbamate; antimetabolite prodrug

Mechanism of Action: Metabolites bind to thymidylate synthetase, inhibiting the formation of uracil from thymidylate and reducing the cell's ability to produce DNA. It also prevents cell division by hindering the formation of RNA by causing nuclear transcription enzymes to mistakenly incorporate its metabolites in the process of RNA transcription.

Indications: Treatment of metastatic breast, colon, or rectal cancers

Dosing: 2500 mg/m^2 PO daily in two divided doses with food for 2 weeks. Treatment followed by a 1-week rest period. Treatment repeated every 3 weeks.

Interrupt for grade 2 nausea, vomiting, diarrhea, stomatis, or hand-foot syndrome.

Dose reduced for renal dysfunction.

Administration: Oral preparation:

Administer after meals with plenty of water.

Divide daily dose in half; take 12 hours apart.

Side Effect Profile: Common:

Neutropenia

Anemia

Thrombocytopenia

Hand-foot syndrome

Less Common:

Nausea and vomiting

Anorexia and diarrhea

Stomatitis

Nursing Implications: Follow CBC count closely. Assess ANC, WBC, Hgb/Hct, and platelet count prior to drug administration. Transfuse with red blood cells as ordered. Patient teaching/nurse assessment: (1) self-assessment of infection, bleeding, fatigue; notify MD or RN T > 100.5°F; signs/symptoms of infection, bleeding; energy-conserving activities, self-care strategies to manage fatigue. Monitor bilirubin at baseline and before each cycle because dose modifications are necessary with hyperbilirubinemia. Folic acid should be avoided while taking drug. Administer antiemetic prior to chemotherapy. Divide daily dose in half; take 12 hours apart and teach about hand-foot syndrome.

Drug Name: Carboplatin (Paraplatin)

Class: Alkylating agent (heavy metal complex)

Mechanism of Action: A second-generation platinum analog. The cytotoxicity is identical to that of the parent, cisplatin. Cell cycle phase nonspecific. Reacts with nucleophilic sites on DNA, causing predominantly intrastrand and interstrand cross links rather than DNA-protein cross links. These cross links are similar to those formed with cisplatin but are formed later.

Indications: Palliative treatment of patients with ovarian carcinoma recurrent after prior chemotherapy, including patients who have been previously treated with cisplatin.

Dosing: As a single agent, 360 mg/m^2 on day 1, cycle repeated every 4 weeks; *or* 300 mg/m^2 on day 1 combined with cyclophosphamide for advanced ovarian cancer, cycle repeated every 4 weeks. Drug administration may have to be delayed if neutrophil count is less than 2000 mm^3 or platelet count is less than 100,000 mm^3.

Drug dose reduction for urine creatinine clearance < 60 ml/min. Because carboplatin has predictable pharmacokinetics based on the drug's excretion by the kidneys, area under the curve (AUC) dosing is now recommended for this drug. The Calvert formula is used where the total dose (mg) = (target AUC) × (glomerular filtration rate [GFR] + 25).

The GFR is approximated by the urine creatinine clearance, either estimated or actual, and can be calculated by hand. The target AUC dose is determined by the treatment plan depending on the type of malignancy and for previously treated patients receiving single-agent carboplatin (see package insert).

Administration: IV bolus over 30 minutes to 1 hour. May also be given as a continuous infusion over 24 hours. Reconstitute with sterile water for injection, D$_5$W, or NS. Dilute further in D$_5$W or NS. The solution is chemically stable for 24 hours; discard solution after 8 hours because of the lack of bacteriostatic preservative.

Side Effect Profile: Common:

Neutropenia

Anemia

Thrombocytopenia

Nephrotoxicity in high doses but does not have the renal toxicity seen with cisplatin

Hypersensitivity reaction

Less Common:

Nausea and vomiting

Anorexia and diarrhea

Hepatic dysfunction

Stomatitis

Nursing Implications: Assess ANC, WBC, Hgb/Hct, and platelet count prior to drug administration; administer antiemetic prior to chemotherapy, and review patient prescription for antiemetic administration at home. Transfuse with red blood cells as ordered. Patient teaching/nurse assessment: (1) self-assessment of infection, bleeding, fatigue; notify MD or RN T > 100.5°F, signs/symptoms of infection, bleeding; energy-conserving activities, self-care strategies to manage fatigue; (2) try to increase fluid intake and call RN or MD if nausea/vomiting severe or unresolved in 24 hours or if unable to take oral fluids. Monitor urine creatinine clearance.

Drug Name: Carmustine (BiCNU, BCNU)

Class: Alkylating agent (nitrosourea)

Mechanism of Action: Alkylates DNA in the same manner as classic mustard agents by causing cross-strand breaks. Also, carbamoylates cellular proteins of nucleic acid synthesis. Is cell cycle phase nonspecific. Causes DNA strand breaks and cross links so cell cannot replicate and dies; crosses blood-brain barrier.

Indications: Brain cancer, Hodgkin's disease, lymphoma, multiple myeloma

Dosing: 75–100 mg/m² IV daily for 2 days *or* 200–225 mg/m² every 6 weeks *or* 40 mg/m²/day on 5 successive days

Administration: Discard solution 2 hours after mixing. Administer via volutrol over 45–120 minutes as tolerated by patient. Add sterile alcohol (provided with drug) to vial, and then add sterile water for injection. May be further diluted with 100–250 ml D$_5$W or NS.

Drug is an irritant; avoid extravasation. Pain at the injection site or along the vein is common. Treat by applying ice pack above the injection site and decreasing the infusion flow rate.

Patient may act inebriated because of the alcohol diluent and may experience flushing.

Side Effect Profile: Common:

Neutropenia (nadir 41–46 days), cumulative

Thrombocytopenia (nadir 26–34 days), cumulative

Pulmonary fibrosis

Nausea and vomiting

Anorexia

Less Common:

Nephrotoxicity

Confusion

Lethargy

Visual changes

Liver dysfunction

Nursing Implications: Assess ANC, WBC, Hgb/Hct, and platelet count prior to drug administration; increased myelosuppression when given with cimetidine. Can decrease the pharmacologic effects of phenytoin.

Review patient prescription for antiemetic administration at home in between dosing. Patient teaching: (1) self-assessment of infection, fatigue; notify MD or RN T > 100.5°F, signs/symptoms of infection; energy-conserving activities, self-care strategies to manage fatigue; (2) try to increase fluid intake and call RN or MD if nausea/vomiting severe or unresolved in 24 hours or if unable to take oral fluids. Monitor before treatment and periodically during treatment: pulmonary function studies and renal and liver function tests.

Drug Name: Chlorambucil (Leukeran)

C

Class: Alkylating agent

Mechanism of Action: Alkylates DNA by causing strand breaks and cross links in the DNA; is a derivative of a nitrogen mustard

Indications: Chronic lymphocytic leukemia, lymphoma

Dosing: 0.1–0.2 mg/kg/day (4–8 mg/m^2/day) to initiate treatment *or* 14 mg/m^2/day for 5 days with a repeat every 21–28 days depending on platelet count and WBC

Administration: Oral preparation

Simultaneous administration of barbiturates may increase toxicity of chlorambucil because of hepatic drug activation.

Side Effect Profile: Common:

Severe nausea and vomiting

Neutropenia

Thrombocytopenia

Anemia

Uncommon:

Pulmonary fibrosis

Neurotoxicity

Nursing Implications: Assess ANC, WBC, Hgb/Hct, and platelet count prior to drug administration; administer aggressive antiemetics prior to chemotherapy. Review patient prescription for antiemetic administration at home in between dosing. Patient teaching: (1) self-assessment of infection, fatigue; notify MD or RN T > 100.5°F, signs/symptoms of infection; energy-conserving activities, self-care strategies to manage fatigue; (2) try to increase fluid intake and call RN or MD if nausea/vomiting severe or unresolved in 24 hours or if unable to take oral fluids.

Drug Name: Cisplatin (cisplatinum, CDDP, platinum, Platinol)

Class: Heavy metal that acts like alkylating agent

Mechanism of Action: Inhibits DNA synthesis by forming interstrand and intrastrand cross links and by denaturing the double helix, preventing cell replication; is cell cycle phase nonspecific and has chemical properties similar to that of bifunctional alkylating agents.

Indications: Testicular and ovarian cancers

Dosing: 50–120 mg/m^2 every 3–4 weeks *or* 15–20 mg/m^2 × 5, repeated every 3–4 weeks

Radiosensitizing effect: administer 1–3 times per week at doses of 15–50 mg/m^2 (total weekly dose of 50 mg/m^2) with concomitant radiotherapy

High dose (investigational): 200 mg/m^2 given in 250 ml of 3% sodium chloride (hypertonic)

Administration: Avoid aluminum needles when administering because precipitate will form.

IV infusion over 2–6 hours, use vesicant precautions.

Add sterile water to develop a concentration of 1 mg/ml. Further dilute solution with 250 ml or more of NS or D$_5$W 1/2 NS. Never mix with D$_5$W because precipitate will form. Refrigerate lyophilized drug but *not* reconstituted drug because precipitate will form.

Side Effect Profile: Common:

Neutropenia

Anemia

Thrombocytopenia

Nausea and vomiting

Neurotoxicity

Nephrotoxicity

Cardiotoxicity

Less Common:

Fatigue

Delayed hypersensitivity

Nursing Implications: Assess ANC, WBC, Hgb/Hct, and platelet count prior to drug administration; administer aggressive antiemetics prior to drug administration.

Review with patient the prescription for antiemetic administration at home if nausea arises and call RN or MD if it does not resolve in 24 hours.

Hydrate vigorously before and after administering drug. Urine output should be at least 100–150 ml/h. Mannitol or furosemide diuresis may be needed to ensure this output. Hypersensitivity reactions have occurred, manifested by wheezing, flushing, hypotension, and tachycardia. Usually occurs within minutes of starting infusion. Treat with epinephrine, corticosteroids, antihistamines. Decreases the pharmacologic effects of phenytoin.

Patient teaching/nurse assessment: (1) neuropathy, such as numbness and tingling of tips of fingers and toes, and whether this interferes with ability to function or ADLs; (2) self-assessment of infection, fatigue; notify MD or RN T > 100.5°F, signs/symptoms of infection; energy-conserving activities, self-care strategies to manage fatigue.

Drug Name: Cladribine (Leustatin, 2-CdA)

Class:	Antimetabolite
Mechanism of Action:	Selectively damages normal and malignant lymphocytes and monocytes that have large amounts of deoxycytidine kinase but small amounts of deoxynucleotidase. The drug, a chlorinated purine nucleoside, enters passively through the cell membrane, is phosphorylated into the active metabolite 2-CdATP, and accumulates in the cell. 2-CdATP interferes with DNA synthesis and prevents repair of DNA strand breaks in both actively dividing and normal cells. The process may involve programmed cell death (apoptosis).
Indications:	Indicated for the treatment of active hairy-cell leukemia
Dosing:	IV administration. Dilute in 0.9% sodium chloride injection. Diluted drug stable at room temperature for at least 24 hours in normal light.
	Continuous infusion: 0.09 mg/kg/day for 7 days for one course of therapy of hairy-cell leukemia.
	Single daily dose: add calculated drug dose to 500 ml of 0.9% sodium chloride injection and administer over 24 hours; repeat daily for 7 days.
	7-Day continuous infusion by ambulatory infusion pump: add calculated drug dose for 7 days to infusion reservoir using a sterile 0.22-μm hydrophilic syringe filter. Then add, using a 0.22-μm filter, sufficient sterile bacteriostatic 0.9% sodium chloride injection containing 0.9% benzyl alcohol to produce 100 ml in the infusion reservoir. **Do not use 5% dextrose because it accelerates degradation of drug.**
Administration:	Dilute in minimum of 100 ml. BUT **unstable in 5% dextrose; should not be used as diluent or infusion fluid.**
	Administer as continuous infusion over 24 hours for 7 days.
	Store unopened vials in refrigerator and protect from light.
	Drug may precipitate when exposed to low temperatures. Allow solution to warm to room temperature and shake vigorously. DO NOT HEAT OR MICROWAVE.
	Contraindicated in patients with known hypersensitivity to drug.
	Administer with caution in patients with renal or hepatic insufficiency.
	Embryotoxic; women of childbearing age should use contraception.
Side Effect Profile:	Common:
	Neutropenia
	Anemia

Thrombocytopenia

Elevated LFTs (ALP, AST, ALT)

Nausea and vomiting

Less Common:

Proteinuria

Hematuria

Pain

Fever

Rash

Dyspnea

Constipation or diarrhea

Bleeding

Alopecia

Infection

Tachycardia

Headaches

Rare:

Chills

Diaphoresis

Malaise

Dizziness

Insomnia

Purpura

Petechiae

Epistaxis

Cough

Nursing Implications: Assess CBC, ANC, WBC, Hgb/Hct, and platelet count prior to drug administration; administer antiemetic prior to chemotherapy, and review patient prescription for antiemetic administration at home. Transfuse with red blood cells, or administer erythropoietin per MD order. Teach patient about diet, and instruct to alternate rest and activity; stress reduction/relaxation techniques may improve energy level. Patient teaching: self-assessment of infection, bleeding, fatigue; notify MD or RN T > 100.5°F, although recognize that drug may cause fever alone, signs/symptoms of infection, bleeding; energy-conserving activities, self-care strategies to manage fatigue. Instruct patient of bleeding, and transfuse platelets per physician order. Teach self-assessment of signs/symptoms of infection and bleeding.

Assess for fever, chills, diaphoresis during visits; assess signs/symptoms of infection. Assess skin for cutaneous changes, such as rash or changes at injection site, and any associated symptoms such as pruritis. Discuss with physician. Instruct patient in self-care measures, including avoiding abrasive skin products and clothing, avoiding tight-fitting clothing, use of skin emolients appropriate to specific skin alteration, measures to avoid scratching involved areas. Consider venous access device if skin is at risk for reaction. Encourage patient to report onset of change in bowel habits (diarrhea or constipation) and assess factors contributing to changes. Teach patient self-assessment, how to report this, and measures to reduce fever. Anticipate laboratory and x-ray tests to rule out infection and perform according to physician order. Administer or teach patient self-administration of antidiarrheal medication or cathartic as ordered. Teach patient diet modification regarding foods that minimize diarrhea or constipation. Assess baseline pulmonary status, including breath sounds, presence of cough, shortness of breath. Instruct patient to report symptoms of cough, shortness of breath, other abnormalities. Encourage small, frequent feedings of cool, bland foods and liquids. Teach to record diet history for 2–3 days and weekly weights. If patient has decreased appetite, assess food preferences (encourage or discourage) and suggest use of spices. Assess baseline cardiac status, including apical heart rate, presence of peripheral edema. Instruct patient to report rapid heart beat or swelling of ankles.

Drug Name: Cyclophosphamide (Cytoxan)

Class: Alkylating agent

Mechanism of Action: Causes cross linkage in DNA strands thus preventing DNA synthesis and cell division. Cell cycle phase nonspecific.

Indications: Breast cancer, adjuvant therapy

Dosing: IV administration: 400 mg/m^2 over 5 days *or* 500–1500 mg/m^2 q 3–4 weeks.

Oral administration: 100 mg/m^2 PO for 14 days.

High dose with BMT (investigational): 1.8–7 g/m^2 in combination with other cytotoxic agents.

Administration: Oral preparation

Dilute vials with sterile water. Shake well. Allow solution to clear if lyophilized preparation not used. Do not use solution unless crystals are fully dissolved.

Oral administration: administer in morning or early afternoon to allow adequate excretion time. Take with meals.

IV administration: for doses > 500 mg, pre- and posthydration to total 500–3000 ml is needed to ensure adequate urine output and to avoid hemorrhagic cystitis. Administer drug over at least 20 minutes for doses > 500 mg.

Mesna given with high-dose cyclophosphamide to prevent hemorrhagic cystitis. Solution is stable for 24 hours at room temperature or for 6 days if refrigerated.

Rapid infusion may cause dizziness, nasal stuffiness, rhinorrhea, sinus congestion during or after infusion.

Drug is mutagenic and teratogenic. Amenorrhea often occurs in females, and testicular atrophy, possibly with reversible oligospermia/azoospermia, occurs in males. Drug is excreted in breast milk.

Side Effect Profile: Common:

Severe nausea and vomiting

Neutropenia

Thrombocytopenia

Anemia

Uncommon:

Pulmonary fibrosis

Neurotoxicity

Nursing Implications: Assess CBC, WBC with differential, platelet count, and signs/symptoms of infection and bleeding prior to treatment. Premedicate with antiemetics prior to drug administration and continue prophylactically for 24 hours, at least for the first cycle. Encourage small feedings of bland foods and liquids. Teach patient about antiemetic administration at home. Patient teaching: (1) self-assessment of infection, fatigue; notify MD or RN T > 100.5°F, signs/symptoms of infection; energy-conserving activities, self-care strategies to manage fatigue; (2) try to increase fluid intake and call RN or MD if nausea/vomiting severe or unresolved in 24 hours or if unable to take oral fluids. Test urine for occult blood.

Monitor BUN and creatinine prior to drug dose and as drug is excreted by the kidneys. Assess for signs/symptoms of hematuria, urinary frequency, or dysuria; instruct patient to report these if they occur. Instruct patient to drink at least 3 liters of fluid daily and empty bladder every 2–3 hours and at bedtime. If high-dose treatment, vigorous hydration is necessary prior to drug administration. Bladder irrigation per protocol. Instruct patient to take oral cyclophosphamide early in the day to prevent drug accumulation in bladder during the night.

Discuss impact of hair loss on patient and strategies to minimize it (i.e., wig, scarf, cap) prior to drug administration. Assess patient's/partner's sexual patterns and reproductive goals. Discuss strategies to preserve sexual and reproductive health including contraception and sperm banking. Mothers should not breast feed.

Assess patients receiving high-dose cyclophosphamide: monitor serum Na+, osmolality, urine osmolality, and electrolytes; strictly monitor I/O, total body fluid balance, and daily weight.

Screen patients for secondary malignancies.

Assess patients receiving high-dose or continuous low-dose cyclophosphamide for signs/symptoms of pulmonary dysfunction. Assess lung sounds

C

prior to drug administration and periodically during treatment. Teach patient to report dyspnea, cough, or any abnormalities.

Drug Name: Cytarabine, cytosine arabinoside (Ara-C, Cytosar-U, arabinosyl cytosine)

Class: Antimetabolite

Mechanism of Action: Antimetabolite (pyrimidine analog) that is incorporated into DNA, slowing its synthesis and causing defects in the linkages in new DNA fragments. Also, cells exposed to cytarabine in the S phase reinitiate DNA synthesis when the drug is removed, resulting in erroneous duplication of the early portions of the DNA strands. Most effective when cells are undergoing rapid DNA synthesis.

Indications: Leukemia

Dosing: Leukemia: 100 mg/m^2/day IV continuous infusion for 5–10 days; 100 mg/m^2 every 12 hours for 1–3 weeks IV or SC

Head and neck: 1 mg/kg every 12 hours for 5–7 days IV or SC

High dose: 2–3 mg/m^2 IV

Differentiation: 10 mg/m^2 SC every 12 hours for 15–21 days

Intrathecal: 20–30 mg/m^2

Administration: Doses of 100–200 mg can be given SC.

Doses less than 1 g: administer via volutrol over 10–20 minutes.

Doses over 1 g: administer over 2 hours.

Thrombophlebitis or pain at the injection site should be treated with warm compresses.

Dizziness has occurred with too rapid IV infusions.

Use with caution if hepatic dysfunction exists.

May decrease bioavailability of digoxin when given in combination.

Side Effect Profile: Common:

Neutropenia

Anemia

Thrombocytopenia

Hand-foot syndrome

Less Common:

Nausea and vomiting

Anorexia and diarrhea

Stomatitis

Skin involvement: rash and alopecia

Neurotoxicity

Tumor lysis syndrome

Nursing Implications: Follow CBC count closely. Assess ANC, WBC, Hgb/Hct, and platelet count prior to drug administration. Transfuse with red blood cells as ordered.

Patient teaching/nurse assessment: (1) self-assessment of infection, bleeding, fatigue; notify MD or RN T > 100.5°F, signs/symptoms of infection, bleeding; energy-conserving activities, self-care strategies to manage fatigue. Monitor bilirubin at baseline and before each cycle because dose modifications are necessary with hyperbilirubinemia.

Drug Name: Cytarabine liposome injection (DepoCyt)

Class: Antimetabolite

Mechanism of Action: Drug is converted to the metabolite ara-CTP intracellularly. Ara-CTP is thought to inhibit DNA polymerase, thereby affecting DNA synthesis. Incorporation into DNA and RNA may also contribute to cytarabine cellular toxicity.

Indications: Intrathecal treatment of lymphomatous meningitis only

Dosing: To be given as follows:

Induction therapy: DepoCyt 50 mg administered intrathecally (intraventricular or lumbar puncture) every 14 days for two doses (weeks 1 and 3).

Consolidation therapy: DepoCyt 50 mg administered intrathecally (intraventricular or lumbar puncture) every 14 days for three doses (weeks 5, 7, and 9) followed by one additional dose at week 13.

Maintenance therapy: DepoCyt 50 mg administered intrathecally (intraventricular or lumbar puncture) every 28 days for 4 doses (weeks 17, 21, 25, and 29).

If drug-related neurotoxicity develops, the dose should be reduced to 25 mg. If toxicity persists, treatment with DepoCyt should be terminated.

Administration: Drug is to be withdrawn immediately before use and should not be used more than 4 hours from the time of withdrawal from vial.

DepoCyt should be administered directly into the CSF over 1–5 minutes. Patients should lie flat for 1 hour after administration.

Must be administered with concurrent dexamethasone. Patients should be started on dexamethasone 4 mg bid either PO or IV for 5 days beginning on the day of DepoCyt injection.

Do not use inline filters with DepoCyt; administer directly into CSF.

Side Effect Profile: Common:

Nausea and vomiting

Headache

Nursing Implications: Administer antiemetics as ordered.

Encourage small frequent feedings.

Teach self-administration of antiemetic therapy.

Administer pain medication as necessary and monitor for chemical arachnoiditis.

Drug Name: Dacarbazine (DTIC-Dome, imidazole carboxamide)

Class: Alkylating agent

Mechanism of Action: Unclear but appears to be an agent that methylates nucleic acids (particularly DNA), causing cross linkage and breaks in DNA strands. This inhibits RNA and DNA synthesis. Also interacts with sulf-hydryl groups in proteins. Generally, cell cycle phase nonspecific.

Indications: Treatment of malignant melanoma

Dosing: 375 mg/m^2 every 3–4 weeks *or*

150–250 mg/m^2/day for 5 days, repeat every 3–4 weeks *or*

800–900 mg/m^2 as a single dose every 3–4 weeks

Administration: Administer via pump over 20 minutes or give via IV push over 2–3 minutes. Stable for 8 hours at room temperature or for 72 hours if refrigerated. Store lyophilized drug in refrigerator and protect from light. Drug decomposition is denoted by a change in color from yellow to pink.

Irritant—avoid extravasation.

Pain may occur above site. Usually unrelieved by slowing IV but may be relieved by applying ice to painful area. May cause venospasm; slow rate if this occurs.

Anaphylaxis has occurred with infusion of dacarbazine.

Drug interactions: increased drug metabolism with concurrent administration of dilantin, phenobarbital; potential increased toxicity with azathioprine and 6-MP.

Side Effect Profile: Common:

Nausea and vomiting

Neutropenia

Thrombocytopenia

Urticaria, erythema, facial flushing

Anemia

Uncommon:

Flu-like syndrome

Photosensitivity

Alopecia

Teratogenic

Nursing Implications: Assess CBC, WBC with differential, platelet count, and signs/symptoms of infection and bleeding prior to treatment. Premedicate with antiemetics prior to drug administration and continue prophylactically for 24 hours, at least for the first cycle. Encourage small feedings of bland foods and liquids. Teach patient about antiemetic administration at home. Patient teaching: (1) self-assessment of infection, fatigue; notify MD or RN T > 100.5°F, signs/symptoms of infection; energy-conserving activities, self-care strategies to manage fatigue; (2) try to increase fluid intake and call RN or MD if nausea/vomiting severe or unresolved in 24 hours or if unable to take oral fluids.

Discuss impact of hair loss on patient and strategies to minimize it (i.e., wig, scarf, cap) prior to drug administration. Assess patient's/partner's sexual patterns and reproductive goals. Discuss strategies to preserve sexual and reproductive health including contraception and sperm banking. Mothers should not breast feed.

Assess patients receiving high-dose cyclophosphamide: monitor serum Na$^+$, osmolality, urine osmolality, and electrolytes; strictly monitor I/O, total body fluid balance, and daily weight.

Screen patients for secondary malignancies.

Assess patients receiving high-dose or continuous low-dose cyclophosphamide for signs/symptoms of pulmonary dysfunction. Assess lung sounds prior to drug administration and periodically during treatment. Teach patient to report dyspnea, cough, or any abnormalities.

D

Drug Name: Dactinomycin (actinomycin D, Cosmegen)

Class:	Antitumor antibiotic isolated from streptomyces fungus
Mechanism of Action:	Binds to guanine portion of DNA and blocks the ability of DNA to act as a template for both DNA and RNA. At lower drug doses, the predominant action inhibits RNA, whereas at higher doses, both RNA and DNA are inhibited. Cell cycle specific for G_1 and S phases.
Indication:	Kidney cancer
Dosing:	10–15 µg/kg/day for 5 days every 3–4 weeks
	15–30 µg/kg/week, 400–600 µg/m²/day for 5 days IV
	Frequency and schedule may vary according to protocol and age
Administration:	Usually given IV push via sidearm of running IV.
	Drug is a vesicant. Give through a running IV to avoid extravasation, which may develop into ulceration, necrosis, and pain.
	Skin changes—radiation recall phenomenon. Skin discoloration along vein used for injection.
Side Effect Profile:	Common:
	Neutropenia (delayed, cumulative)
	Thrombocytopenia (delayed, cumulative)
	Nausea and vomiting
	Fatigue
	Alopecia
	Stomatitis
	Anorexia

Less Common:

Flu-like syndrome

Stomatitis

Hepatotoxic and renal toxicity

Nursing Implications: Assess ANC, WBC, Hgb/Hct, and platelet count prior to drug administration; administer aggressive antiemetics prior to drug administration; review with patient the prescription for antiemetic administration at home in between dosing. Patient teaching: (1) self-assessment of infection, fatigue; notify MD or RN T > 100.5°F, signs/symptoms of infection; energy-conserving activities, self-care strategies to manage fatigue; (2) try to increase fluid intake and call RN or MD if nausea/vomiting severe or unresolved in 24 hours or if unable to take oral fluids. Monitor before treatment and periodically during treatment: renal and liver function tests.

D

Drug Name: Daunorubicin citrate liposome injection (DaunoXome)

Class: Anthracycline antibiotic that is isolated from streptomycin products, in particular the rhodomycin products, and encapsulated in a liposome

Mechanism of Action: No clearly defined mechanism. Intercalates DNA, therefore blocking DNA, RNA, and protein synthesis. Binds to DNA and inhibits DNA replication and DNA-dependent RNA synthesis. Drug is encapsulated within liposomes (lipid vesicles) and is preferentially delivered to solid tumor sites. The liposomal encapsulated drug is protected from chemical and enzymatic degradation, protein binding, and uptake by normal tissues while circulating in the blood. The exact mechanism for selective targeting of tumor sites is unknown but is believed to be related to increased permeability of the tumor neovasculature. Once delivered to the tumor, the drug is slowly released and exerts its antineoplastic action.

Indications: Kaposi's sarcoma

Dosing: 40 mg/m^2/day IV bolus over 60 minutes every 2 weeks

Administration: IV bolus over 60 minutes, repeated every 2 weeks.

Do not use an inline filter.

Drug is an irritant, not a vesicant.

Dose should be reduced in patients with renal or hepatic dysfunction.

Hold dose if absolute granulocyte count is < 750 cells/mm^3.

Drug is embryotoxic, so female patients should use contraceptive measures as appropriate.

Back pain, flushing, and chest tightness may occur during the first 5 minutes of drug administration and resolve with cessation of the infusion. Most patients do not experience recurrence when the infusion is restarted at a slower rate.

Drug indicated in the treatment of Kaposi's sarcoma. Activity reported to be equivalent to treatment with ABV (doxorubicin, vincristine, bleomycin) but with less alopecia, cardiotoxicity, and neurotoxicity.

Side Effect Profile: Common:

Neutropenia

Thrombocytopenia

Nausea and vomiting

Anemia and fatigue

Cardiotoxic

Stomatitis

Nursing Implications: Assess ANC, WBC, Hgb/Hct, and platelet count prior to drug administration; administer aggressive antiemetics prior to drug administration; review with patient the prescription for antiemetic administration at home in between dosing. Patient teaching: (1) self-assessment of infection, fatigue; notify MD or RN T > 100.5°F, signs/symptoms of infection; energy-conserving activities, self-care strategies to manage fatigue; (2) try to increase fluid intake and call RN or MD if nausea/vomiting severe or unresolved in 24 hours or if unable to take oral fluids. Monitor cardiac dose.

Drug Name: Daunorubicin hydrochloride (Cerubidine, daunomycin)

Class: Anthracycline antibiotic isolated from streptomycin products, in particular the rhodomycin products

Mechanism of Action: No clearly defined mechanism. Intercalates DNA, therefore blocking DNA, RNA, and protein synthesis. Binds to DNA and inhibits DNA replication and DNA-dependent RNA synthesis.

Indication: Acute myelogenous leukemia

Dosing: 30–60 mg/m²/day IV for 3 consecutive days

Administration: Give IV push through the sidearm of a freely flowing IV or as a bolus over 1–2 hours or as a continuous infusion over 24 hours. Must be given via a central line if given via bolus or continuous infusion because drug is a potent vesicant.

Give through running IV to avoid extravasation.

Moderate to severe nausea and vomiting occur in 50% of patients within first 24 hours.

Causes discoloration of urine (pink to red for up to 48 hours after administration).

Side Effect Profile: Common:

Neutropenia

Thrombocytopenia

Anemia

Less Common:

Nausea and vomiting

Fatigue

Alopecia

Stomatitis

Anorexia

Flu-like syndrome

Nursing Implications: Assess ANC, WBC, Hgb/Hct, and platelet count prior to drug administration; administer aggressive antiemetics prior to drug administration; review with patient the prescription for antiemetic administration at home in between dosing. Patient teaching: (1) self-assessment of infection, fatigue; notify MD or RN T > 100.5°F, signs/symptoms of infection; energy-conserving activities, self-care strategies to manage fatigue; (2) try to increase fluid intake and call RN or MD if nausea/vomiting severe or unresolved in 24 hours or if unable to take oral fluids.

Cardiac toxicity—dose limit at 550 mg/m^2. Patients may exhibit irreversible congestive heart failure (CHF). Acute toxicity may be seen within hours after administration. This is unrelated to cumulative dose and may manifest symptoms of pump or conduction function. Rarely, transient EKG abnormalities, CHF, and pericardial effusion (whole syndrome referred to as myocarditis-pericarditis syndrome) may occur, which may lead to demise of patient.

Drug Name: Decitabine (5-aza-2-deoxycitidine)

Class: Antimetabolite

Mechanism of Action: Prevents cell from making DNA and causing cell death; in addition, can cause hypomethylation of genes that were silenced, leading to differentiate and then death.

Indication: Being studied in myelodysplastic syndrome and chronic myelogenous leukemia

Dosing: Per protocol

Side Effect Profile: Common:

Bone marrow depression

Nausea

Vomiting

Stomatitis

Nursing Implications: Assess ANC, WBC, Hgb/Hct, and platelet count prior to drug administration. Patient teaching: (1) self-assessment of infection, fatigue; notify MD or RN T > 100.5°F, signs/symptoms of infection; energy-conserving activities, self-care strategies to manage fatigue; (2) try to increase fluid intake and call RN or MD if nausea/vomiting severe or unresolved in 24 hours or if unable to take oral fluids.

Drug Name: Dexrazoxane for injection (Zinecard)

Class: Cardioprotector

Mechanism of Action: Enters easily through cell membranes, but the exact mechanism of cardiac cell protection is unclear. A possible mechanism is that the drug becomes a chelating agent within the cell and interferes with iron-mediated free radical formation that otherwise would cause cardiotoxicity from anthracyclines. Drug is a derivative of edetic acid (EDTA).

Indication: Cardioprotection from anthracycline antibiotics

Dosing: 10:1 ratio of dexrazoxane to doxorubicin (i.e., 500 mg/m^2 of dexrazoxane to 50 mg/m^2 of doxorubicin)

Administration: Give slow IV push or IV bolus <30 minutes prior to beginning doxorubicin.Drug is indicated for reduction of the incidence and severity of cardiomyopathy associated with doxorubicin in women with metastatic breast cancer who have received a cumulative doxorubicin dose of 300 mg/m^2 and who would benefit from continuing doxorubicin.

Drug may reduce the response from fluorouracil, doxorubicin, cyclophosphamide (FAC) chemotherapy when given concurrently on the first cycle of therapy (48% response rate versus 63% without the drug, and shorter time to disease progression).

Side Effect Profile: Common:

Neutropenia

Thrombocytopenia

Anemia

Hepatic and renal alterations

Pain at injection site

Nursing Implications: Assess ANC, WBC, Hgb/Hct, and platelet count prior to drug administration. Patient teaching: (1) self-assessment of infection, fatigue; notify MD or RN T > 100.5°F, signs/symptoms of infection; energy-conserving activities, self-care strategies to manage fatigue; (2) try to increase fluid intake and call RN or MD if nausea/vomiting severe or unresolved in 24 hours or if unable to take oral fluids. Monitor liver kidney function tests. Monitor site and use measures to reduce the discomfort at injection site.

Drug Name: Docetaxel (Taxotere)

Class: Taxoid, mitotic spindle poison

Mechanism of Action: Enhances microtubule assembly and inhibits tubulin depolymerization, thus arresting cell division in metaphase. Cell cycle specific for M phase.

Indication: Indicated for the treatment of (1) locally advanced or metastatic breast cancer after failure of prior chemotherapy and (2) locally advanced or metastatic non–small-cell lung cancer (NSCLC) after failure of prior platinum-based chemotherapy.

Contraindicated in patients with history of severe hypersensitivity reactions to docetaxel or to other drugs formulated with polysorbate 80; drug should

D

not be used in patients with neutrophil counts of < 1500 cells/mm^3. Drug should not be used in pregnant or breast-feeding women; women of childbearing age should use effective birth control measures.

Dosing:

Breast cancer: 60–100 mg/m^2 IV as a 1-hour infusion every 3 weeks

NSCLC: 75 mg/m^2 as a 1-hour infusion every 3 weeks

Premedication regimen with corticosteroids: for example, dexamethasone 8 mg bid for 3 days, starting 1 day prior to docetaxel to reduce risk of fluid retention and hypersensitivity reactions

Administration:

Assess patient's ANC and treat only if ANC > 1500/mm^3; assess liver function studies and, if abnormal, discuss with physician.

Use only glass or polypropylene bottles or polypropylene or polyolefin plastic bags for drug infusion, and administer infusion ONLY through polyethylene-lined administration sets.

Patient should receive corticosteroid premedication (e.g., dexamethasone 8 mg bid) for 3 days beginning 1 day before drug administration to reduce the incidence and severity of fluid retention and hypersensitivity reactions.

Administer drug infusion over 1 hour.

Radiosensitizing effect.

Theoretically, CYP3A4 inhibitors, such as ketoconazole, erythromycin, troleandomycin, cyclosporine, terfenadine, and nifedipine, can inhibit docetaxel metabolism and result in elevated serum levels of docetaxel; use together with caution or not at all.

Theoretically, CYP3A4 inducers, such as anticonvulsants and St. John's Wort, may increase metabolism and decrease serum levels of docetaxel.

Docetaxel generally should not be administered to patients with bilirubin $>$ upper limit of normal (ULN) or to patients with AST and/or ALT $> 1.5 \times$ ULN concomitant with alkaline phosphatase $> 2.5 \times$ ULN. Patients treated with elevated bilirubin or abnormal transaminases plus alkaline phosphatase have an increased risk of grade 4 neutropenia, febrile neutropenia, severe stomatitis, infections, severe thrombocytopenia, severe skin toxicity, and toxic death. Serum bilirubin, AST, ALT, and alkaline phosphatase should be obtained and reviewed by the treating physician before each cycle of docetaxel treatment.

Dose modifications during treatment: (1) Patients with breast cancer dosed initially at 100 mg/m^2 who experience febrile neutropenia, ANC < 500/mm^3 for > 1 week, or severe or cumulative cutaneous reactions should have dose reduced to 75 mg/m^2. If reactions continue at the reduced dose, further reduce to 55 mg/m^2 or discontinue drug. Patients dosed initially at 60 mg/m^2 who do not experience febrile neutropenia, ANC < 500/mm^3 for > 1 week, severe cutaneous reactions, or severe peripheral neuropathy during drug therapy may tolerate higher drug doses and may be dose escalated. Patients who develop $>$ grade 3 peripheral neuropathy should have drug discontinued.

(2) Patients with NSCLC dosed initially at 75 mg/m^2 who experience febrile neutropenia, ANC < 500/mm^3 for > 1 week, severe or cumulative cutaneous reactions, or other nonhematologic toxicity of grades 3 or 4 should have treatment withheld until toxicity resolves and then have dose reduced to 55 mg/m^2; patients who develop > grade 3 peripheral neuropathy should discontinue docetaxel chemotherapy.

Patients should receive 3-day dexamethasone premedication.

Administration of docetaxel in Europe is not subject to United States Federal Drug Administration recommendations—non-PVC containers and tubing are not required.

Incomplete cross resistance between paclitaxel and docetaxel in many tumor types.

Studies ongoing to determine effectiveness of docetaxel 30–45 mg/m^2 weekly in metastatic breast cancer because the drug given in this fashion may act as an antiangiogenesis agent and also provides dose-dense therapy, which provides less opportunity for malignant cells to develop resistant clones. Weekly dose schedules being studied are 3 weeks of treatment, 1 week off or 6 weeks of treatment, and 2 weeks off, with drug being administered as a 30-minute infusion. Most common side effects when drug is given this way are asthenia, anemia, fluid retention, nail toxicity, and hyperlacrimation. Corticosteroid premedication is often dexamethasone 4 or 8 mg PO q 12 hours for three doses beginning on the day before treatment.

Side Effect Profile: Common:

Hypersensitivity and anaphylaxis

Neutropenia

Anemia

Alopecia

Nausea and vomiting

Myalgias

Arthralgias

Fatigue

Peripheral neuropathy

Neuropathy

Less Common:

Stomatitis

Elevated LFTs

Hypotension

Hyperlacrimation

Thrombocytopenia

Nursing Implications: Assess ANC, WBC, Hgb/Hct, and platelet count prior to drug administration; administer antiemetics and medications to prevent hypersensitivity reactions prior to drug administration. Review with patient the prescription for antiemetic administration at home if nausea arises, and call RN or MD if it does not resolve in 24 hours. Assess patient closely during first few infusions for signs/symptoms of hypersensitivity reaction. Patient teaching/nurse assessment: (1) neuropathy, such as numbness and tingling of tips of fingers and toes, and whether this interferes with ability to function or do ADLs; (2) self-assessment of infection, fatigue; notify MD or RN T > 100.5°F, signs/symptoms of infection; energy-conserving activities, self-care strategies to manage fatigue; (3) strategies to reduce painful neuropathy if present.

Drug Name: Doxorubicin hydrochloride (Adriamycin, Rubex)

Class: Anthracycline antibiotic isolated from streptomycin products, in particular from the rhodomycin products

Mechanism of Action: Antitumor antibiotic—no clearly defined mechanism. Binds directly to DNA base pairs (intercalates) and inhibits DNA and DNA-dependent RNA synthesis, as well as protein synthesis. Cell cycle specific for S phase.

Indication: Metastatic ovarian cancer, breast cancer

Dosing: 30–75 mg/m^2 IV every 3–4 weeks

20–45 mg/m^2 IV for 3 consecutive days

For bladder instillation: 3–60 mg/m^2

For intraperitoneal instillation: 40 mg in 2 liters dialysate (no heparin)

Continuous infusion: varies with individual protocol

Administration: Give IV push through the sidearm of a freely flowing IV or as a bolus over 1–2 hours or as a continuous infusion over 24 hours.

Must be given via a central line if given via bolus or continuous infusion because drug is a potent vesicant. Give through running IV to avoid extravasation and tissue necrosis. Give through central line if drug is to be given by continuous infusion.

Causes discoloration of urine (from pink to red) for up to 48 hours.

Skin changes: may cause recall phenomenon—recalls reaction to previously irradiated tissue.

Cardiac toxicity: dose limit at 550 mg/m^2. Patients may exhibit irreversible CHF. May see acute toxicity in hours or days after administration. This is unrelated to cumulative dose and may manifest symptoms of pump or conduction function. Rarely, transient EKG abnormalities, CHF, and pericardial effusions (whole syndrome referred to as myocarditis-pericarditis syndrome) may occur, which may lead to demise of patient.

Vein discoloration. Increased pigmentation in black patients.

When given with barbiturates, there is increased plasma clearance of doxorubicin.

When given with cyclophosphamide, there is risk of hemorrhage and cardiotoxicity.

When given with mitomycin, there is increased risk of cardiotoxicity. There is decreased oral bioavailability of digoxin when given together. When given with mercaptopurine, there is increased risk of hepatotoxicity. Abnormalities in liver function require dose modification.

Side Effect Profile: Common:

Neutropenia

Thrombocytopenia

Anemia

Cardiotoxicity

Nausea and vomiting

Fatigue

Teratogenic, mutagenic, and carcinogenic

Stomatitis

Anorexia

Nursing Implications: Assess ANC, WBC, Hgb/Hct, and platelet count prior to drug administration; administer aggressive antiemetics prior to drug administration; review with patient the prescription for antiemetic administration at home in between dosing. Patient teaching: (1) self-assessment of infection, fatigue; notify MD or RN T > 100.5°F, signs/symptoms of infection; energy-conserving activities, self-care strategies to manage fatigue; (2) try to increase fluid intake and call RN or MD if nausea/vomiting severe or unresolved in 24 hours or if unable to take oral fluids.

Cardiac toxicity—dose limit at 550 mg/m². Patients may exhibit irreversible CHF. Acute toxicity may be seen within hours after administration. This is unrelated to cumulative dose and may manifest symptoms of pump or conduction function. Rarely, transient EKG abnormalities, CHF, and pericardial effusion (whole syndrome referred to as myocarditis-pericarditis syndrome) may occur, which may lead to demise of patient.

Drug Name: Doxorubicin hydrochloride liposomal injection (Doxil)

Class: Anthracycline antibiotic isolated from streptomycin products, in particular from the rhodomycin products. Drug is encapsulated in liposomes that have surface-bound methoxypolyethylene glycol to protect the pilosome from detection by blood phagocytes and prolong circulation time.

Mechanism of Action: Antitumor antibiotic—no clearly defined mechanism. Binds directly to DNA base pairs (intercalates) and inhibits DNA and DNA-dependent RNA synthesis, as well as protein synthesis. Cell cycle specific for S phase.

Indication: Treatment of metastatic carcinoma of the ovary refractory to paclitaxel and platinum-based chemotherapy

AIDS/Kaposi's sarcoma

Dosing:	50 mg/m^2 IV q 4 weeks $\times$ 4 cycles
	20 mg/m^2 IV over 30 minutes q 3 weeks
	Dose reduce for palmar-plantar erythrodysesthesia, hematologic toxicity, or stomatitis
Administration:	Ovarian cancer: administer at an initial rate of 1 mg/min to minimize risk of infusion reaction; if no reaction, increase rate to complete administration over 1 hour
	AIDS/Kaposi's sarcoma: administer IV over 30 minutes through patent IV.
	Monitor for infusion reaction if drug is infused too rapidly.
	Do not use inline filter.
	Dose reduce for hepatic dysfunction.
	Drug is an irritant, not a vesicant.
	Cardiac toxicity: dose limit at 550 mg/m^2. Patients may exhibit irreversible CHF. May see acute toxicity in hours or days after administration. This is unrelated to cumulative dose and may manifest symptoms of pump or conduction function. Rarely, transient EKG abnormalities, CHF, and pericardial effusions (whole syndrome referred to as myocarditis-pericarditis syndrome) may occur, which may lead to demise of patient.
	Do not administer IM or SC.
Side Effect Profile:	Common:
	Neutropenia
	Thrombocytopenia
	Anemia and fatigue
	Cardiotoxicity
	Hypersensitivity to liposomal components
	Nausea and vomiting
	Anorexia
	Hand-foot syndrome
	Teratogenic, mutagenic, and carcinogenic
	Stomatitis
Nursing Implications:	Assess ANC, WBC, Hgb/Hct, and platelet count prior to drug administration; administer aggressive antiemetics prior to drug administration; review with patient the prescription for antiemetic administration at home in between dosing. Patient teaching: (1) self-assessment of infection, fatigue; notify MD or RN T > 100.5°F, signs/symptoms of infection; energy-conserving activities, self-care strategies to manage fatigue; (2) try to increase fluid intake and call RN or MD if nausea/vomiting severe or unresolved in 24 hours or if unable to take oral fluids.
	Cardiac toxicity—dose limit at 550 mg/m^2. Patients may exhibit irreversible CHF. Acute toxicity may be seen within hours after administration. This is unrelated to cumulative dose and may manifest symptoms of pump or

D

conduction function. Rarely, transient EKG abnormalities, CHF, and pericardial effusion (whole syndrome referred to as myocarditis-pericarditis syndrome) may occur, which may lead to demise of patient.

Drug Name: Eniluracil (776C85) investigational

Class:	Dihydropyrimidine dehydrogenase (DPD) inhibitor
Mechanism of Action:	By inhibiting DPD, eniluracil permits higher dose and longer sustained serum levels of fluorouracil (5-FU) because DPD is the rate-limiting enzyme in the degradation of 5-FU.
Indication:	Advanced breast cancer
Dosing:	Per protocol; dose reduce for hematologic or gastrointestinal toxicity
Administration:	Take with large amounts of water at least 1 hour before and after eating. Eniluracil dose is in 10:1 ratio with 5-FU. Concurrent oral eniluracil and oral 5-FU are well tolerated with low toxicity profile.
Side Effect Profile:	Common: Thrombocytopenia Neutropenia Anemia and fatigue Nausea and vomiting Stomatitis
Nursing Implications:	Follow CBC count closely. Assess ANC, WBC, Hgb/Hct, and platelet count prior to drug administration. Patient teaching/nurse assessment: (1) self-assessment of infection, bleeding, fatigue; notify MD or RN T > 100.5°F, signs/symptoms of infection, bleeding; energy-conserving activities, self-care strategies to manage fatigue. Monitor bilirubin at baseline and before each cycle because dose modifications are necessary with hyperbilirubinemia. Folic acid should be avoided while taking drug. Administer antiemetic prior to chemotherapy.

E

Drug Name: Epirubicin hydrochloride (Farmorubicin(e), Farmorubicina, Pharmorubicin, Ellence)

Class:	Antitumor antibiotic
Mechanism of Action:	Antitumor antibiotic—no clearly defined mechanism. Binds directly to DNA base pairs (intercalates) and inhibits DNA and DNA-dependent RNA synthesis, as well as protein synthesis. Cell cycle specific for S phase.
Indication:	Adjuvant therapy in patients with positive axillary lymph nodes after resection of primary breast cancer
Dosing:	60–90 mg/m^2 as a single dose q 3 weeks; dose may be divided over 2–3 days. 120 mg/m^2 every 3 weeks or 45 mg/m^2 for 3 consecutive days every 3 weeks.

20 mg as a single weekly dose.

Intravesicle: 50 mg weekly as a 0.1% solution for 8 weeks; reduce dose for chemical cystitis.

Administration: Give IV push through a free-flowing line of NS or D_5W over 3–5 minutes or by bolus over 30 minutes.

Dose reduce with liver dysfunction or bone marrow compromise or when given with other antineoplastics.

Do not exceed total cumulative dose of 0.9–1 g/m^2 because of risk of cardiotoxicity. Cardiac toxicity may occur at lower cumulative doses, whether or not cardiac risk factors are present.

May cause severe myelosuppression.

Has caused secondary leukemia in a small number of patients.

Drug is a potent vesicant. Give through a running IV to avoid extravasation and tissue necrosis.

Skin changes: may cause recall phenomenon—recalls reaction to previously irradiated tissue.

Causes discoloration of urine (from pink to red color) for up to 48 hours.

Side Effect Profile: Common:

Neutropenia

Thrombocytopenia

Anemia

Cardiotoxicity

Nausea and vomiting

Fatigue

Alopecia

Stomatitis

Anorexia

Mutagenic, teratogenic, and carcinogenic

Nursing Implications: Assess ANC, WBC, Hgb/Hct, and platelet count prior to drug administration; administer aggressive antiemetics prior to drug administration; review with patient the prescription for antiemetic administration at home in between dosing. Patient teaching: (1) self-assessment of infection, fatigue; notify MD or RN T > 100.5°F, signs/symptoms of infection; energy-conserving activities, self-care strategies to manage fatigue; (2) try to increase fluid intake and call RN or MD if nausea/vomiting severe or unresolved in 24 hours or if unable to take oral fluids.

Cardiac toxicity—dose limit at 550 mg/m^2. Patients may exhibit irreversible CHF. Acute toxicity may be seen within hours after administration. This is unrelated to cumulative dose and may manifest symptoms of pump or conduction function. Rarely, transient EKG abnormalities, CHF, and pericardial effusion (whole syndrome referred to as myocarditis-pericarditis syndrome) may occur, which may lead to demise of patient.

Drug Name: Estramustine phosphate (Estracyte, Emcyt)

Class: Alkylating agent

Mechanism of Action: At usual therapeutic concentrations, estramustine acts as a weak alkylator. A chemical combination of mechlorethamine and estradiol phosphate, estramustine is believed to selectively enter cells with estrogen receptors, where the drug acts as an alkylating agent because of bischlorethyl side-chain and liberated estrogens.

Indications: Palliative treatment of prostate cancer

Dosing: 600 mg/m² (15 mg/kg) PO daily in three divided doses (range, 10–16 mg/kg/day in most studies, with evaluation after 30–90 days)

Administration: Oral

Administer with food or antacids to decrease gastrointestinal side effects.

IV preparation is a vesicant; avoid extravasation.

Transient perineal itching and pain after IV administration.

Side Effect Profile: Common:

Neutropenia

Thrombocytopenia

Nausea and vomiting

Thrombophlebitis

Rare:

Gynecomastia

Skin reactions

Alopecia

Nursing Implications: Assess ANC, WBC, Hgb/Hct, and platelet count prior to drug administration; administer antiemetics prior to chemotherapy if given IV; otherwise, review patient prescription for antiemetic administration at home in between dosing. Patient teaching: (1) self-assessment of infection, fatigue; notify MD or RN T > 100.5°F, signs/symptoms of infection; energy-conserving activities, self-care strategies to manage fatigue; (2) try to increase fluid intake and call RN or MD if nausea/vomiting severe or unresolved in 24 hours or if unable to take oral fluids.

Drug Name: Estrogens: diethylstilbestrol (DES), diethylstilbestrol diphosphate (Stilphostrol, stilbestrol diphosphate), ethinyl estradiol (Estinyl), conjugated equine estrogen (Premarin), chlorotrianisene (Tace)

Class: Hormones

Mechanism of Action: Unknown. Estrogens change the hormonal milieu of the body.

Indication: Used in the treatment of prostate cancer

Dosing: DES—prostate cancer: 1–3 mg PO daily; breast cancer: 5 mg PO tid.

Diethylstilbestrol diphosphate—prostate cancer: 50–200 PO tid, 0.5–1.0 g IV daily for 5 days, then 250–1000 mg each week.

Chlorotrianisene—1–10 PO tid.

Ethinyl estradiol—0.5–1.0 mg PO tid.

Administration: Oral

Long-term dosage of DES in males has been associated with cardiovascular deaths. Maximum dose should be 1 mg tid for prostate cancer.

Can cause inaccurate laboratory results (liver, adrenal, thyroid).

Causes rapid rise in serum calcium in patients with bony metastases; watch for symptoms of hypercalcemia.

Side Effect Profile: Common:

Gastric irritation

Hyperglycemia

Sodium and water retention

Fluid and electrolyte imbalance

Immunosuppression

Less Common:

Cushing's syndrome

Osteoporosis

Decreased bone mineral density

Bone fractures

Steroid-induced psychosis: ranging from emotional lability, insomnia, mood swings, and euphoria to psychosis

Nursing Implications: Observe patient for these side effects and taper doses; do not withdraw steroids rapidly. Teach patient that these side effects may occur and to report them. Assess patient coping with mood changes and provide emotional support; discontinue drug if psychoses occurs.

Drug Name: Etoposide (VP-16, Vepesid)

Class: Plant alkaloid, a derivative of the mandrake plant (mayapple plant)

Mechanism of Action: Inhibits DNA synthesis in S and G_2 so that cells do not enter mitosis. Causes single-strand breaks in DNA. Cell cycle specific for S and G_2 phases.

Indications: Small-cell lung cancer

Dosing: 50–100 mg/m^2 IV qd $\times$ 5 (testicular cancer) q 3–4 weeks

75–200 mg/m^2 IV qd $\times$ 3 (small-cell lung cancer) q 3–4 weeks

PO dose is twice IV dose

Administration: IV infusion: over 30–60 minutes to minimize risk of hypotension and bronchospasm (wheezing). In some instances, a test dose may be infused slowly (0.5 ml in 50 NS) and the remaining drug infused if no untoward reaction occurs after 5 minutes.

Stability: drug must be diluted with either 5% dextrose injection, USP, or 0.9% sodium chloride solution and is stable 96 hours in glass and 48 hours in plastic containers at room temperature (77°F, 25°C) under normal fluorescent light at a concentration of 0.2 mg/ml.

Inspect for clarity of solution prior to administration.

PO administration: may give as a single dose if ≤ 400 mg; otherwise, divide dose.

Reduce drug dose by 50% if bilirubin > 1.5 mg/dl and by 75% if bilirubin > 3.0 mg/dl.

Synergistic drug effect in combination with cisplatin.

Radiation recall may occur when combined therapies are used.

Side Effect Profile: Common:

Hypersensitivity and anaphylaxis

Neutropenia

Thrombocytopenia

Less Common:

Anemia

Peripheral neuropathy

Constipation

Alopecia

Nausea and vomiting

Stomatitis

Nursing Implications: Assess ANC (> 1500 cells/mm^3), WBC, Hgb/Hct, platelet count (> 100,000 cells/mm^3), and LFTs, as well as signs and symptoms of peripheral neuropathy before drug administration and periodically during treatment. Patient teaching: (1) self-assessment of infection, bleeding, fatigue; notify MD or RN T > 100.5°F, signs/symptoms of infection, bleeding; energy-conserving activities, self-care strategies to manage fatigue; (2) strategies to prevent constipation and to report it right away if it develops; (3) inform that numbness and tingling of fingertips and toes may develop and to report it if it develops.

Drug Name: Exemestane (Aromasin)

Class: Steroidal aromatase inhibitor

Mechanism of Action: Aromatase converts adrenal and ovarian androgens into estrogens peripherally in postmenopausal women. Exemestane acts as a false substrate and binds irreverably to aromatase enzyme, making it inactive.

Indication: Advanced breast cancer

Dosing: 25-mg tablets PO daily

Side Effect Profile: Common:

Fatigue

Hot flashes, increased sweating, and pain

Nursing Implications: Observe patient for these side effects. Teach patient that these side effects may occur and to report them. Assess patient coping with mood changes and provide emotional support.

Drug Name: Floxuridine (FUDR, 5-FUDR, 5-fluoro-2′-deoxyuridine)

Class: Antimetabolite

Mechanism of Action: Antimetabolite (fluorinated pyrimidine) that is metabolized to 5-fluorouracil (5-FU) when given by IV bolus or metabolized to 5-FUDR-MP when smaller doses are given by continuous infusion intra-arterially. FUDR-MP is 4 times more effective in inhibiting the enzyme thymidine synthetase than 5-FU, and this prevents the synthesis of thymidine, an essential component of DNA, resulting in interruption of DNA synthesis and cell death. Other FUDR metabolites inhibit RNA synthesis. Drug is cell cycle specific, with activity during the S phase.

Indication: Intra-arterial treatment of liver metastases from colon cancer

Dosing: Intra-arterially by slow infusion pump: 0.3 mg/kg/day (range, 0.1–0.6 mg/kg/day) *or*

5–20 mg/m^2/day every day for 14–21 days

Administration: Usually administered by slow intra-arterial infusion using a surgically placed catheter or percutaneous catheter in a major artery.

Drug usually given for 14 days, then heparinized saline is given for 14 days to maintain line patency. Dose reductions or infusion breaks may be necessary depending on toxicity. FDA approved for intrahepatic arterial infusion only.

Side Effect Profile: Common:

Nausea and vomiting

Less Common:

Hand-foot syndrome

Neutropenia

Thrombocytopenia

Rash or dermatitis

Nursing Implications: Observe patient for these side effects. Teach patient that these side effects may occur and to report them. Assess patient coping and monitor infusion catheter.

Drug Name: Fludarabine phosphate (Fludara, FLAMP)

Class: Antimetabolite

Mechanism of Action: Interferes with DNA synthesis by inhibiting ribonucleotide reductase.

Indication: Palliative treatment of patients with B-cell lymphocytic leukemia who have not responded or have progressed during treatment with at least one standard alkylating agent–containing regimen.

Dosing:	20–30 mg/m² IV over 30 minutes daily for 5 days; cycle resumes every 28 days except with bone marrow or other toxicity
	or
	20 mg/m² loading dose (bolus), then 30 mg/m² continuous infusion for 48 hours
Administration:	Administer as an IV bolus or continuous infusion.
	Use drug with caution in patients with advanced age, renal insufficiency, bone marrow impairment, or neurologic deficiency.
	Severe risk of pulmonary toxicity when fludarabine is given with pentostatin.
	May cause tumor lysis syndrome (TLS). Hydrate and use allopurinol to prevent TLS.
	Do not use in patients with known hypersensitivity to fludarabine.
Side Effect Profile:	Common:
	Neutropenia
	Thrombocytopenia
	Anemia and fatigue
	Neuropathies
	Less Common:
	Nausea and vomiting
	Pulmonary toxicity and dyspnea
	Teratogenicity
Nursing Implications:	Assess CBC, ANC, WBC, Hgb/Hct, and platelet count prior to drug administration; administer antiemetic prior to chemotherapy, and review patient prescription for antiemetic administration at home. Transfuse with red blood cells or administer erythropoietin per MD order. Teach patient about diet and instruct to alternate rest and activity; stress reduction/relaxation techniques may improve energy level. Patient teaching: self-assessment of infection, bleeding, fatigue; notify MD or RN T > 100.5°F, although recognize that drug may cause fever alone, signs/symptoms of infection, bleeding; energy-conserving activities, self-care strategies to manage fatigue. Instruct patient of bleeding and transfuse platelets per MD order.
	Assess baseline pulmonary status, including breath sounds, presence of cough, shortness of breath. Instruct patient to report symptoms of cough, shortness of breath, other abnormalities. Encourage small, frequent feedings of cool, bland foods and liquids. Teach patient to record diet history for 2–3 days and weekly weights. If patient has decreased appetite, assess food preferences (encourage or discourage) and suggest use of spices.

F

Drug Name: 5-Fluorouracil (fluorouracil, Adrucil, 5-FU, Efudex [topical])

Class:	Pyrimidine antimetabolite
Mechanism of Action:	Acts as a "false" pyrimidine, inhibiting the formation of an enzyme (thymidine synthetase) necessary for the synthesis of DNA. Also incorporates into

RNA, causing abnormal synthesis. Methotrexate given prior to 5-fluorouracil (5-FU) results in synergism and enhanced efficacy.

Indication: Treatment of cancers of the colon and rectum, in combination with leucovorin

Dosing: 12–15 mg/kg IV once a week *or*

12 mg/kg IV every day for 5 days every 4 weeks *or*

500mg/m^2 IVP 60 min into a 2 hour infusion of leucovorin weekly × 6, repeated every 8 weeks (Roswell Park regimen)

Hepatic infusion: 22 mg/kg in 100 ml D$_5$W infused into hepatic artery over 8 hours for 5–21 consecutive days

Head and neck: 1000 mg/m^2/day as continuous infusion for 4–5 days

Administration: Given IV push or bolus (slow drip) or as continuous infusion.

Given topically as cream.

Patients who have had adrenalectomy may need higher doses of prednisone while receiving 5-FU, or dose of 5-FU may be reduced in postadrenalectomy patients.

Reduce dose in patients with compromised hepatic, renal, or bone marrow function and malnutrition.

Inspect solution for precipitate prior to continuous infusion.

When given with cimetidine, there are increased pharmacologic effects of fluorouracil.

When given with thiazide diuretics, there is increased risk of myelosuppression.

Side Effect Profile: Common:

Neutropenia

Anemia

Thrombocytopenia

Less Common:

Nausea and vomiting

Anorexia and diarrhea

Stomatitis

Skin changes, alopecia

Ocular changes (photophobia) and cerebellar ataxia

Nursing Implications: Follow CBC count closely. Assess ANC, WBC, Hgb/Hct, and platelet count prior to drug administration. Patient teaching/nurse assessment: (1) self-assessment of infection, bleeding, fatigue; notify MD or RN T > 100.5°F; signs/symptoms of infection, bleeding; energy-conserving activities, self-care strategies to manage fatigue. Monitor bilirubin at baseline and before each cycle because dose modifications are necessary with hyperbilirubinemia. Folic acid should be avoided while taking drug. Administer antiemetic prior to chemotherapy.

Drug Name: Flutamide (Eulexin)

Class: Antiandrogen

Mechanism of Action: Exerts its effect by inhibiting androgen uptake or by inhibiting nuclear binding of androgen in target tissues or both.

Indication: Treatment of metastatic prostate cancer

Dosing: 250 mg every 8 hours

Administration: Oral

Side Effect Profile: Common:

Decreased libido

Hot flashes

Nausea, vomiting, and diarrhea

Nursing Implications: Observe patient for these side effects. Teach patient that these side effects may occur and to report them. Assess patient coping with mood changes and provide emotional support.

Drug Name: Fulvestrant injection (Faslodex)

Class: Estrogen downregulator

Mechanism of Action: Estrogen receptor antagonist, preventing estrogen from stimulating the growth of breast cancer cells

Indication: Treatment of hormone receptor–positive metastatic breast cancer in post-menopausal women with disease progression after antiestrogen therapy

Dosing: 250 mg q month

Administration: IM in buttock

Side Effect Profile: Common:

Hot flushes

Edema

Injection site reaction

Uncommon:

Nausea and vomiting

Constipation or diarrhea

Nursing Implications: Observe patient for these side effects. Teach patient that these side effects may occur and to report them. Assess patient coping and provide emotional support. Rotate IM sites, and in small-muscled women, divide injection into two injections, each 2.5 ml.

Drug Name: Ftorafur (tegafur) and uracil (UFT, Orzel) investigational

Class: Pyrimidine antimetabolite (tegafur) plus uracil

Mechanism of Action: Acts as a "false" pyrimidine, inhibiting the formation of an enzyme (thymidine synthetase) necessary for the synthesis of DNA. Also incorporates into

RNA, causing abnormal synthesis and suppression of tumor cell replication. Uracil is thought to inhibit the degradation of 5-FU.

Indication: Treatment of colon cancer

Dosing: 200 mg/m²/day with 5 or 50 mg leucovorin for 28 days per cycle

300–350 mg/m²/day in three divided doses 8 hours apart for 28 days

Administration: Oral

Side Effect Profile: Common:

Injection site irritation

Abdominal and back pain

Gastrointestinal: nausea, vomiting, and diarrhea

Hot flashes

Nursing Implications: Observe patient for these side effects. Teach patient that these side effects may occur and to report them. Assess patient coping and provide emotional support.

Drug Name: Gemcitabine (Gemzar)

Class: Antimetabolite

Mechanism of Action: Nucleoside analog, and mimics a natural building block of DNA. It is cell cycle specific for S phase. Drug inhibits DNA polymerase, and through intracellular phosphorylation, it inhibits DNA synthesis.

Indications: Indicated for (1) first-line treatment of inoperable locally advanced (stage IIIA or IIIB) or metastatic (stage IV) NSCLC in combination with cisplatin; (2) first-line, single-agent therapy for the treatment of locally advanced (stage II or stage III) or metastatic (stage IV) pancreatic cancer; and (3) first-line treatment of patients with metastatic breast cancer after failure of prior anthracycline-containing adjuvant chemotherapy (unless anthracyclines were clinically contraindicated) in combination with paclitaxel.

Dosing: Lung cancer: 21-day cycle: 1250 mg/m² IV over 30 minutes, days 1 and 8; *or* 28-day cycle: 1000 mg/m² IV over 30 minutes, days 1, 8, and 15; each with cisplatin 100 mg day 1 *following* gemcitabine administration

Pancreatic cancer: 1000 mg/m² IV over 30 minutes weekly up to 7 weeks (or until toxicity necessitates dose reduction or delay), then followed by a 1-week break; continue weekly × 3, 1 week off, repeated q 4 weeks

Breast cancer: 21-day cycle: 1250 mg/ m² IV over 30 minutes, days 1 and 8 *following* paclitaxel 175 mg/m² IV infusion over 3 hours

Administration: IV, as a single agent, or before cisplatin or after paclitaxel.

When combined with paclitaxel, ANC should be ≥ 1500 cells/mm³ and platelets ≥ 100,000 cells/mm³ prior to each cycle.

Dose reduce based on ANC and platelet count.

Infusion time > 60 minutes or more frequently than weekly increases toxicity.

Side Effect Profile: Common (> 50%):

Neutropenia

Anemia

Elevated LFTs (ALP, AST, ALT)

Nausea and vomiting

Less Common (10–50%):

Thrombocytopenia

Proteinuria

Hematuria

Pain

Fever

Rash

Dyspnea

Constipation or diarrhea

Bleeding

Alopecia

Infection

Rare (< 10%):

Pulmonary toxicity

Hepatotoxicity

Hemolytic uremic syndrome

Nursing Implications: Assess ANC, WBC, Hgb/Hct, and platelet count prior to drug administration; administer antiemetic prior to chemotherapy, and review patient prescription for antiemetic administration at home. Transfuse with red blood cells as ordered. Patient teaching: self-assessment of infection, bleeding, fatigue; notify MD or RN T > 100.5°F, although recognize that drug may cause fever alone, signs/symptoms of infection, bleeding; energy-conserving activities, self-care strategies to manage fatigue.

Drug Name: Goserelin acetate

Class: Synthetic analog of luteinizing hormone-releasing hormone (LHRH)

Mechanism of Action: Inhibits pituitary gonadotropin so that a chemical orchiectomy is achieved in 2–4 weeks.

Indications: (1) Palliative treatment of advanced prostate cancer; (2) in combination with flutamide in stage B2–C prostate cancer

Dosing: 3.6 mg SC q 28 days or 10.8 mg SC q 3 months

Administration: SC

When given for stage B2–C prostate cancer in combination with flutamide, begin 8 weeks prior to radiation therapy and continue throughout radiotherapy.

Side Effect Profile: Common (> 50%):

Hot flashes

Sexual dysfunction

Decreased erections

Less Common (10–50%):

Osteoporosis

Decreased bone mineral density

Bone fractures

Rare (< 10%):

Hypersensitivity reaction

Hypercalcemia

Pain related to initial flare of bony metastatic lesions

Hypo- or hypertension

Gynecomastia

Constipation or diarrhea

Fever, chills, tenderness

Anxiety, depression, headache

Nursing Implications: Observe patients with bony metastases closely during first 2 weeks following initial therapy because tumor flare may occur. Teach patient that these side effects may occur and to report them. Assess patient coping with changes in sexuality, and provide emotional support; refer for counseling as appropriate. Discuss regular examination of bone density.

Drug Name: Hydroxyurea (Hydrea, Droxia)

Class: Antimetabolite

Mechanism of Action: Inhibits DNA synthesis; increases amount of fetal hemoglobin in red blood cells, which decreases sickling

Indications: Treatment of (1) chronic myelogenous leukemia in chronic phase; (2) radiosensitizer (primary brain tumors, head and neck cancer, cancer of the cervix or uterus, NSCLC); and (3) treat sickle-cell anemia in patients with > three sickle cell crises in the previous year

Dosing: (1) 500–3000 mg (20–30 mg/kg/day) PO daily (reduce dose if renal dysfunction)

(2) 80 mg/kg PO every third day of RT

(3) 15 mg/kg/day PO increased by 5 mg/kg every 12 weeks, to maximum dose of 35 mg/kg/day

Administration: Oral, monitor blood counts and dose reduce in renal dysfunction

Side Effect Profile: Common:

Leukopenia

Less Common:

Thrombocytopenia

Anemia

Rare:

Nausea

Vomiting

Dizziness

Headache

Confusion

Nursing Implications: Assess CBC at baseline and periodically during therapy. Teach patient that side effects may happen and to notify MD or RN if they occur; self-assessment of signs/symptoms of infection, measures to avoid infection.

Drug Name: Idarubicin (Idamycin)

Class: Antitumor antibiotic

Mechanism of Action: Interferes with DNA and RNA synthesis so that cell dies

Indications: Acute myeloid leukemia

Dosing: 12 mg/m^2/day IV push × 3 in combination with cytosine arabinoside 100 mg/m^2 continuous infusion for 7 days, or 25 mg/m^2 IV push followed by cytosine arabinoside 200 mg/m^2 continous infusion for 5 days

Administration: IV push through a freely flowing IV line using vesicant precautions

Side Effect Profile: Common (> 50%):

Leukopenia

Thrombocytopenia

Anorexia

Less Common (10–50%):

Cardiotoxicity

Nausea and vomiting

Stomatitis

Rare (< 10%):

Diarrhea

Hepatitis

Nursing Implications: Assess ANC, WBC, Hgb/Hct, and platelet count prior to drug administration; administer antiemetic prior to chemotherapy, and review patient prescription for antiemetic administration at home. Teach patient that urine will be pink for up to 48 hours after drug administration. Patient teaching: self-assessment of infection, bleeding, fatigue; notify MD or RN T > 100.5°F; signs/symptoms of infection, bleeding; energy-conserving activities, self-care strategies to manage fatigue.

Drug Name: Idoxifene (investigational)

Class: Selective estrogen receptor modulator

Mechanism of Action: Blocks estrogen stimulation in estrogen receptor–positive breast cancer

Indications: Investigational, per protocol

Dosing: Per protocol

Administration: Oral

Side Effect Profile: Common:

Menopausal symptoms

Less Common:

Nausea and vomiting

Rare:

Tiredness

Lethargy

Weakness

Nursing Implications: Teach patient that side effects may happen and to notify MD or RN if they do not resolve with symptom management strategies.

Drug Name: Ifosfamide (IFEX)

Class: Alkylating agent

Mechanism of Action: Destroys DNA by cross linking strands together

Indications: Third-line chemotherapy for germ cell testicular cancer

Dosing: 700 mg–2 g/m²/day for 5 days or 2400 mg/m² for 3 days or as a continuous infusion 1200 mg/m²/day for 5 days

Administration: IV with mesna, a bladder protector

Side Effect Profile: Common (> 50%):

Hemorrhagic cystitis if mesna not used

Nausea and vomiting

Mild neutropenia

Alopecia

Less Common (10–50%):

Phlebitis

Skin changes

Rare (< 10%):

Elevated LFTs

Thrombocytopenia

Anemia

Nursing Implications: Assess ANC, WBC, Hgb/Hct, platelet count prior to drug administration, and urine for presence of blood; administer antiemetic prior to chemotherapy, and review patient prescription for antiemetic administration at home. Administer mesna prior to ifosfamide or together, if given via a continuous infusion, and ensure that mesna is given following ifosfamide administration. Teach patient to report pink or red urine. Patient teaching: self-assessment of infection, bleeding, fatigue; notify MD or RN T > 100.5°F, signs/symptoms of infection, bleeding; energy-conserving activities, self-care strategies to manage fatigue.

Drug Name: Irinotecan (Camptosar)

Class: Topoisomerase I inhibitor

Mechanism of Action: Active metabolite SN-38 prevents repair of previous, reversible single-strand DNA breaks by binding to topoisomerase I, an enzyme that relaxes tension in the DNA helix so strands can split apart to be copied during cell division. This causes cell death.

Indications: (1) First-line treatment in combination with 5-FU and leucovorin for patients with metastatic colon and rectal cancers; (2) treatment of patients with colon or rectal cancer who have progressed.

Dosing: (1) 125 mg/m^2 IV over 90 minutes on days 1, 8, 15, and 22, then 2-week rest, repeated q 6 weeks; (2) 350 mg/m^2 IV over 90 minutes q 3 weeks; (3) 125 mg/m^2 IV over 90 minutes on days 1, 8, 15, and 22, together with leucovorin 20 mg/m^2 IV bolus immediately after irinotecan on days 1, 8, 15, and 22, and 5-FU 500 mg/m^2 IV bolus immediately after leucovorin on days 1, 8, 15, and 22, then 2-week rest, repeated q 6 weeks.

Dose reduce based on ANC, grade of diarrhea, or other toxicity (see package insert).

Administration: IV bolus over 90 minutes; drug is an irritant, so avoid infiltration. If infiltration occurs flush site with sterile water and then apply ice.

Side Effect Profile: Common (> 50%):

Early diarrhea (cholinergic, within 24 hours)

Late diarrhea, occurring > 24 hours after the drug dose

Neutropenia

Anemia

Nausea and vomiting

Less Common (10–50%):

Pulmonary effects (dyspnea, infiltrates, cough)

Rare (< 10%):

Thrombocytopenia

Nursing Implications: Assess ANC, WBC, Hgb/Hct, and platelet count prior to drug administration; assess bowel elimination pattern and whether diarrhea occurred during prior treatment cycle. Administer antiemetic prior to chemotherapy, and review patient prescription for antiemetic administration at home. Administer red blood cells as ordered. Patient teaching: (1) teach patient that diarrhea may occur 24 hours or later after treatment and may be deadly; teach patient self-administration of loperamide (Imodium) 4 mg at first sign of diarrhea and continue 2 mg q 2 hours until 12 hours after diarrhea has stopped; call RN or MD immediately if diarrhea does not stop within 24 hours or if unable to take oral fluids; increase oral intake to 2–3 liters a day; (2) self-assessment of infection, fatigue; notify MD or RN T > 100.5°F, signs/symptoms of infection; energy-conserving activities, self-care strategies to manage fatigue; (3) self-administration of parenteral erythropoietin growth factor and neutrophil growth factor, if ordered.

Drug Name: Letrozole (Femara)

Class: Nonsteroidal aromatase inhibitor

Mechanism of Action: Binds to aromatase enzyme so that androgens are not converted to estrogen, thus suppressing serum estradiol levels and removing estrogen stimulus of breast cancer cell growth and replication.

Indications: (1) First-line treatment of postmenopausal women with hormone receptor–positive or unknown locally advanced or metastatic breast cancer; (2) treatment of advanced breast cancer in postmenopausal women with disease progression following antiestrogen therapy. (3) extended adjuvant therapy.

Dosing: 2.5 mg PO qd

Administration: Oral, without regard to meals

Side Effect Profile: Common (> 50%):

None

Less Common (10–50%):

Hot flushes

Bone pain

Rare (< 10%):

Musculoskeletal pain

Arthralgias

Headache

Fatigue

Chest pain

Nursing Implications: Teach patient that these side effects may occur, self-care strategies to minimize discomfort, and to report side effects if they are not effectively managed; teach patient to continue to take the drug even though she feels well.

Drug Name: Leuprolide acetate (Lupron, Lupron Depot, Viadur)

Class: Antihormone

Mechanism of Action: Luteinizing hormone-releasing hormone analog that suppresses the secretion of follicle-stimulating hormone in the pituitary gland; this reduces luteinizing hormone, which causes testosterone levels to become reduced

Indications:	Palliative treatment of advanced prostate cancer
Dosing:	1 mg q day SC; Lupron Depot: 30 mg (q 4 months), 22.5 mg (q 3 months), 7.5 mg (q 1 month); Viadur Implant 65 mg (q 12 months)
Administration:	SC (q day); IM (depot); SC (implant)
Side Effect Profile:	Common (> 50%):
	Hot flushes
	Less Common (10–50%):
	Nausea
	Decrease in bone density
	Rare (< 10%):
	Impotence
	Musculoskeletal pain
	Arthralgias
	Headache
	Fatigue
	Gynecomastia
Nursing Implications:	Observe patients with bony metastases closely during first 2 weeks following initial therapy because tumor flare may occur. Teach patient that these side effects may occur, self-care strategies to minimize discomfort, and to report side effects if they are not effectively managed; teach patient to continue to take the drug even though he feels well. Assess coping to changes in sexuality and provide emotional support; refer for counseling as appropriate. Discuss regular examination of bone density.

Drug Name: Lomustine (CCNU)

Class:	Alkylating agent (nitrosourea)
Mechanism of Action:	Causes DNA strand breaks and cross links so cell cannot replicate and dies; crosses blood-brain barrier.
Indications:	Hodgkin's disease: second-line therapy following recurrence or progression on first-line therapy; brain tumors (primary or metastatic): following surgery and/or RT primary therapy.
Dosing:	130 mg/m^2 PO × 1 q 6 weeks; 100 mg/m^2 PO q 6 weeks if given in combination with other chemotherapy agents or as a dose reduction based on prior cycle nadir counts
Administration:	Oral, on an empty stomach at bedtime
Side Effect Profile:	Common (> 50%):
	Neutropenia (nadir 41–46 days), cumulative
	Thrombocytopenia (nadir 26–34 days), cumulative
	Nausea and vomiting
	Anorexia

Less Common (10–50%):

Diarrhea

Rare (< 10%):

Lung fibrosis

Renal dysfunction

Confusion

Lethargy

Visual changes

Liver dysfunction

Nursing Implications: Assess ANC, WBC, Hgb/Hct, and platelet count prior to drug administration; teach patient to take capsule at bedtime on an empty stomach, about 30 minutes after taking an antiemetic. Review patient prescription for antiemetic administration at home in between dosing. Patient teaching: (1) self-assessment of infection, fatigue; notify MD or RN T > 100.5°F, signs/symptoms of infection; energy-conserving activities, self-care strategies to manage fatigue; (2) try to increase fluid intake and call RN or MD if nausea/vomiting severe or unresolved in 24 hours or if unable to take oral fluids. Monitor before treatment and periodically during treatment: pulmonary function studies and renal and liver function tests.

Drug Name: Mechlorethamine hydrochloride (nitrogen mustard)

Class:	Alkylating agent
Mechanism of Action:	Causes DNA strand breaks and cross links so cell cannot replicate and dies
Indications:	Hodgkin's disease
Dosing:	6 mg/m^2 IV push on days 1 and 8 q 28 days as part of MOPP regimen
Administration:	IV push through patent, freely flowing IV; use vesicant precautions
Side Effect Profile:	Common (> 50%):

Severe nausea and vomiting

Neutropenia

Thrombocytopenia

Less Common (10–50%):

Chills, fever

Diarrhea

Weakness

Drowsiness

Headache

Rare (< 10%):

Ringing in ears

Deafness

M

Nursing Implications: Assess ANC, WBC, Hgb/Hct, and platelet count prior to drug administration; administer aggressive antiemetics prior to chemotherapy. Review patient prescription for antiemetic administration at home in between dosing. Patient teaching: (1) self-assessment of infection, fatigue; notify MD or RN T > 100.5°F, signs/symptoms of infection; energy-conserving activities, self-care strategies to manage fatigue; (2) try to increase fluid intake and call RN or MD if nausea/vomiting severe or unresolved in 24 hours or if unable to take oral fluids.

Drug Name: Megestrol acetate (Megace)

Class:	Hormone
Mechanism of Action:	Alters hormonal stimulation of malignant cell
Indications:	(1) Breast cancer; (2) endometrial cancer
Dosing:	(1) 40 mg PO qid or 160 mg qd; (2) 80 mg PO qid
Administration:	Oral, without regard to meals
Side Effect Profile:	Common (> 50%):
	Increased appetite
	Less Common (10–50%):
	Fluid retention
	Nausea
	Rare (< 10%):
	Allergic reactions
	Jaundice
	Hypertension

Nursing Implications: Teach patient that these side effects may occur, self-care strategies to minimize discomfort, and to report side effects if they are not effectively managed; teach patient to continue to take the drug even though he or she feels well.

Drug Name: Melphalan hydrochloride (Alkeran)

Class:	Alkylating agent
Mechanism of Action:	Causes DNA strand breaks and cross links so cell cannot replicate and dies
Indications:	Palliative treatment of (1) multiple myeloma and (2) nonresectable epithelial ovarian cancer
Dosing:	6 mg/m² PO qd × 5 repeated q 6 weeks, with prednisone; IV high dose with stem-cell rescue (investigational)
Administration:	Oral, on empty stomach; IV (investigational)
Side Effect Profile:	Common (> 50%):
	Neutropenia
	Thrombocytopenia

Immune suppression

Severe nausea and vomiting (high dose, IV)

Less Common (10–50%):

Nausea and vomiting (low dose, oral)

Rare (< 10%):

Anorexia

Severe hypersensitivity reaction (high dose, IV)

Secondary malignancy (acute leukemia)

Pulmonary fibrosis

Alopecia

Nursing Implications: Assess ANC, WBC, Hgb/Hct, and platelet count prior to drug administration; administer aggressive antiemetics prior to chemotherapy if given IV; otherwise, review patient prescription for antiemetic administration at home in between dosing. Patient teaching: (1) self-assessment of infection, fatigue; notify MD or RN T > 100.5°F, signs/symptoms of infection; energy-conserving activities, self-care strategies to manage fatigue; (2) try to increase fluid intake and call RN or MD if nausea/vomiting severe or unresolved in 24 hours or if unable to take oral fluids.

Drug Name: Mercaptopurine (Purinethol, 6-MP)

Class: Antimetabolite

Mechanism of Action: False nucleotide incorporated into DNA so cell cannot divide and dies

Indications: Leukemia

Dosing: 100 mg/m^2 PO qd × 5

Administration: Oral, with or without food

Side Effect Profile: Common (> 50%):

Leukopenia

Less Common (10–50%):

Thrombocytopenia

Anemia

Hepatotoxicity

Rare:

Nausea and vomiting

Stomatitis

Rash

Nursing Implications: Assess ANC, WBC, Hgb/Hct, and platelet count prior to drug administration; review patient prescription for antiemetic administration at home if needed. Patient teaching: (1) self-administration of drug; (2) self-assessment of infection, fatigue; notify MD or RN T > 100.5°F, signs/symptoms of infection;

energy-conserving activities, self-care strategies to manage fatigue; (3) drink 2–3 liters of fluid on day of therapy and day after to flush kidneys.

Drug Name: Methotrexate (Mexate, Folex, amethopterin)

Class: Antimetabolite

Mechanism of Action: Folic acid antagonist, preventing DNA synthesis and cell replication so cell dies

Indications: (1) Choriocarcinoma (hydatiform mole); (2) acute lymphocytic leukemia; (3) intrathecal leukemia; (4) osteogenic sarcoma; (5) lymphoma

Dosing: (1) 15–30 mg PO/IM qd × 5, repeated up to 5 times as needed; (2) 3.3 mg/m^2 with prednisone 60 mg/m^2 PO qd until remission, then maintenance 15 mg/m^2 twice a week (PO/IM); (3) 12 mg intrathecally with systemic leucovorin rescue; (4) 12 g/m^2 IV after serum alkalinization and hydration, with systemic leucovorin rescue starting 24 hours after drug q 6 hours for 10 doses; (5) 100–500 mg/m^2 IV

Administration: PO, IM, IV; moderate, high, and intrathecal doses require leucovorin rescue of normal cells

Side Effect Profile: Common (> 50%):

Anorexia

Sun sensitivity

Diarrhea

Stomatitis

Renal toxicity if urine not alkalinized in high-dose therapy

Less Common (10–50%):

Nausea and vomiting

Hepatotoxicity

Rare (< 10%):

Leukopenia

Thrombocytopenia

Anemia

Allergic pneumonitis

Alopecia

Dermatitis

Dizziness

Malaise

Nursing Implications: Assess ANC, WBC, Hgb/Hct, platelet count, BUN, creatinine, and LFTs prior to drug administration; administer antiemetics if medium to high dose.

Review patient prescription for antiemetic administration at home in between dosing. If high dose, ensure leucovorin available, and urine pH > 7.0 prior to drug administration. Patient teaching: (1) self-assessment of infection, fatigue; notify MD or RN T > 100.5°F; signs/symptoms of infection; energy-conserving activities, self-care strategies to manage fatigue; (2) increase fluid intake to 2–3 liters a day on day of treatment and for 3–4 days afterwards; (3) if medium to high dose, take oral leucovorin q 6 hours × 10, exactly on time.

Drug Name: Methyl-CCNU (semustine, MeCCNU, investigational)

Class: Alkylating agent (nitrosourea)

Mechanism of Action: Causes DNA strand breaks and cross links so cell cannot replicate and dies; crosses blood-brain barrier

Indications: Investigational

Dosing: Per protocol, 150–200 mg/m^2 PO × 1 q 6 weeks

Administration: Oral, take at bedtime on empty stomach

Side Effect Profile: Common (> 50%):

Neutropenia

Thrombocytopenia

Severe nausea and vomiting

Less Common (10–50%):

Fatigue

Rare (< 10%):

Stomatitis

Hepatotoxicity

Renal dysfunction

Lethargy

Ataxia

Visual changes

Pulmonary fibrosis

Nursing Implications: Assess ANC, WBC, Hgb/Hct, and platelet count prior to drug administration; teach patient to take capsule at bedtime on an empty stomach, about 30 minutes after taking an antiemetic and sedative. Review patient prescription for antiemetic administration at home in between dosing. Patient teaching: (1) self-assessment of infection, fatigue; notify MD or RN T > 100.5°F, signs/symptoms of infection; energy-conserving activities, self-care strategies to manage fatigue; (2) try to increase fluid intake and call RN or MD if nausea/vomiting severe or unresolved in 24 hours or if unable to take oral fluids. Monitor before treatment and periodically during treatment: pulmonary function studies and renal and liver function tests.

Drug Name: Mitomycin (mitomycin C, mutamycin)

Class: Antitumor antibiotic

Mechanism of Action: Cross links DNA strands so DNA cannot be copied and cell dies

M

Indications:	In combination with other agents, for the treatment of disseminated adenocarcinoma of the stomach or pancreas
Dosing:	2 mg/m^2 IV qd × 5 or 5–20 mg/m^2 IV push q 6–8 weeks
Administration:	IV push through patent, freely flowing IV line with vesicant precautions
Side Effect Profile:	Common (> 50%):
	Neutropenia (delayed, cumulative)
	Thrombocytopenia (delayed, cumulative)
	Nausea and vomiting
	Fatigue
	Alopecia
	Anorexia
	Less Common (10–50%):
	Hair breakage
	Stomatitis
	Rare (< 10%):
	Hemolytic uremic syndrome
	Interstitial pneumonitis
Nursing Implications:	Assess ANC, WBC, Hgb/Hct, and platelet count prior to drug administration; administer aggressive antiemetics prior to drug administration; review with patient prescription for antiemetic administration at home in between dosing. Patient teaching: (1) self-assessment of infection, fatigue; notify MD or RN T > 100.5°F, signs/symptoms of infection; energy-conserving activities, self-care strategies to manage fatigue; (2) try to increase fluid intake and call RN or MD if nausea/vomiting severe or unresolved in 24 hours or if unable to take oral fluids. Monitor before treatment and periodically during treatment: renal and liver function tests and pulmonary function studies if dyspnea or symptoms arise.

Drug Name: Mitoxantrone (Novantrone)

Class:	Antitumor antibiotic
Mechanism of Action:	Attaches to strands of DNA so strands cannot separate and DNA cannot be synthesized; the cell dies
Indications:	Acute leukemia
Dosing:	12 mg/m^2 IV qd × 3 in combination with cytosine arabinoside 100 mg/m^2/day continuous infusion × 7 days
Administration:	IV push into freely flowing IV line or as IV bolus
Side Effect Profile:	Common (> 50%):
	Neutropenia
	Blue urine for 24 hours

Less Common (10–50%):

Nausea and vomiting

Alopecia

Blue sclera

Rare (< 10%):

Thrombocytopenia

Cardiotoxicity

Stomatitis

Nursing Implications: Assess ANC, WBC, Hgb/Hct, and platelet count prior to drug administration; review with patient the prescription for antiemetic administration at home if nausea arises, or instruct patient to alert the RN. Patient teaching/nurse assessment: (1) urine will be blue-green for 24 hours; sclera may be blue tinged; (2) self-assessment of infection, fatigue; notify MD or RN T > 100.5°F, signs/symptoms of infection; energy-conserving activities, self-care strategies to manage fatigue; (3) try to increase fluid intake and call RN or MD if nausea/vomiting severe or unresolved in 24 hours or if unable to take oral fluids.

Drug Name: Nilutamide (Nilandron)

Class:	Antiandrogen
Mechanism of Action:	Binds irreversibly to adrenal androgen receptors, thereby preventing androgen binding. Testosterone effects are blocked and do not stimulate the prostate cancer cells.
Indications:	Advanced prostate cancer following castration
Dosing:	300 mg/day × 30 days, then 150 mg/day, beginning the day of or the day after castration
Administration:	Oral, without regard to means
Side Effect Profile:	Common (> 50%):

None

Less Common (10–50%):

Hot flushes

Difficulty adapting to the dark

Rare (< 10%):

Interstitial pneumonitis

Hepatitis

Nausea

Constipation

Abnormal vision

Increased liver function enzymes

Anorexia

Angina

Nursing Implications: Teach patients: (1) that these side effects may occur, self-care strategies to minimize discomfort, and to report the side effects if they are not effectively managed; (2) to continue to take the drug even though he feels well; (3) to wear tinted glasses so the transition from light to dark is easier; also, to be cautious driving at night or through tunnels; (4) to call MD immediately if the patient develops breathing difficulty or yellowing of the skin or sclerae.

Drug Name: Oxaliplatin (Eloxatin)

Class: Alkylating agent, cisplatin analog

Mechanism of Action: Causes cross linking of DNA strands so DNA cannot be replicated and cell dies

Indications: (1) Adjuvant colon cancer; (2) first-line treatment for metastatic colon or rectal cancers

Dosing: (1) FOLFOX4: day 1: oxaliplatin 85 mg/m^2 IV over 2 hours, at same time as leucovorin 200 mg/m^2, followed by 5-fluorouracil (5-FU) 400 mg/m^2 IV push, then 5-FU 600 mg/m^2 IV infusion over 22 hours; day 2: leucovorin 200 mg/m^2, followed by 5-FU 400 mg/m^2 IV push, then 5-FU 600 mg/m^2 IV infusion over 22 hours, repeated q 2 weeks

(2) FOLFOX4 or FOLFOX6: oxaliplatin 85–100 mg/m^2 IV over 2 hours, at same time as leucovorin 200–400 mg/m^2 IV over 2 hours, followed by 5-FU 400 mg/m^2 IV push, then 5-FU 2.4–3.0 g/m^2 IV infusion over 46 hours, repeated q 2 weeks, in combination with bevacizumab

Administration: IV infusion over 2–6 hours, use vesicant precautions

Side Effect Profile: Common (> 50%):

Neutropenia

Anemia

Cold-induced acute neurotoxicity

Persistent or cumulative neurotoxicity

Nausea and vomiting

Less Common (10–50%):

Fatigue

Delayed hypersensitivity

Rare (< 10%):

Pharyngolaryngeal dysesthesia

Nursing Implications: Assess ANC, WBC, Hgb/Hct, and platelet count prior to drug administration; administer aggressive antiemetics prior to drug administration.

Review with patient the prescription for antiemetic administration at home if nausea arises, and instruct patient to call RN or MD if it does not resolve in 24 hours. Patient teaching/nurse assessment: (1) neuropathy, such as numbness and tingling of tips of fingers and toes, and whether this interferes with ability to function or do ADLs; (2) self-assessment of infection, fatigue; notify MD or RN T $> 100.5°F$, signs/symptoms of infection; energy-conserving activities, self-care strategies to manage fatigue; (3) avoid touching cold objects or drinking/eating cold food for 2–5 days after oxaliplatin administration.

Drug Name: Paclitaxel (Taxol)

Class: Taxoid, mitotic inhibitor

Mechanism of Action: Causes cell to make mitotic apparatus earlier than normal, and it can't break apart, so cell dies

Indications: (1) first-line advanced ovarian cancer in combination with cisplatin; (2) treatment of previously treated advanced ovarian cancer; (3) adjuvant treatment of lymph node–positive breast cancer given sequentially to doxorubicin-containing combination therapy; (4) treatment of recurrent or metastatic breast cancer following failure of initial or adjuvant chemotherapy; (5) first-line therapy in combination with cisplatin for NSCLC that is unresectable or appropriate for radiotherapy; (6) AIDS-related Kaposi's sarcoma

Dosing: (1) 175 mg/m^2 IV over 3 hours followed by cisplatin 75 mg/m^2 q 3 weeks or other regimens; (2) 135–175 mg/m^2 IV over 3 hours q 3 weeks; (3) 175 mg/m^2 IV over 3 hours q 3 weeks $\times$ 4 cycles, in combination with doxorubicin-containing regimen (response in estrogen receptor–negative women); (4) 175 mg/m^2 IV over 3 hours q 3 weeks (ASCO 2004 showed q week dosing to be superior to q 3 week dosing); (5) 135 mg/m^2 IV over 24 hours, followed by cisplatin 75 mg/m^2 q 3 weeks; (6) 135 mg/m^2 IV over 3 hours q 3 weeks or 100 mg/m^2 IV over 3 hours q 2 weeks

Carboplatin may be substituted at a different dose for cisplatin; paclitaxel must be given BEFORE cisplatin.

If given in combination with doxorubicin or liposomal doxorubicin, give doxorubicin BEFORE paclitaxel.

Significant increase in cardiotoxicity risk if given with doxorubicin for cumulative doxorubicin doses > 380 mg/m^2

Administration: IV over 1–24 hours following premedication with dexamethasone, diphenhydramine, and H$_2$ antagonist to prevent hypersensitivity reactions to Cremophor oil (vehicle of drug as insoluble)

Side Effect Profile: Common ($> 50\%$):

Neutropenia

Anemia

Alopecia

Nausea and vomiting

Myalgias

Arthralgias

Peripheral neuropathy

Diarrhea

Neuropathic pain

Less Common (10–50%):

Cardiotoxicity

Stomatitis

Elevated LFTs

Rare (< 10%):

Hypersensitivity reactions

Hypotension

Arrythmia

Thrombocytopenia

Nursing Implications: Assess ANC, WBC, Hgb/Hct, and platelet count prior to drug administration; administer antiemetics and medications to prevent hypersensitivity reactions prior to drug administration. Review with patient the prescription for antiemetic administration at home if nausea arises, and instruct patient to call RN or MD if it does not resolve in 24 hours. Assess patient closely during first few infusions for signs/symptoms of hypersensitivity reaction. Patient teaching/nurse assessment: (1) neuropathy, such as numbness and tingling of tips of fingers and toes, and whether this interferes with ability to function or do ADLs; (2) self-assessment of infection, fatigue; notify MD or RN T > 100.5°F, signs/symptoms of infection; energy-conserving activities, self-care strategies to manage fatigue; (3) strategies to reduce painful neuropathy if present. Monitor cardiac function study and liver function studies at baseline and periodically during therapy.

Drug Name: Pegasparaginase

Class: Miscellaneous agent (enzyme)

Mechanism of Action: Modified L-asparaginase, an enzyme which hydrolyzes serum asparagine, a nonessential amino acid for both leukemic and normal cells, but normal cells can synthesize their own, and leukemic cells starve

Indications: Acute lymphocytic leukemia

Dosing: 2500 U/m^2 every 14 days (adults)

Administration: IV or IM (preferred because of lower incidence of allergic reactions)

Side Effect Profile: Common (> 50%):

Elevated LFTs

Less Common (10–50%):

Acute hypersensitivity reaction, especially if given IV

Lethargy

Drowsiness

Somnolence

Anemia

Rare ($<$ 10%):

Leukopenia

Thrombocytopenia

Nursing Implications: Assess for signs/symptoms of acute hypersensitivity when drug is being given for first and second times, and be prepared for management of hypotension and bronchospasm with epinephrine. Teach patient that side effects may occur and to report them.

Drug Name: Pemetrexate (Alimta)

Class:	Antimetabolite
Mechanism of Action:	Interferes with DNA synthesis so DNA is not replicated and cell dies
Indications:	Unresectable malignant pleural mesothelioma in combination with cisplatin
Dosing:	500 mg/m^2 IV over 10 minutes q 21 days, cisplatin 75 mg/m^2 IV q 21 days

Folic acid 350–1000 µg PO beginning 1 week prior to treatment and continuing throughout and after treatment

Vitamin B$_{12}$ 1000 µg IM 1 week prior to initial treatment then q three cycles thereafter

Dexamethasone 4 mg PO day before, day of, and day after treatment to help prevent skin rash

Dose reduce for hepatic failure

Administration: IV over 10 minutes

Side Effect Profile: Common ($>$ 50%):

Nausea

Vomiting

Fatigue

Less Common (10–50%):

Neutropenia

Thrombocytopenia

Anemia

Fever

Diarrhea

Stomatitis

Rash

Rare ($<$ 10%):

Infection

Nursing Implications: Assess (1) compliance with folic acid and vitamin B$_{12}$ administration prior to initial and subsequent treatments; (2) ANC ($\geq$ 1500 cells/mm^3), WBC, Hgb/Hct, platelet count ($\geq$ 100,000 cells/mm^3) prior to drug administration; administer antiemetics and medications to prevent rash prior to drug administration. Review with patient the prescription for antiemetic administration at home if nausea arises, and instruct patient to call RN or MD if it does not resolve in 24 hours. Patient teaching: self-assessment of infection, fatigue; notify MD or RN T > 100.5°F, signs/symptoms of infection; energy-conserving activities, self-care strategies to manage fatigue.

Drug Name: Pentostatin (Nipent)

Class:	Antitumor antibiotic
Mechanism of Action:	Inhibits adenosine deaminase, which is found in high amounts in lymphocytes. Preferentially induces apoptosis (programmed cell death).
Indications:	Hairy-cell leukemia, first line, or in patients unresponsive to interferon alfa
Dosing:	4 mg/m^2 IV q 2 weeks for 3–6 months, dose reduce for renal dysfunction
Administration:	IV
Side Effect Profile:	Common (> 50%):
	Neutropenia
	Thrombocytopenia
	Nausea and vomiting
	Less Common (10–50%):
	Neurotoxicity (dose related)
	Conjunctivitis (irreversible)
	Rare (< 10%):
	Cardiac effects (angina, CHF, arrhythmia)
	Changes in vision
	Stomatitis
	Renal dysfunction
	Thrombophebitis
	Hepatotoxicity
Nursing Implications:	Assess ANC, WBC, Hgb/Hct, and platelet count prior to drug administration; administer antiemetic prior to chemotherapy, and review patient prescription for antiemetic administration at home. Patient teaching: self-assessment of infection, bleeding, fatigue; notify MD or RN T > 100.5°F, although recognize that drug may cause fever alone, signs/symptoms of infection, bleeding; energy-conserving activities, self-care strategies to manage fatigue. Teach that neurotoxicity may occur and to report headache, lethargy, seizures, and conjunctivitis right away.

Drug Name: Plicamycin (mithramycin)

Class:	Antitumor antibiotic
Mechanism of Action:	Interferes with synthesis of DNA, causing cell death
Indications:	(1) Testicular cancer; (2) hypercalcemia

Dosing: (1) 25–30 µg/kg IV over 4–6 hours, alternating days until toxicity occurs

                                  (2) 25 µg/kg IV over 4–6 hours

Administration: IV over 4–6 hours to minimize emesis, avoid extravasation

Side Effect Profile: Common (> 50%):

Severe nausea and vomiting

Alopecia

Leukopenia

Immunosuppression

Stomatitis

Less Common (10–50%):

Thrombocytopenia

Coagulopathy

Anemia

Hypocalcemia

Taste alterations

Rare (< 10%):

CNS effects (crosses blood-brain barrier)

Nursing Implications: Assess ANC, WBC, Hgb/Hct, and platelet count prior to drug administration; administer antiemetic prior to chemotherapy, and review patient prescription for antiemetic administration at home. Patient teaching: self-assessment of infection, bleeding, fatigue; notify MD or RN T > 100.5°F, signs/symptoms of infection, bleeding; energy-conserving activities, self-care strategies to manage fatigue.

Drug Name: Procarbazine hydrochloride (Matulane)

Class: Miscellaneous agent

Mechanism of Action: Interferes with DNA and RNA, causing cell death

Indications: Hodgkin's disease, malignant brain tumor

Dosing: 100 mg/m^2 PO qd $\times$ 7–14 days q 4 weeks, in combination with other drugs, such as MOPP regimen

Administration: Oral, taken 30 minutes after antiemetic at bedtime

Side Effect Profile: Common (> 50%):

Neutropenia

Thrombocytopenia

Severe nausea and vomiting

Less Common (10–50%):

Anemia

Lethargy

Nightmares

Insomnia

Nervousness

Hallucinations

Rare ($<$ 10%):

Diarrhea

Ataxia

Paresthesias

Nursing Implications: Assess ANC, WBC, Hgb/Hct, and platelet count prior to drug administration. Teach patient: (1) drug administration and to administer antiemetic prior to drug; (2) self-assessment of infection, bleeding, fatigue; notify MD or RN T $>$ 100.5°F, signs/symptoms of infection, bleeding; energy-conserving activities, self-care strategies to manage fatigue; (3) to avoid other CNS-depressing drugs, alcohol, or MAO inhibitors while taking drug; (4) to report paresthesias, neuropathy, confusion right away.

Drug Name: Prolifeprosan 20 with carmustine (BCNU) implant (Gliadel)

Class:	Alkylating agent (carmustine)
Mechanism of Action:	Implanted in surgical cavity where chemotherapy is absorbed locally by residual brain tumor cells, and tumor cells die
Indications:	Newly diagnosed, high-grade malignant glioma, in conjunction with surgery and RT
Dosing:	8 wafers or 61.6 mg of carmustine
Administration:	Implanted wafer after surgical resection of malignant glioma
Side Effect Profile:	Common ($>$ 50%):
	Postoperative seizures
	Less Common (10–50%):
	Healing abnormalities (CSF leaks, wound effusions)
	Rare ($<$ 10%):
	Depression
	Cerebral edema
	Insomnia
	Ataxia
	Hypertension
Nursing Implications:	Assess patient postoperatively for seizures, along with other neurologic vital signs after craniectomy. Teach patient about drug, and provide emotional support.

Drug Name: Raltitrexed (Tomudex, investigational)

Class:	Antimetabolite
Mechanism of Action:	Interferes with DNA synthesis, so cell dies

Indications:	Investigational
Dosing:	3 mg/m^2 IV q 3 weeks per protocol, hold if creatinine clearance < 25 ml/min
Administration:	IV bolus over 15 minutes
Side Effect Profile:	Common (> 50%):
	Neutropenia
	Anemia
	Asthenia
	Fatigue
	Less Common (10–50%):
	Thrombocytopenia
	Diarrhea
	Nausea and vomiting
	Stomatitis
	Rare (< 10%):
	Constipation
	Anorexia
Nursing Implications:	Assess ANC, WBC, Hgb/Hct, and platelet count prior to drug administration; administer antiemetic prior to chemotherapy, and review patient prescription for antiemetic administration at home. Patient teaching: self-assessment of infection, bleeding, fatigue; notify MD or RN T > 100.5°F, signs/symptoms of infection, bleeding; energy-conserving activities, self-care strategies to manage fatigue. Transfuse red blood cells as ordered.
	Teach self-injection of erythropoietin growth factor if ordered.

Drug Name: Streptozocin (Zanosar)

Class:	Alkylating agent (nitrosourea)
Mechanism of Action:	Cross linking between DNA strands prevents cell replication and causes cell death
Indications:	Pancreatic cancer
Dosing:	500 mg/m^2 IV qd × 5, q 3–4 weeks, or 1500 mg/m^2 IV q week
Administration:	IV infusion over 1 hour
Side Effect Profile:	Common (> 50%):
	Neutropenia
	Renal dysfunction
	Nausea and vomiting
	Hepatotoxicity
	Less Common (10–50%):
	Hypoglycemia
	Leukopenia

Thrombocytopenia

Anemia

Rare ($<$ 10%):

Secondary malignancies

Nursing Implications: Assess ANC, WBC, Hgb/Hct, platelet count, BUN, creatinine, and LFTs prior to drug administration and periodically during treatment. Administer antiemetic prior to chemotherapy, and review patient prescription for antiemetic administration at home. Patient teaching: self-assessment of infection, bleeding, fatigue; notify MD or RN T $>$ 100.5°F, signs/symptoms of infection, bleeding; energy-conserving activities, self-care strategies to manage fatigue.

Drug Name: Tamoxifen citrate (Nolvadex)

Class: Antiestrogen

Mechanism of Action: Blocks estrogen receptor in breast cancer cells, so cell cannot be stimulated by estrogen

Indications: (1) Metastatic breast cancer in estrogen receptor–positive women; (2) adjuvant treatment of lymph node–positive, postmenopausal women in combination with total or segmental mastectomy, RT, and axillary dissection; (3) treatment of women with DCIS; (4) risk reduction in high-risk women (Gail model $\geq$ 1.67%)

Dosing: (1, 2): 20–40 mg PO qd $\times$ 5 years; (3, 4): 20 mg PO qd $\times$ 5 years

Administration: Oral, without regard to meals, at the same time every day

Side Effect Profile: Common ($>$ 50%):

Hot flashes

Less Common (10–50%):

Vaginal discharge

Transient tumor flare with tumor pain

Fluid retention

Nausea

Irregular menses

Weight loss

Skin changes

Rare ($<$ 10%):

Endometrial cancer

Uterine sarcoma

Thromboembolism with pulmonary and cerebral emboli

Cerebral vascular accident

Visual changes

Depression

Rash

Tumor flare

Vaginal bleeding

Nursing Implications: Assess patient with metastatic breast cancer during drug introduction to identify symptoms associated with flare reaction. Teach patient that these side effects may occur and self-care strategies to minimize discomfort and to report side effects if they are not effectively managed; teach patient to continue to take the drug even though she feels well and to report vaginal bleeding, pain in the calf, or difficulty breathing right away.

Drug Name: Temozolomide (Temodar)

Class: Alkylating agent

Mechanism of Action: Prodrug, metabolized into active cytotoxic metabolite that crosses blood-brain barrier; forms cross linkages between DNA strands, also RNA, leading to cell death

Indications: Treatment of patients with refractory anaplastic astrocytoma, following first-line treatment with a nitrosourea and procarbazine

Dosing: 150 mg/m^2/day $\times$ 5 q 28 days initially, then titrated to nadir counts to keep ANC to 1000–1500 cells/mm^3 and platelet count to 50,000–100,000 cells/mm^3

Administration: Oral, on an empty stomach with a full glass of water, following antiemetic 30 minutes prior to dose

Side Effect Profile: Common (> 50%):

Neutropenia

Thrombocytopenia

Nausea and vomiting

Less Common (10–50%):

Headache

Asthenia

Fatigue

Peripheral edema

Constipation

Diarrhea

Anemia

Stomatitis

Anorexia

Lethargy

Ataxia

Rare (< 10%):

Visual changes

Skin rash

Alopecia

Nursing Implications: Assess ANC, WBC, Hgb/Hct, and platelet count prior to drug administration. Teach patient: (1) drug administration at the same time each day and to administer antiemetic prior to drug; (2) self-assessment of infection, bleeding, fatigue; notify MD or RN T > 100.5°F, signs/symptoms of infection, bleeding; energy-conserving activities, self-care strategies to manage fatigue; (3) CNS symptoms that may occur and to report them, such as ataxia.

Drug Name: Thioguanine (Tabloid, 6-thioguanine)

Class:	Antimetabolite
Mechanism of Action:	Inhibits synthesis of DNA so that cell cannot replicate and cell dies
Indications:	Acute nonlymphocytic leukemias
Dosing:	100 mg/m^2 PO q 12 hours for 5–10 days, often in combination with cytosine arabinoside
Administration:	Oral, on an empty stomach, about 30 minutes after antiemetic medicine
Side Effect Profile:	Common (>50%)

Nausea and vomiting

Leukopenia

Thrombocytopenia

Less Common (10–50%):

Loss of vibratory sense and unsteady gait

Rare (< 10%):

Veno-occlusive disease of the liver

Anorexia

Stomatitis

Hepatoxicity

Nursing Implications: Assess ANC, WBC, Hgb/Hct, and platelet count prior to drug administration. Teach patient: (1) drug administration at the same time each day and to administer antiemetic prior to drug; (2) self-assessment of infection, bleeding, fatigue; notify MD or RN T > 100.5°F, signs/symptoms of infection, bleeding; energy-conserving activities, self-care strategies to manage fatigue; (3) to notify MD right away if abdominal pain (RUQ), rapid weight gain, yellowing of the skin or eyes, or swelling of the hands, feet, face, or abdomen (veno-occlusive disease) occur.

Drug Name: Thiotepa (Thioplex, triethylenethiophosphoramide)

Class:	Alkylating agent
Mechanism of Action:	Forms cross linkages between DNA strands so that DNA cannot be copied, cell cannot replicate, and cell dies

Indications:	Adenocarcinoma of the breast, adenocarcinoma of the ovary, superficial papillary bladder cancer, controlling intracavitary effusions
Dosing:	Parenteral: 8 mg/m² IV qd × 5, q 3–4 weeks; *or* 0.3–0.4 mg/kg IV q 1–4 weeks, depending on WBC count
	Intravesicular: 60 mg in 60 ml sterile water q week for 3–4 weeks
Administration:	IV or intravesicular
Side Effect Profile:	Common (> 50%):
	Neutropenia
	Thrombocytopenia
	Less Common (10–50%):
	Nausea and vomiting
	Dizziness
	Headache
	Fever
	Rare (< 10%):
	Secondary malignancy (acute nonlymphocytic leukemia)
	Hypersensitivity reaction
	Anorexia
Nursing Implications:	Assess ANC, WBC, Hgb/Hct, and platelet count prior to drug administration; administer antiemetic prior to drug administration, and review with patient the self-administration of antiemetic if needed and if receiving high-dose IV. Teach patient self-assessment of infection, bleeding, fatigue; notify MD or RN T > 100.5°F, signs/symptoms of infection, bleeding; energy-conserving activities, self-care strategies to manage fatigue (including patients who receive intravesicular administration because drug is systemically absorbed).

Drug Name: Topotecan hydrochloride for injection (Hycamtin)

Class:	Topoisomerase I inhibitor
Mechanism of Action:	Prevents repair of previous, reversible single-strand DNA breaks by binding to topoisomerase I, an enzyme that relaxes tension in the DNA helix so strands can split apart to be copied during cell division. This causes cell death.
Indications:	(1) Metastatic ovarian cancer after failure of initial or subsequent chemotherapy; (2) small-cell lung cancer after failure of first-line chemotherapy
Dosing:	1.5 mg/m² IV on days 1–5 q 21 days
Administration:	IV over 30 minutes
Side Effect Profile:	Common (> 50%):
	Neutropenia
	Thrombocytopenia
	Anemia

Less Common (10–50%):

Sepsis

Nausea and vomiting

Constipation

Diarrhea

Alopecia

Dyspnea

Headache

Rash

Rare ($< 10\%$):

Parasthesia

Elevated LFTs

Nursing Implications: Assess ANC (> 1500 cells/mm^3), WBC, Hgb/Hct, platelet count ($> 100{,}000$ cells/mm^3), and LFTs prior to drug administration and periodically during treatment; administer antiemetic prior to chemotherapy, and review patient prescription for antiemetic administration at home. Patient teaching: (1) self-assessment of infection, bleeding, fatigue; notify MD or RN T $> 100.5°$F, signs/symptoms of infection, bleeding; energy-conserving activities, self-care strategies to manage fatigue; (2) potential drug interactions.

Drug Name: Toremifene citrate (Fareston)

Class: Antiestrogen (SERM)

Mechanism of Action: Tamoxifen analog, estrogen antagonist that blocks estrogen receptor in malignant cell, thus blocking the hormonal stimulus for the cell to divide

Indications: Treatment of metastatic breast cancer in postmenopausal women with estrogen receptor–positive or unknown disease; unknown whether this agent is superior to tamoxifen and whether it has less side effects in terms of causing endometrial malignancy

Dosing: 60 mg PO qd

Administration: Oral, without regard to meals, at the same time every day

Side Effect Profile: Common ($> 50\%$):

None

Less Common (10–50%):

Nausea

Vaginal discharge

Elevated LFTs

Hot flashes

Sweating

Edema

Rare ($< 10\%$):

Cardiac effects, including myocardial infarction

Stroke

Blood clots

Tumor flare

Vaginal bleeding

Hypercalcemia

Depression

Nursing Implications: Assess patient with metastatic breast cancer during drug introduction to identify symptoms associated with flare reaction. Teach patient that these side effects may occur, self-care strategies to minimize discomfort, and to report side effects if they are not effectively managed; teach patient to continue to take the drug even though she feels well and to report vaginal bleeding, pain in the calf, or difficulty breathing right away.

Drug Name: Trimetrexate (Neutrexin)

Class: Antimetabolite

Mechanism of Action: Interferes with DNA synthesis so DNA cannot be replicated, the cell cannot divide, and it dies

Indications: *Pneumocystis carinii* pneumonia

Dosing: 45 mg/m^2 IV qd over 60–90 minutes for 21 days, with leucovorin rescue of normal cells 20 mg/m^2 IV over 5–10 minutes or PO q 6 hours for days of trimetrexate treatment plus 72 hours after trimetrexate last dose

Administration: IV over 60–90 minutes in D$_5$W only, incompatible with 0.9% NS and leucovorin; hold dose if serum creatinine is $\geq$ 2.5 mg/dl

Side Effect Profile: Common (> 50%):

None

Less Common (10–50%):

Neutropenia

Thrombocytopenia

Rare (< 10%):

Stomatitis

Nausea and vomiting

Alopecia

Dyspnea

Nursing Implications: Assess baseline ANC and platelet count and monitor during therapy; dose reduce as necessary per package insert; ensure leucovorin given exactly on time; teach patient that side effects may occur and to report them.

Drug Name: Valrubicin (Valstar)

Class: Antitumor antibiotic

Mechanism of Action: Semisynthetic analog of doxorubicin; inhibits topoisomerase II so DNA cannot replicate and malignant cells die

Indications:	Bladder cancer
Dosing:	800 mg q week for 6 weeks; discontinue if no response after 3 months
Administration:	Intravesicular
Side Effect Profile:	Common (> 50%):

Symptoms of bladder irritation (dysuria, urgency)

Less Common (10–50%):

Bladder spasm

Hematuria

Pain in bladder

Incontinence

Cystitis

UTI

Rare (< 10%):

Nocturia

Urinary retention

Chest pain

Peripheral edema

Headache

Malaise

Rash

Weakness

Nursing Implications: Teach patient that side effects may occur and to report them. Discuss symptom management strategies with patient, and teach patient to report symptoms that persist.

Drug Name: Vinblastine (Velban)

Class:	Vinca alkaloid, mitotic inhibitor
Mechanism of Action:	Binds to mitotic tubules, so mitosis is arrested in metaphase
Indications:	Cancers of the testes, breast, bladder, lung, kidney, and prostate and lymphoma and melanoma
Dosing:	0.1 mg/kg q week *or* 6 mg/m² IV q week; dose reduce for hepatic dysfunction
Administration:	IV push through freely flowing IV line using vesicant precautions
Side Effect Profile:	Common (> 50%):

Neutropenia

Thrombocytopenia

Less Common (10–50%):

Anemia

Peripheral neuropathy

Constipation

Alopecia

Rare ($< 10\%$):

Nausea and vomiting

Stomatitis

Nursing Implications: Assess ANC (> 1500 cells/mm^3), WBC, Hgb/Hct, platelet count ($> 100,000$ cells/mm^3), LFTs, and signs and symptoms of peripheral neuropathy prior to drug administration and periodically during treatment. Patient teaching: (1) self-assessment of infection, bleeding, fatigue; notify MD or RN T $>$ 100.5°F, signs/symptoms of infection, bleeding; energy-conserving activities, self-care strategies to manage fatigue; (2) strategies to prevent constipation and to report it right away if it develops; (3) inform that numbness and tingling of fingertips and toes may develop and to report it if it develops.

Drug Name: Vincristine (Oncovin)

Class: Vinca alkaloid, mitotic inhibitor
Mechanism of Action: Binds to mitotic tubules, so mitosis is arrested in metaphase
Indications: Multiple myeloma, lung cancer, lymphoma, leukemia
Dosing: 0.4–1.4 mg/m^2 q week
Administration: IV push via patent, freely flowing IV using vesicant precautions
Side Effect Profile: Common ($> 50\%$):

Peripheral neuropathy

Less Common (10–50%):

Constipation

Alopecia

Impotence

Rare ($< 10\%$):

Neutropenia

Thrombocytopenia

Nursing Implications: Assess ANC, WBC, Hgb/Hct, platelet count, LFTs, and signs and symptoms of peripheral neuropathy prior to drug administration and periodically during treatment. Patient teaching: (1) self-assessment of infection, bleeding, fatigue; notify MD or RN T $>$ 100.5°F, signs/symptoms of infection, bleeding; energy-conserving activities, self-care strategies to manage fatigue; (2) strategies to prevent constipation and to report it right away if it develops; (3) inform that numbness and tingling of fingertips and toes may develop and to report it if it develops.

Drug Name: Vinorelbine tartrate (Navelbine)

Class: Mitotic inhibitor, semisynthetic vinca alkaloid
Mechanism of Action: Binds to mitotic tubules, so mitosis is arrested in metaphase

Indications:	Lung cancer, lymphoma
Dosing:	30 mg/m^2 IV q week or in combination with cisplatin; dose reduce for hepatic dysfunction
Administration:	IV push via patent, freely flowing IV at injection site furthest from IV site using vesicant precautions
Side Effect Profile:	Common ($>$ 50%):
	Neutropenia
	Transient increase in LFTs
	Less Common (10–50%):
	Thrombocytopenia
	Anemia
	Peripheral neuropathy
	Nausea and vomiting
	Stomatitis
	Phlebitis
	Rare ($<$ 10%):
	Alopecia
Nursing Implications:	Assess ANC ($>$ 1500 cells/mm^3), WBC, Hgb/Hct, platelet count ($>$ 100,000 cells/mm^3), LFTs, and signs and symptoms of peripheral neuropathy prior to drug administration and periodically during treatment. Patient teaching: (1) self-assessment of infection, bleeding, fatigue; notify MD or RN T $>$ 100.5°F, signs/symptoms of infection, bleeding; energy-conserving activities, self-care strategies to manage fatigue; (2) strategies to prevent constipation and to report it right away if it develops; (3) inform that numbness and tingling of fingertips and toes may develop and to report it if it develops.

References

AstraZeneca Pharmaceutical. 2000. Arimidex (anastrozole). Package insert.

Bristol Myers Squibb Oncology. Taxol. http://www.bms.com/products.

Celgene Corporation. 2000. Thalidomide. Package insert.

Federal Drug Administration. Idamycin. http://www.fda.gov/cder/foi/appletter/2002/50661slr007ltr.pdf.

Glaxo Smith Kline. Hycamptin. http://us.gsk.com/products/assets/us_hycamtin.pdf.

Hancock, C.M. 2003. Fulvestrant antiestrogen for treatment of breast cancer. *Clinical Journal of Oncology Nursing* 7(2):201–202.

Law, A., Kennedy, P., Pellittea, P., et al. 2004. Concurrent paclitaxel, carboplatin, and radiotherapy with subcutaneous amifostine in advanced squamous cell head and neck cancer (SECHN). Preliminary results of a phase II study. *J Clin Oncol* 22 (Suppl): 145, Abstract 5564.

Lilly Oncology. Alimta. http://pi.lilly.com/us/alimta-pi.pdf.

Lilly Oncology. 2003. Gemzar (gemcitabine). Package insert.

McLeod, D.G. 1997. Tolerability of Nonsteroidal antiandrogens in the treatment of advanced prostate cancer. *Oncologist* 2:18–27.

MedImmune. Neutrexin. http://www.medimmune.com/products/providers/neutrexin.asp.

Novartis. Femara (letrozole). Package insert. http://www.pharma.us.novartis.com/product/pi/pdf/Femara.pdf.

Novartis Oncology. 2002. Aredia (pamidronate disodium). Package insert.

Orion Corporation. Fareston. http://www.fareston.com/pdfs/Prescribing_Info.pdf.

Pfizer. Camptosar package insert. http://www.pfizer.com/download/uspi_camptosar.pdf.

Roche Pharmaceutical. 2003. Xeloda (capecitabine). Package insert.

Savient Pharmaceuticals. 2003. Oxandrin (oxandrolone). Package insert.

Schering Corporation. 2003. Temodar (temozolomide). Package insert

Schering Oncology. Temodar. http://www.temodar.com.

Sicor Pharmaceuticals. Thiotepa. http://www.sicor.com/products/fdp/4303-01.html.

SuperGen Pharmaceuticals. 1998. Nipent (pentostatin). Package insert.

TAP Pharmaceuticals. Lupron Depot. http://www.lupron.com/prostate/PackageInsert.asp.

Visvanathan, K., and Davidson, N.E. 2003. Aromatase inhibitors as adjuvant therapy in breast cancer. *Oncology* 17(3):335–342.

Wilkes, G.M., and Barton-Burke, M. 2005. *Oncology nursing drug handbook*. Sudbury, MA: Jones and Bartlett Publishers.

Biologic Therapy for Cancer Treatment

Paula M. Muehlbauer, R.N., M.S.N., O.C.N.®

Introduction and Overview

The field of biotherapy has evolved greatly over the past century. As our knowledge of the immune system has increased, so has the development of biologic agents. Indeed, biotherapy has become a mainstay of cancer therapy along with surgery, radiation therapy, and chemotherapy in the past decade. Biotherapy has emerged as part of the armamentarium that is used against neoplastic diseases and as supportive care of more traditional therapies such as chemotherapy.

The purpose of this chapter is to provide a review of those biologic therapies that are currently approved by the US Food and Drug Administration (FDA) for cancer therapy. Cytokines that are used as supportive care in cancer therapy will be covered as well. Newer agents continue to enter clinical trials in this rapidly expanding field. A separate section will address some of the most promising and exciting biologics currently under investigation.

Historical Perspective

To fully understand how biotherapy developed as a cancer treatment, one must go back to the 1800s. Generally defined, biotherapy is therapy that uses the immune system, including the cells and molecules that act as messengers between the various immune cells, to invoke an immune response to fight cancer (Rieger 2001). One of the earliest known accounts of biotherapy concerns a New York surgeon, Dr. William Coley, who observed a connection between severe infection and the regression of tumors in some of his patients. Dr. Coley developed toxins called "Coley's toxins" from attenuated or weakened forms of bacteria, which he injected into solid tumors. He hoped these bacterial substances would induce an immune response and have an effect on the cancer cell similar to the natural immune response he witnessed in his infected cancer patients (Rieger 2001; Tomaszewski *et al*. 1995). These bacterial substances are believed to have included *Streptococcus pyogens* with *Serratia marcesens* and *Bacillus prodigiosus*. However, no standard doses or administration or treatment duration guidelines were followed in these early efforts. Of importance was a lack of replication of his results, which were mixed, although Dr. Coley reports long-term survival of several patients who had inoperable cancer (Coley 1898; Coley 1911; Rieger 2001). The active ingredient in Coley's toxins is thought to be endotoxin from the bacterial cell wall, which induces tumor necrosis factor (TNF) and other cytokines (Wheeler 1996).

Despite these criticisms, Coley's work is considered the basis of current cytokine therapy. In the early 1960s to the 1970s, clinical trials using nonspecific immune modulators, such as bacille Calmette-Guérin (BCG), *Corynebacterium parvum*, and levamisole, were conducted in a range of tumor types. The best responses were obtained in patients with a low tumor burden. Poor clinical outcomes were also attributed to the use of impure agents and inconsistent experimental procedures. The results were neither generalizable nor predictive of human response despite responses seen in the animal models (Rieger 2001).

In the 1970s, we gained a better understanding of how the human immune system works, which led to the discovery of certain cytokines such as interleukin-2 (IL-2). The 1980s brought advances in biotechnology, which helped advance the use of biotherapy as a true cancer treatment. One of these discoveries, the introduction of recombinant DNA technology, the reproduction and cloning of parts of the DNA molecule, made it possible to produce large quantities of biologic agents to use for therapeutic purposes (Rieger 2001; Schwartzentruber 2000; Tomaszewski *et al.* 1995). As a result, numerous clinical trials were initiated using various biologics that are in use today. In the past 15 years, FDA approval has been obtained for many categories of biologics. New uses for biologic therapy are underway, including use for many cancer types as well as nononcologic diseases such as rheumatic disorders (Shanahan *et al.* 2003). A timeline of the historical development of biotherapy is outlined in Table 4.1.

Tumor Immunology

Basic knowledge of tumor immunology is helpful when trying to understand biologic therapy. Humoral (antibody mediated or B cell) and cellular (T cell) immune systems comprise the two major components of the immune system. It is believed that cell-mediated immunity provides the primary immune response in tumors. There are two types of responses, namely innate and adaptive immunity. Innate immunity allows the body to distinguish between normal or self and nonself, such as

infection, malignancies, or transplanted organs. With innate immunity, a nonspecific immune effect transpires that harnesses macrophages and natural killer (NK) cells to eliminate the offending organism. Innate immunity is not antigen specific and results in no immunologic memory.

Adaptive immunity is antigen dependent and starts when the phagocytized antigen is presented to B lymphocytes or T lymphocytes. Adaptive immunity has two unique aspects, which are specificity and immunologic memory. The T lymphocytes recognize antigens once they are processed and presented by the antigen-presenting cells. The T cells signal B cells to produce antibodies with specificity against that foreign substance. Innate and adaptive immunity play a part in the immune response to tumors. Although many cell types are involved in antitumor activity, T cells are the most important in developing antitumor activity (Siemens and Ratliff 2001; Hyde 1992; Rieger 2001; Bremers and Parmiani 2000).

Antigen presentation initiates the immune pathway to generate a tumor-specific T-cell response. Antigen is first encountered by antigen-presenting cells (APC) such as macrophages, dendritic cells, monocytes, Kupffer's cells, and Langerhans' cells. Of these cells, dendritic cells are largely responsible for initiating T-cell immunity. Dendritic cells capture, process, and present antigens to T lymphocytes. This is accomplished by internalizing the antigen and splitting it into smaller fragments called peptides. These peptides are combined with major histocompatibility complex (MHC) molecules in the cell and are moved to the cell surface for presentation to T cells for immune recognition. Two basic T cells, CD4[+] helper T cells and CD8[+] cytotoxic T cells, use a T-cell receptor (TCR) to recognize antigens on the target cell surface (Darrow *et al.* 1995). The CD8[+] cytotoxic T cells (Tc) recognize antigen in conjunction with class I MHC molecules and CD4[+] T helper (Th) cells in conjunction with class II MHC molecules. This activity usually occurs simultaneously. For complete T-cell activation, there needs to be a costimulatory signal resulting from the interaction

TABLE 4.1 Timeline of Key Events in the Development of Biotherapy	
Late 1800s to mid-1900s	Impure vaccines Coleyís toxins Interferon discovered (1957)
1960s to early 1970s	Clinical trials of the use of bacterial agents to nonspecifically stimulate the immune system; examples: bacilli Calmette-Guérin and *Corynebacterium parvum* Early immunotherapy trials Limitations of studies related to: ■ Impure agents ■ Variability in experimental procedures ■ Incongruence between animal and human studies ■ Lack of generalizable results
Late 1970s to mid-1980s	Major technical advances Increased understanding of immune system Advances in genetic engineering Continued advances in molecular biology Ability to mass produce biologic proteins and antibodies ■ Recombinant DNA technology ■ Hybridoma technology Advances in laboratory methods and processes and computer systems Single-agent cytokine studies initiated Biologic response modifier program initiated by the National Cancer Institute First biologic agent (interferon-α) approved by the US Food and Drug Administration
Late 1980s to present	Discovery and isolation of a variety of immune system products Numerous agents recombinantly produced for clinical trials Multisite clinical trials initiated; some ongoing Initiation of clinical trials of combination cytokine therapy Initiation of clinical trials of combination cytokine therapy and chemotherapy Regulatory approval for all categories of biologic agents

Source: Used with permission. Rieger, P.T. 2001. *Biotherapy: A comprehensive overview* (ed 2). Sudbury, MA: Jones and Bartlett Publishers p. 4.

of the CD28$^+$ molecule on the T-cell surface with the ligand B7. Cytokines, such as IL-2 and interferon gamma are then secreted from triggered CD4$^+$ cells, which help activated CD8$^+$ cells grow and differentiate into cytotoxic T cells. The cytotoxic T cells then kill target cells expressing the original antigen that elicited this response (Hyde 1992; Darrow *et al.* 1995).

Tumor Escape Mechanisms

Despite a complex immune system, tumors are able to escape immune recognition for a variety of reasons. Possible mechanisms of tumor escape include variability in expression of antigen by tumors, poor antigen processing, and presentation or loss of antigen expression (Matzku and Zoller 2001; Marincola 2000; Restifo 2000; Schreiber 1999).

Other theories for poor immune recognition of tumors may be attributed to disease-associated alterations, including apoptosis, signaling defects of T cells, and immunologic aging. Immunologic aging involves alterations in T-cell functions, causing decline in T-cell proliferation, generation of T-killer cells, production of IL-2, signal transduction in lymphocytes, and an overall decline in function of other immune cells such as B cells, dendritic cells, and natural killer cells.

In the presence of an infection, inflammation triggers the innate immune response that activates monocytes, macrophages, and dendritic cells. Unlike an infectious process, tumors do not give off inflammatory warning signals to stimulate an immune response. Without these warning signals, the immune system may not be fully activated (Marincola 2000; Restifo 2000).

Tumors have unstable genomes causing them to become heterogeneous for expressing tumor-associated antigens. The tumor cells can mutate and escape immune recognition. This inadequate immune response, known as tolerance, may be in response to only minor differences between the tumor cell and normal cell. Because the differences are slight, no destructive immune reaction to an antigen occurs (Matzku and Zoller 2001; Restifo 2000; Hyde 1992).

Tumors produce immunosuppressive mechanisms inhibiting growth factors that would normally stimulate an immune response. One example is the production of cytokines, such as IL-10 and IL-18, by tumors, which limits the efficacy of immune surveillance including macrophage-mediated antigen presentation. Also, expression of Fas ligand by tumors may lead to the destruction of lymphocytes, allowing tumors to escape immune recognition (Matzku and Zoller 2001; Marincola 2000; Restifo 2000; Lokich 1997).

Biologic therapy as a cancer treatment attempts to harness the immune system to fight the disease. The administration of natural immune substances in large amounts may induce cancer regression. Additionally, by targeting tumor antigens, a therapeutic response may be obtained that would otherwise not be possible because of the limitations of the human immune system.

Interleukin-2 (IL-2)

IL-2 is a cytokine produced by activated helper T cells and first described as a T-cell growth factor in 1976 (Schwartzentruber 2000). Bindon and colleagues were the first to report use of IL-2 as cancer treatment in 1983. At that time, they used natural IL-2 derived from stimulated normal lymphocytes in two patients with melanoma (Schwartzentruber 2000; Bindon *et al.* 1983). Broad-based use of IL-2 was not possible until recombinant IL-2 (rIL-2) was available. The gene for IL-2 was discovered and expressed in *Escherichia coli*, producing a new molecule with properties similar to natural IL-2 (Schwartzentruber 2000).

Second only to the interferons, IL-2 has been at the forefront of biologic therapies (Sharp 1995). IL-2 was discovered in 1976 by Drs. Gallo, Ruscetti, and Morgan (Tushinski and Mulé 1995). A number of phase II trials demonstrated that IL-2 could mediate profound, durable tumor responses in patients with metastatic melanoma and renal carcinoma (Rosenberg *et al.* 1998; Fyfe *et al.* 1995; Rosenberg *et al.* 1994; Atkins *et al.* 1993; Rosenberg *et al.* 1989).

Biologic Activity

Interleukins as a group function primarily by signaling or communicating with the various lymphocytes. Each interleukin is assigned a number in the order of approval by the International Congress of Immunology. The therapeutic effect of interleukins is through interactions with the patient's immune system (Gale and Sorokin 2001; Wheeler 1996).

IL-2 is derived from T cells. IL-2 activates lymphocytes and macrophages and stimulates lymphokine secretion (Hyde 1992; Noble and Goa 1997). Primarily, IL-2 induces proliferation of antigen-stimulated T cells, activates cytotoxic T lymphocytes (CD8$^+$) and natural killer cells, and is a cofactor for the growth and differentiation of B cells. Immunoglobulins are produced by stimulating B lymphocytes. An immunomodulator, IL-2 acts to mediate the secretion of many other cytokines and various immune functions such as humoral and cell-mediated immunity (Wheeler 1996; Tushinski and Mulé 1995; Lotze 1995).

Indications for the Use of IL-2

In 1992, the FDA approved the use of high-dose (HD) intravenous (IV) IL-2 for the treatment of patients with metastatic renal cell carcinoma and, in 1998, for the treatment of patients with metastatic melanoma (Chiron Corporation 2000). Various routes and doses of IL-2 are presently prescribed in community settings or are under study in a host of clinical trials for a variety of malignancies (Mavroukakis et al. 2001; Rosenberg et al. 1998; Rosenberg 1997; Keilholz et al. 1997; Ghezzi et al. 1997; Davey et al. 1997; Sharp 1995). The effectiveness of IL-2 is based on stimulation of the host's own cytotoxic immunologic response, making it an ideal cytokine to test with other tumors.

Recently, studies have indicated that IL-2 may be used to enhance the immune system as a therapeutic strategy in patients with HIV. Patients with HIV infection develop health problems when their CD4$^+$ T-cell counts decline. IL-2 directly expands the CD4$^+$ T-cell pool predominantly in naïve CD4$^+$ T cells not yet exposed to their antigen versus memory CD4$^+$ T cells (Napolitano 2003; Lu et al. 2003; Morris 1998). IL-2 can induce proinflammatory cytokine production that might enhance HIV-1 expression in latently infected cells (Morris 1998). Fauci has suggested an explanation for this paradox: latently infected cells, once stimulated, reject the virus and then undergo cell death (Morris 1998). If IL-2 is given at the same time that highly active antiretroviral therapy is administered, the released virus can be prevented from replicating and contaminating other cells. Therefore, over time, the reservoir of latently infected cells decreases (Morris 1998). Lu et al. (2003) report that the major pathogens in AIDS patients are cytomegalovirus and *Pneumocystis jiroveci* to which patients have been previously exposed and developed memory responses. They conclude that a major benefit of IL-2 therapy may be to maintain the memory inventory because this may be sufficient for preventing opportunistic infections in most patients until the CD4$^+$ cell count drops below 200/μl. Hence, IL-2 therapy may be beneficial if it is started in the early stages of HIV infection by maintaining and expanding the stock of CD4$^+$ cells and thus preventing the occurrence of opportunistic infections.

IL-2 is not FDA approved in the United States as treatment for HIV, although it is approved for use in Europe in patients with low CD4$^+$ cell counts. Currently, two ongoing phase III clinical trials are studying the clinical benefits of IL-2 in HIV. The ESPRIT study consists of patients with initial CD4$^+$ counts of 300/μl or higher, and the SILCAAT study contains patients with initial CD4$^+$ counts of 50 to 299/μl (Napolitano 2003). Dosing of IL-2 in clinical trials includes subcutaneous (SC) injections of 9 to 15 MIU/day (4.5 or 7.5 MIU twice daily) for 5 days every 4 to 8 weeks. If IL-2 therapy leads to prolonged increases in CD4$^+$ cell counts, the dosing interval may be extended to 12 months or longer. Patients experience manageable toxicities that are not as severe as with higher doses. Doses less than 6 MIU/day are not as effective in raising CD4$^+$ cell counts (Napolitano 2003; Conrad 2003).

IL-2: Other Directions

Many different combinations of IL-2 therapy continue to be tested. One combination that seemed promising was IL-2 plus interferon-alfa (IFN-α).

Preclinical data in animals suggests that IL-2 works synergistically with IFN-α to produce greater immunologic effects. French researchers Tourani et al. (2003) tested the efficacy of outpatient SC IL-2 (5 days/wk, 9 and 18 MIU/day) plus IFN-α (3 days/wk, 6 MIU/day) over a 12-week induction period in patients with metastatic renal cell carcinoma (RCC) in a multicenter, phase II trial (n = 122). Patients with objective responses or stable disease were randomized to maintenance treatment or consolidation therapy. Forty-one patients were alive at the median follow-up time of 32 months (range, 4 to 55$^+$ months). The trial was closed at the 12th sequential analysis when it showed a 21% response rate, which is similar to IL-2 alone. Severe toxicities resulted in treatment delay, dose reduction, or treatment termination in 27% of patients. The authors concluded that the combination was no better than SC IL-2 alone in patients with metastatic RCC, and the results were consistent with other trials with similar combinations (McDermott et al. 2001; Atzpodien et al. 1995; Ravaud et al. 1994). A nice review of multiple trials using similar combinations can be found in Dutcher (2002) and Noble and Goa (1997).

A question that has been bandied about for years is whether IL-2 in the adjuvant setting would be beneficial; however, high dose (HD) IL-2 would be too toxic in the adjuvant setting. The possible synergistic combination of SC IL-2 and IFN-α may be of benefit is this setting. A study by Hauschild et al. (2003) investigated melanoma patients with intermediate- or high-risk primary melanoma after resection of the primary tumor. After resection, these patients were randomized to either observation or a combination regimen of SC low-dose (LD) IL-2 (9 MIU/m^2/day) plus IFN-α (3 MIU/m^2/day) for 48 weeks on variable days of the week. Follow-up (median, 79.4 months) of 223 randomized patients revealed no effect on disease-free survival or overall survival. At 5 years, disease-free survival in the surgery plus treatment group and in the surgery plus observation arm was 70.1% and 69.9%, respectively.

Other areas of study with IL-2 include biochemotherapy and hematologic malignancies (Mitchell 2003; Slavin et al. 2003; Buzaid 2002; Flaherty et al. 2001). Buzaid (2002) reports results from two meta-analyses suggesting improved response rates for combinations involving cisplatin, IL-2, and IFN-α. The response rates from the first analysis of 631 patients showed a 45% response rate in patients treated with biochemotherapy and a 21% and 15% response rate when treated with IL-2 and IFN-α or IL-2 alone, respectively. However, there was no significant difference in survival between the groups, which averaged 10.5 months. The second meta-analysis analyzed 154 studies encompassing 7000 patients; this study reports a response rate of 47% for patients who received cisplatin, dacarbazine, IL-2, and IFN-α. However, there is no mention of overall survival and how it compares with IL-2 alone. Phase III studies comparing biochemotherapy with immunotherapy alone or chemotherapy alone are underway, but preliminary results are mixed. Toxicities are substantial and include expected side effects from IL-2 and IFN-α as well as chemotherapy-related toxicities such as peripheral neuropathy (Buzaid 2002).

Methods of Administration

The only US FDA–approved regimen for IL-2 is as HD IV bolus administration. However, it is also given IV in lower doses (Yang and Rosenberg 1997). Many clinicians also administer IL-2 by the SC route because of the cost and dose-limiting toxicities seen with IV infusion. Many doses in the assorted methods of administration are under investigation, and the treatment of patients with regimens not approved by the FDA should be viewed as experimental. IL-2 is given alone or in combination with chemotherapy, vaccines, or other biotherapy in many research studies (Mavroukakis et al. 2001).

Yang et al. (2003) conducted a three-arm randomized study comparing response rates and overall survival of patients with metastatic RCC receiving HD or one of two LD IL-2 regimens. Patients were randomized to receive 720,000 IU/kg HD IV bolus (n = 156) or 72,000 IU/kg LD IV bolus (n = 150) every 8 hours. The third arm (n = 117) of LD patients were administered SC IL-2. The response rate with HD IV IL-2 was 13%, and the response rate in the LD arms was similar at 10%. Patients who were complete responders in the HD IV arm had more durable responses than patients in the LD arms. The authors concluded that major tumor regression and response durability was more likely to occur in the HD IV IL-2 arm compared with either of the LD IL-2 arms. However, there was no overall difference in survival for patients with metastatic RCC in either arm. Yang *et al.* (2003) state that the LD regimens are viable options for patients with significant comorbidities and for physicians with minimal experience managing HD IV IL-2–related side effects.

Kammula *et al.* (1998) reviewed the safety trends in administering HD IV IL-2 therapy over a 12-year period. In this series, they evaluated the toxicities, the maximum number of doses of IL-2 administered, and objective response rates of 1241 patients with metastatic cancer treated with HD IV IL-2 during their first cycle of therapy. Patients were on clinical trials, which may have included concurrent treatment with other cytokines, lymphokine-activated killer (LAK) cells, tumor-infiltrating lymphocytes (TIL), polyethelene glycol-modified (PEG) IL-2, chemotherapy, radiation, monoclonal antibodies, or cancer vaccines. The authors found significant decreases in the number of grade 3 and 4 toxicities with the last 809 patients compared with the initial patients. Of note, the decline in grade 3 and 4 toxicities included line sepsis (18% to 4%), diarrhea (92% to 12%), neuropsychiatric toxicity (grade 4, 19% to 8%), pulmonary intubations (12% to 3%), hypotension (81% to 31%), and grade 4 cardiac ischemia (3% to 0%). The authors surmised that these improvements were most likely reflective of better pretreatment screening strategies, improved therapeutic conditions, early recognition

and treatment of toxicities, and prudent termination of dosing as toxicities warrant. This experience suggests that, with appropriate management of side effects and appropriate patient selection, HD IV IL-2 can be administered safely.

Systemic Side Effects: Nursing and Medical Management

The severity of side effects varies according to the route, dose, and schedule of administration (Schwartzentruber 2000). Frequency of patient monitoring depends on these factors as well as how well the patient tolerates IL-2 (Table 4.2). When given as an IV bolus intermittently, many side effects peak about 2 to 4 hours after dosing. Generally, the side effects diminish as time passes from the last dose. Once IL-2 therapy has been stopped, most toxicities abate and reverse within 48 to 72 hours. Although some side effects are of unknown etiology, several of the most profound toxicities are attributable to IL-2–induced capillary leak syndrome (CLS). With CLS, other cytokines are stimulated, such as tumor necrosis factor alpha (TNF-α) and IL-5; complement activation is generated; neutrophils are activated; and endothelial-cell antigens are stimulated. Symptoms of CLS include generalized edema, hypotension, oliguria, pleural effusions, pulmonary congestion, and ascites. These symptoms will be further elucidated throughout this chapter (Mavroukakis *et al.* 2001; Schwartzentruber 2001; Schwartzentruber 2000; Schwartz *et al.* 2002; Dutcher *et al.* 2001). Table 4.3 provides a quick reference summary of IL-2 side effects, causes, and interventions.

Constitutional Symptoms

The most common side effects that occur with all methods of IL-2 administration are flu-like symptoms. Within 30 minutes to 2 hours after the first dose of IL-2, patients may experience chills and rigors that tend to abate with subsequent doses. Initially, these symptoms can be treated with warm blankets, but if this is ineffective, symptoms may be relieved with the administration of 25 to 50 mg of IV meperidine. Other flu-like symptoms may

TABLE 4.2 Guidelines for Monitoring Patients Receiving Interleukin-2 Therapy

Parameter to Monitor	Frequency		
	Inpatient		Outpatient
	Not Requiring Vasopressors	Requiring Intensive Care Unit/ Vasopressors	
Vital signs	Every 4 hours	Every 1 hour	As needed
Intake and output	Every 8 hours	Every 1 hour	Not strictly measured
Weight	Daily	Daily	Daily
Mental status	Every 8 hours	Every 4 hours	Daily
Intravenous site/ injection site	Every 8 hours Change peripheral IV every 3rd day	Every 8 hours Change peripheral IV every 3rd day	Daily
Complete blood count and differential	Daily	Twice daily	Weekly
Electrolytes, blood urea nitrogen, creatinine, glucose	Daily	Twice daily	Weekly
AST, ALT, alkaline phosphates, bilirubin	Daily	Daily	Weekly
Albumin, CA^+, Mg^+, phosphorus	Daily	Daily	Each course
Creatinine phosphokinase	Daily	Daily	Weekly
Prothrombin time, partial thromboplastin time	Every 3rd day	Every 3rd day	Weekly
Thyroid-stimulating hormone and free T_4	Each cycle	Each cycle	Each course
Urinalysis	Each cycle	Each cycle	Each course
Electrocardiogram	Each cycle	Each cycle	Each course
Chest x-ray	Each cycle	Each cycle	Each course

ALT, alanine aminotransferase; AST, aspartate aminotransferase

NOTE: These guidelines recommend the **minimum** requirements. Good nursing and medical judgment will dictate more frequent monitoring as indicated.

Source: Used with permission. Schwartzentruber, D.J. 2000. Interleukin 2: Clinical applications: Principles of administration and management of side effects. In: Rosenberg, S.A. (Ed). *Principles and Practice of Biologic Therapy of Cancer* (ed 3). Philadelphia: Lippincott Williams & Wilkins pp. 35–36.

include headaches, malaise, arthralgias, myalgias, anorexia, and abdominal discomfort. Many of these symptoms can be prophylactically treated with indomethacin, acetaminophen, and ranitidine starting the night before the first dose of IL-2 and continuing until 24 hours after IL-2 therapy stops (Schwartzentruber 2001; Mavroukakis et al. 2001; Schwartz *et al.* 2002; Dutcher *et al.* 2001). To help alleviate fatigue, patients should be encouraged to ambulate when possible and not spend all day in bed. This is especially important upon discharge. Strategies for managing cancer- and treatment-related fatigue include moderate daily increases in exercise, adequate hydration

TABLE 4.3 IL-2 Toxicities: Causes and Interventions

System	Signs/Symptoms	Pathophysiology	Interventions
Cardiovascular	Peripheral edema Hypotension Tachycardia Weight gain Ascites Arrhythmias	Capillary leak syndrome (CLS): Shift of fluid from **intravascular** spaces to **interstitial** spaces induces increase in heart rate and decrease in blood pressure	Monitor blood pressure ≥ q4h Fluid boluses as ordered Daily weights Strict intake and output (I & 0) Daily labs to follow electrolytes
Pulmonary	Crackles Dyspnea/SOB Increased RR Hypoxia Nasal/sinus congestion	CLS	Assess breath sounds q4h or more if needed Assess breath sounds **before** and **after** fluid boluses Baseline O_2 saturation and prn O_2 therapy prn
Gastrointestinal	Anorexia Nausea/vomiting Mucositis Diarrhea Ileus	Unknown	Antiemetics: prophylactic and around the clock Antidiarrheals Diligent oral care Perirectal care H_2 blocker Nutrition counseling Antacids
Renal	Oliguria Increased creatinine Increased BUN	1. CLS: decreased intravascular volume 2. Cumulative effect of IL-2; direct action on the kidneys	Fluid boluses Dopamine at low dose (2–4 µcg/kg/min) Foley catheter
Hematologic	Anemia Thrombocytopenia Lymphocytopenia	1. Anemia partially R/T bone marrow suppression 2. Cumulative IL-2 doses	Daily CBC with differential Assess for petechiae, bruises Guiac stools, emesis as indicated Monitor temperatures Assess for potential sites of infection including skin, perirectal and oral mucosa
Flu-like symptoms	Fever Chills Malaise Arthalgias Fatigue	1. May be R/T direct IL-2 effect on the hypothalamic regulatory centers 2. Fever may be caused by circulating TNF-α levels induced by IL-2	Prophylactic anti-inflammatory agents Warm blankets for chills Demerol for chills
Hepatic	Elevated bilirubin Elevated ALT, AST, LDH	Manifested as reversible cholestasis	Monitor liver function tests daily

(Continued)

TABLE 4.3 (Continued)

System	Signs/Symptoms	Pathophysiology	Interventions
Integumentary	Pruritus Erythematous rash Skin dry, peeling, and desquamation	Unknown	Nonalcohol-based skin lotions Oatmeal baths Mild soaps Anti-itching meds
Neurologic	Confusion Fatigue Somnolence Irritation/agitation Hallucinations Vivid dreams Anxiety Sleep disturbances	1. IL-2 penetrates the blood-brain barrier, resulting in increased brain water content 2. Altered sleep patterns/deprivation	Assess neuro status q8h and prn Teach relaxation techniques Music therapy Assess for subtle changes in personality Limit antianxiety and sleep medications in later stages of treatment Discontinuation of therapy Airway protection if somnolent
Psychosocial	Fear Tearfulness Depression Mood swings	Unknown/unclear	Emotional support Teach relaxation techniques Provide safe environment Involve social worker and psychiatrist liaison as indicated Reassure family and patient

SOB, shortness of breath; RR, respiratory rate; prn, as needed; BUN, blood urea nitrogen; R/T, related to; CBC, complete blood cell count; TNF-α, tumor necrosis factor alpha.

and nutrition, balancing rest with activities, and possibly employing distraction techniques (Curt 2000; Portenoy and Itri 1999; Winningham 1991; Piper 1991; Aistars 1987). For those patients receiving SC regimens of IL-2 for longer periods of time, education and support for managing fatigue is particularly important.

Gastrointestinal

It is not uncommon for most patients receiving IL-2 to experience some gastrointestinal distress such as nausea, vomiting, diarrhea, and anorexia. Patients experiencing these symptoms are advised not to eat or to eat small, frequent meals. Dry, cold,

or salty foods tend to cause less nausea than spicy, greasy, or overly sweet foods. Nausea is treated prophylactically with antiemetics, such as ondansetron or granisetron, and with droperidol, prochlorperazine, lorazepam, or phenergan for breakthrough nausea and vomiting (Mavroukakis et al. 2001; Schwartzentruber 2001; Schwartz et al. 2002; Dutcher et al. 2001; Sharp 1995). It may take a combination of these agents to obtain relief. It is important to be aware of the different pharmacologic classes of antiemetics to avoid overlap with a similar agent. If initial antiemetic therapy fails, it is recommended that an agent from another class be added or that the initial agent be increased to the maximum accepted dosage range or a combination of both (ASHP 1999). For example, if a patient is receiving scheduled ondansetron, a 5-HT3 antagonist, and continues to experience nausea, a dopaminergic antagonist antiemetic, such as prochlorperazine, should be added. Another gastrointestinal side effect suffered may be gastric upset, or reflux, which may be relieved with antacids.

Some patients experience diarrhea, which can occasionally reach grade 3 or 4 toxicity. With the first loose stool or with an increase in bowel movements, patients are given antidiarrheals such as imodium, kaopectate, or lomotil. If the diarrhea is severe and does not abate with these medications, codeine or tincture of opium may be administered, although cautiously. It is essential to assess the patient's abdomen for distention, pain, and bowel sounds when using these medications because they can aggravate an intestinal ileus. Because of the psychotropic effects of codeine and tincture of opium, a neurologic assessment needs to be done prior to administering and throughout treatment (Schwartzentruber 2001; Mavroukakis et al. 2001; Schwartz et al. 2002; Dutcher et al. 2001). Patients are instructed to avoid caffeine, alcohol, and foods high in roughage and to increase their intake of pectin-containing foods, such as peeled fruits (apples and pears), and gum fibers contained in foods such as cooked vegetables, white rice, bananas, and oatmeal (Mavroukakis et al. 2001; Viele and Moran 1993).

Cardiopulmonary

IL-2 administration induces a profound increase in vascular permeability known as capillary leak syndrome (CLS), causing a shift of fluid from the intravascular space to the interstitial space (Mier 1993). As the intravascular space becomes depleted, the patient can develop oliguria, tachycardia, and hypotension. Oliguria generally precedes hypotension, so accurate measurement of intake and output is essential. Because of the hypotension that occurs with IL-2, patients are encouraged to stop antihypertensive medications

from the day before therapy until they have recovered from IL-2 side effects. Patients with a history of heart disease or questionable cardiac event or patients who are over the age of 50 years should undergo thallium cardiac stress testing as part of the pretreatment screening process. These precautions have all but eliminated the incidence of myocardial infarction (Schwartzentruber 2001; Kammula et al. 1998).

Myocarditis related to lymphocyte and eosinophil infiltration has been seen in patients receiving IL-2 (Schwartzentruber 2000; Kragel et al. 1990). Clinically, patients may have increased creatine kinase isoenzymes with MB-band elevations. Sometimes, these are not seen until 1 or 2 days post IL-2 therapy and are detected with routine daily laboratory work. Patients are usually asymptomatic but are placed on a cardiac monitor, troponin levels are measured, and electrocardiograms are done. Prior to receiving future doses of IL-2, an exercise ECHO will be performed to rule out myocardial dysfunction. If the ECHO is normal, the patient can receive future cycles of IL-2 (Schwartzentruber 2001; Schwartz et al. 2002).

Cardiac arrhythmias have been observed in 6% of patients, with the majority being supraventricular (atrial fibrillation or tachycardia) in nature. These usually are short in duration and do not cause hemodynamic instability. The prime time for arrhythmias to occur is at the peak of systemic toxicities when multiple fluid, electrolyte, and metabolic abnormalities occur. Treatment consists of discontinuation of therapy for that cycle, correction of electrolyte abnormalities, maintenance of good oxygenation, and diuretics for fluid overload. If indicated, interventions with agents such as digoxin, verapamil, diltiazem, or adenosine are initiated. It is safe for patients to receive subsequent cycles of IL-2 because only small numbers of patients develop cardiac arrhythmias again (Schwartzentruber 2000; White et al. 1994).

Interstitial fluid accumulates throughout the body, including the skin, abdomen, and lungs, leading to profound peripheral edema, ascites, and occasionally pulmonary edema. Patients require increased fluid intake to make up for losses of intravascular volume. It is not uncommon for patients' intake to exceed output by 1 to 3 liters per day, causing patients to gain up to 2 kg per day (Mavroukakis et al. 2001; Schwartzentruber 2000).

Initially, treatment of intravascular fluid loss requires replacement with IV fluids of either normal saline (NS) or lactated ringers (LR). Colloid replacement has not been shown to provide any benefit over crystalloid (Schwartzentruber 2000; Pockaj et al. 1994). The patient is given a fluid bolus of 250 to 500 ml until the blood pressure responds (systolic > 90 mm Hg) or the patient begins to experience lung crackles or decreased O_2 saturation. If the O_2 saturation drops below 95%, fluids should be used prudently. These respiratory symptoms indicate fluid overload and CLS-related interstitial pulmonary edema (White et al. 1994). The patient may become tachypneic and dyspneic and develop lung crackles on auscultation. For these reasons, it is imperative to assess breath sounds both before and after administration of fluid boluses and to limit fluid boluses to 1–2 liters/day. Inability to maintain O_2 saturation above 95% on 4 liters of O_2 via nasal cannula or 40% O_2 via face mask is an indication to discontinue dosing patients on HD IL-2 (Schwartz et al. 2002; Dutcher et al. 2001; Mavroukakis et al. 2001; Schwartzentruber 2000). Because greater experience with IL-2 has been gained, the frequency for intubation for respiratory distress has decreased to about 1%. Patients with preexisting pulmonary disease are at high risk for pulmonary complications requiring intensive-care monitoring. Patients with a history of smoking or with large pulmonary tumor burdens should undergo pretreatment screening with pulmonary function tests (Schwartzentruber 2000).

Up to 50% of patients may continue to experience hypotension and tachycardia despite fluid resuscitation, requiring vasopressor therapy (Rosenberg et al. 1994). The vasopressors of choice are alpha-adrenergic agonists, such as phenylephrine, titrated to counteract the vasodilatory effects of IL-2. The hypotensive effects of IL-2 usually peak 4–6 hours after dosing. If the phenylephrine can be weaned to approximately 0.5 μg/kg/min, it is generally safe to continue IL-2 dosing. Requirements of phenylephrine doses greater than 2.0 μg/kg/min suggest that IL-2 dosing should be discontinued (Schwartzentruber 2000; Mavroukakis et al. 2001; Schwartz et al. 2002; Dutcher et al. 2001).

Renal

Renal dysfunction associated with IL-2 is described as prerenal azotemia. Hypotension and decreased intravascular volume results in reduced renal perfusion and oliguria (Schwartzentruber 2000; Schwartz et al. 2002; Dutcher et al. 2001). Also, IL-2 appears to have a direct toxic effect on the kidneys, further contributing to decreased urinary output, which results in an increase in serum creatinine and blood urea nitrogen. It has been reported that the highest mean peak creatinine value during HD IL-2 is 2.7 mg/dl (Guleria et al. 1994). Patients with renal cell carcinoma (RCC) who have undergone a prior nephrectomy are at a greater risk for dysfunction. Other factors linked with an increased risk of nephrotoxicity include a diagnosis of renal cell carcinoma, older age, male gender, and preexisting hyptertension (Schwartz et al. 2002). Oliguria is initially treated with fluid boluses to increase the circulating fluid volume. After appropriate fluid resuscitation, low-dose dopamine at 2 to 4 μg/kg/min may be initiated to increase renal perfusion, although the value of this intervention has never been studied. Generally, creatinine levels revert to normal within 7 to 14 days, and hemodialysis is rarely necessary. While patients experience these significant fluid shifts and undergo fluid replacement, electrolyte imbalances frequently occur including hypokalemia, hypomagnesemia, hypocalcemia, and hypophosphatemia. Electrolyte levels are monitored daily and replaced as needed (Schwartzentruber 2001).

Neurologic

IL-2 crosses the blood-brain barrier and increases brain water content that may cause the neurologic side effects seen with IL-2 (Schwartzentruber 2000).

These can include lethargy, anxiety, vivid dreams, confusion, sleep disturbances, decreased concentration, mood swings, combativeness, hallucinations, depression, and coma (Sparber and Biller-Sparber 1993; Lerner et al. 1999; Schwartz et al. 2002; Dutcher et al. 2001). Contributing factors may include concomitant medications to treat other side effects, such as meperidine for chills or phenothiazine or lorazepam for nausea (Schwartz et al. 2002). It is important to factor in these medications when monitoring mental status changes. With the first sign of neuropsychiatric toxicity, IL-2 should be discontinued because these effects can worsen for several days before improving (Schwartzentruber 2000). Aspiration becomes a significant threat in the presence of neurotoxicity, and on rare occasions, patients may require intubation to maintain a patent airway. These side effects must be closely monitored for neurologic deterioration and are a prime area for nursing interventions. Reassuring patients and their families that these are normal and reversible side effects helps relieve some of the anxiety that neurotoxicities generate. Reorientation, relaxation techniques, and music therapy can help reduce patients' discomfort. Emotional support by the patient's family, health care providers, and social worker are imperative throughout treatment (Sharp 1995; Sparber and Biller-Sparber 1993; Lerner et al. 1999; Mavroukakis et al. 2001). On rare occasions, more aggressive patient interventions are required to prevent self-harm, such as padding the bedrails or restraining the patient (Mavroukakis et al. 2001). If restraints are warranted, check the institution's policy for monitoring the patient in restraints. Severe behavioral changes may require medication such as haloperidol, which does not have some of the secondary side effects of other sedatives (Schwartzentruber 2000).

Integumentary

IL-2 also affects the skin and mucous membranes. Skin changes include generalized flushing or erythematous rash, pruritis, dry peeling skin, and severe itching, which start within 3 days of initiation of treatment and continue for up to 6 weeks (Schwartz et al. 2002; Gallagher 1995). Patients may also complain of skin burning. In some cases, patients have had skin peel off the palms of their hands and soles of their feet (Schwartzentruber 2000). To help alleviate these discomforts, nonalcohol-based lotions and/or aloe vera gels should be applied liberally. Washing with mild soaps or nonsoap cleansers such as Cetaphil may diminish the intensity of the skin problems. Topical steroids should be avoided (Schwartz et al. 2002; Schwartzentruber 2001). Patients should be instructed to avoid excessive heat and swimming in salt or chlorinated water (Viele and Moran 1993). Patients with severe, uncontrolled itching may be prescribed diphenhydramine HCL or hydroxyzine HCL. Dutcher et al. (2001) recommend gabapentin for severe pruritus because it affects peripheral nerve fibers. Patients may experience varying degrees of mucositis, glossitis, stomatitis, pharyngitis, and altered sense of taste. These are usually managed with frequent, meticulous mouth care and lidobenalox. Patients should be encouraged to avoid extremely hot, cold, or rough foods that might injure the oral mucosa. They should be instructed to try soft or blended foods and to avoid tobacco products and alcoholic beverages because these can also be irritating (Viele and Moran 1993).

Immunologic/Metabolic

Infection can be a lethal complication of IL-2 therapy. Neutrophil function is clearly impaired in patients receiving IL-2. Therefore, IV sites and all mucosal areas including the perirectal area must be assessed frequently because of the increased risk of infection during treatment. Peripheral IV sites should be changed routinely, and meticulous care of central venous catheters must be maintained. Prophylactic antibiotics should be considered for patients with central lines to prevent infection. Long-term indwelling lines are prone to infection and are not used in some institutions in patients receiving IL-2 (Schwartzentruber 2000; Mavroukakis et al. 2001).

Changes in laboratory values reflect other side effects occurring with IL-2 therapy and require regular monitoring. Lymphocytopenia develops rapidly and persists throughout therapy, putting the patient at risk for infection. Once treatment stops, a rapid rebound of lymphocytes above baseline develops and persists for 3 to 7 days before returning to normal. Thrombocytopenia and anemia may occur and require assessment for petechiae, epistaxis, hematuria, guiac-positive stools, and emesis for occult blood loss (Sharp 1995; Schwartzentruber 2000; Mavroukakis *et al.* 2001; MacFarlane *et al.* 1995; Schwartz *et al.* 2002). Elevations can occur in the alkaline phosphatase, ALT, AST, LDH, and total bilirubin and are indicative of the reversible cholestasis commonly observed in patients during IL-2 therapy (Schwartz *et al.* 2002; Schwartzentruber 2000; Sharp 1995; Fisher *et al.* 1989). Thyroid dysfunction has been reported in 13% to 41% of patients receiving monotherapy with IL-2. The majority of these irregularities have been hypothryroidism, which occurs in 35% of patients and is normally subclinical. The incidence increases with the number of courses and duration of treatment. Screening of thyroid function is done routinely with each course. Moderate to severe hypothyroidism is treated with levothyroxine for up to 1 year, at which point the dysfunction typically reverses (Schwartzentruber 2000).

Hypersensitivity Reactions

Patients treated with IL-2 may develop hypersensitivity reactions to contrast dye or medications. This occurs in 10% to 28% of patients and manifests as wheezing, rash, diarrhea, chills, fever, emesis, hypotension, edema, and oliguria shortly after IV contrast (Schwartzentruber 2000; Choyke *et al.* 1992; Zukiwski *et al.* 1990). Hypersensitivity reactions have been seen when using drugs such as furosemide for post–IL-2 diuresis. Supportive measures and diphenhydramine are useful in alleviating symptoms. However, steroids should not be used because they block the effects of IL-2 (Schwartzentruber 2000).

Subcutaneous IL-2

Overall side effects seen in patients receiving SC IL-2 are diminished but not insubstantial. The dose-limiting toxicities observed in patients receiving SC IL-2 are similar to the profile seen in patients receiving IV IL-2, except that the overall intensity and duration of subjective side effects, such as nausea and vomiting, tend to be lower (Davey *et al.* 1997). Constitutional symptoms of fatigue, myalgias, and fever are the most common symptoms patients experience and may have more impact on their quality of life than in patients receiving IV IL-2 (Dutcher *et al.* 2001; Mavroukakis *et al.* 2001; Viele and Moran 1993). Yang *et al.* (2003) report that a quality-of-life (QOL) assessment obtained on patients receiving various routes of administration of IL-2 did not show a significant advantage from a QOL standpoint in patients receiving SC IL-2. The prolonged nature of the treatment (6 weeks), the toxicities, and the inconvenience of SC therapy offset the more intense but short-lived toxicities seen with IV IL-2. Fevers in the range of 38°C to 40°C (100.4°F to 104°F) occur within the first 2 to 8 hours after SC administration and generally peak approximately 4 hours after each injection. Premedication as prescribed can ameliorate these sequelea (Viele and Moran 1993).

Mild hematologic, renal, and hepatic laboratory changes are also observed. Patients' symptoms are treated with oral analgesics, antipyretics, and antiemetics and generally are not treatment limiting (Mavroukakis *et al.* 2001). One recommendation is to administer the dose of IL-2 around dinnertime (6 pm) to take advantage of potential initial fever and chills prior to bedtime. The patient can then sleep throughout the night.

Other considerations for the patient receiving SC IL-2 include the patient's support systems at home, the ability to give a self-injection, the patient's overall general condition, the patient's reliability in calling the medical team when indicated, and the patient's learning abilities (Viele and Moran 1993). However if the patient is referred to a large medical center but lives in a rural area, this may limit access to immediate health care and the availability of IL-2 at the local pharmacy. All of these factors determine one's ability to care for the patient as an outpatient. Several specialty home delivery pharmacies exist, such as Biologics Inc. (1-800-850-4306 or www.biologicstoday.com), that can assist with reimbursement and getting patients' prescribed medications delivered to their home.

Clinical Pathways for Patients Receiving IL-2 Therapy

Outcome guidelines and clinical pathways demonstrate a positive impact on patient outcomes in clinical practice as well as a reduction in costs. This is accomplished by reducing variations in the care provided, facilitating expected outcomes, reducing delays in interventions, and reducing the length of hospital stay (Katterhagen 1996; Coffe et al. 1992). Clinical pathways can function to support the education of the multidisciplinary team and as a platform for the introduction of new and unique treatments. Clinical pathways are most useful for high-volume, high-risk, or high-cost diagnoses, procedures, or treatments. Treating patients with IL-2 can be high risk and high cost and, because of its predictable treatment course, lends itself well to an outcome-based clinical pathway (Coffe et al. 1992; Mavroukakis et al. 2001). Table 4.4 outlines the clinical pathway for patients receiving the standard FDA treatment with HD IL-2. Table 4.5 illustrates a frequently used SC regimen for IL-2. A cycle in these regimens is defined as either up to 5 days of dosing for HD IL-2 or 5 days of treatment with a 2-day rest for 6 weeks for SC IL-2. A course is considered to be two cycles of treatment. These clinical pathways represent a typical or expected treatment schema but must be individualized by the various dosing schemas and based on the patients' needs and the clinical side effects (Mavroukakis et al. 2001).

Eligibility for IL-2

The toxicity associated with HD IL-2 requires judicious and rigorous patient selection. Careful screening of IL-2 candidates must be done prior to initiating therapy. Patients with limited pulmonary function, active cardiac disease, or symptomatic brain metastases are at significant risk for a lethal complication and are rarely eligible for IL-2 administration. IL-2 therapy demands an intact immune system. Pretreatment evaluation includes screening for HIV and other active infections, although the use of IL-2 in low doses is investigational in patients with HIV (Schwartz et al. 2002; Schwartzentruber 2000; Dutcher et al. 2001; Davey et al. 1997). Because the effects of IL-2 on a fetus are unknown, women of childbearing age should undergo a pregnancy test and receive birth control instructions and information on how to prevent pregnancy. Mothers are instructed not to breast feed during IL-2 therapy because of the unknown effects. Screening parameters are included in pretreatment evaluation in the clinical pathways. During the screening process, patients are asked to select a durable power of attorney (DPA) because potential neurologic side effects may impair their ability to make sound decisions during therapy (Mavroukakis et al. 2001).

Acute toxicities are minimized in patients receiving LD IL-2, and therefore, more patients are eligible to receive this therapy. Patients with a poor performance status or respiratory involvement or who, for other medical reasons, may be unable to tolerate HD IL-2 may be eligible to receive LD IL-2. The eligibility criteria are not as clear with this regimen as they are with HD IL-2, and the eligibility decision is primarily the responsibility of the prescribing physician (Mavroukakis et al. 2001).

Dose Modification for IL-2

Patients rarely tolerate all 12 doses of HD IL-2. Therapy is routinely discontinued on the basis of dose-limiting toxicity. Doses are delayed or skipped in patients who are hemodynamically unstable or oliguric and resumed if appropriate interventions stabilize these toxicities. The IL-2 dose should not be reduced. Toxicities that indicate the need to stop a cycle of therapy include: EKG changes indicative

TABLE 4.4 Clinical Pathway for Patients Receiving High-Dose Interleukin-2

Date	Pre-Treatment Evaluation (DATE:)
Site	Clinic

ASSESSMENT & INTERVENTIONS	■ History and physical, noting exact size and location of lesions ■ Complete baseline assessment of all systems ■ Obtain informed consent if patient is participating in an investigational study

LABS	Metabolic panel: (incl. as minimum):
	  ■ electrolytes
	  ■ creatinine
	  ■ BUN
	  ■ glucose
	  ■ AST/SGOT
	  ■ ALT/SGPT
	  ■ total bilirubin
	  ■ CK
	  ■ LDH
	  ■ calcium
	  ■ phosphorus
	  ■ magnesium
	  ■ albumen
	■ CBC, differential
	■ PT/PTT
	■ Urinalysis (each cycle)
	■ TSH, free T_4 (each cycle)
	■ HIV antibody
	■ Hepatitis screen: Hb_sAg, anti-HCV
	■ Beta HCG pregnancy test for women of childbearing age

DIAGNOSTIC TESTS	■ Chest x-ray
	■ EKG
	■ Baseline scans within 6 weeks of starting therapy:
	  ■ Brain MRI with contrast
	  ■ CT of chest, abdomen, and pelvis
	  ■ Bone scan, when indicated
	■ Cardiovascular workup with stress thallium or other stress tests in patients $\geq$ 50 years of age or with ischemic symptoms
	■ PFTs in patients with history of heavy smoking or pulmonary symptoms

TEACHING	■ Assess for social work needs ■ Meet with reimbursement personnel ■ Teaching: including no steroids, IL-2 side effects and management, have patient complete DPA, answer questions ■ Advise regarding the availability of spiritual support ■ Instruct to take acetaminophen 650 mg p.o. and indomethicin 50–75 mg p.o. the evening prior to admission
OUTCOMES	■ Able to describe the purpose of treatment and potential side effects ■ Able to discuss measures to alleviate side effects and prevent complications

(Continued)

TABLE 4.4 (Continued)

(DATE) Approximate Day of cycle (Course/Cycle)	(DATE) Day 1 through 4 Course ☐ /Cycle ☐
SITE	Inpatient

ASSESSMENT & INTERVENTIONS	■ Admission assessment ■ Weight and height on admission and then daily weights, or per institutional preference ■ Pulse oximetry reading on admission ■ Vital signs q2–8h, and at start of IL-2, and as clinically indicated (incl. Neuro checks and breath sounds) ■ Strict I&O q4h ■ Mouth care q2h and prn ■ Initiate skin care per hospital guidelines, avoiding alcohol-containing lotions ■ Mental status checks q8h ■ IV site checks q8h

LABS	Metabolic panel: (incl. as minimum): Daily after starting IL-2
	    ■ electrolytes
	    ■ creatinine
	    ■ BUN
	    ■ glucose
	    ■ AST/SGOT
	    ■ ALT/SGPT [probably not needed]
	    ■ total bilirubin
	    ■ CK
	    ■ LDH [not needed]
	    ■ calcium
	    ■ phosphorus
	    ■ magnesium
	    ■ albumen [not needed]
	■ CBC, daily
	■ PT/PTT as clinically indicated

MEDICATIONS	■ 600,000 IU/kg IV over 15 min q8h (max 12 doses)
	    ■ Doses may be skipped for hemodynamic instability or inadequate urine output
	    ■ Proceed with caution when patient experiences significant hematologic changes
	    ■ May not receive the total 12 doses depending upon toxicities
	■ Initiate supportive therapy immediately upon admission: acetaminophen (650 mg q4h), Indomethacin (50–75 mg q8h), ranitidine (50 mg q8h) or H₂ blocker, continue until 24 hours after completing IL-2
	■ Antiemetics prn: Droperidol, Prochlorperazine, Ondansetron HCL or Granisetron HCL, Lorazepam
	■ Antidiarrheals prn: Loperamide, Diphenoxylate HCL with Atropine, or codeine
	■ Pruritis prn: Hydroxyzine HCL, Diphenhydramine HCL
	■ Mucositis prn: Sodium bicarbonate (6 tsp/1500 ml) swish and swallow, lidobenalox oral

(Continued)

TABLE 4.4 (Continued)

Site	Inpatient	
	■ For hypotension or oliguria, administer fluid boluses per physician's orders ■ For hypotension not responsive to fluid boluses, consider initiating vasopressors (alpha-adrenergic agents) ■ For oliguria not responsive to fluid boluses, consider initiating renal dose dopamine (2–4 µg/kg/min)	
DIAGNOSTIC TESTS	■ Chest x-ray as clinically indicated	
TEACHING	■ Initial assessment of needs and family support ■ Reinforce side effects to report ■ Begin discharge teaching	
OUTCOMES	■ Hemodynamically stable as demonstrated by HR < 120, SBP > 90 mmHg, mean > 50 mmHg ■ Adequate kidney function: urine output ≥ 25 cc/h, or 100 cc/4h ■ Electrolytes normalize after appropriate replacement ■ Safe, with patent airway, if neurologic symptoms occur ■ Skin free of s/s infection, incl. mucous membranes, IV sites, and perianal area ■ Anxiety minimized	

(DATE) Approximate Day	(DATES) Day 5–7 Course ☐ /Cycle ☐	Conclusion of Every Course (2 cycles) to Evaluate for Retreatment and Long-Term Follow-Up*
SITE	Inpatient	Outpatient
ASSESSMENT & INTERVENTIONS	■ Strict I&O q8h or as clinically indicated ■ Daily weights ■ VS q4–8h, unless otherwise clinically indicated (incl. Neuro checks and breath sounds) ■ Mouth care as clinically indicated ■ Taper or discontinue IV fluids ■ Advance diet as tolerated	■ History and physical examination. Measurement of evaluable lesions with physical examination
LABS	Metabolic panel: (incl. as minimum): Daily until discharge and returning to baseline ■ electrolytes ■ creatinine ■ BUN ■ glucose ■ AST/SGOT ■ ALT/SGPT ■ total bilirubin ■ CK ■ calcium	Metabolic panel: (incl. as minimum): ■ electrolytes ■ creatinine ■ BUN ■ glucose ■ AST/SGOT ■ ALT/SGPT ■ total bilirubin ■ CK ■ calcium ■ phosphorus

(*Continued*)

TABLE 4.4 (Continued)

Site	Inpatient	Outpatient
DIAGNOSTIC TESTS	■ phosphorus ■ magnesium ■ albumen ■ CBC, daily ■ PT/PTT if clinically indicated	■ magnesium ■ albumen ■ CBC, differential ■ Urinalysis ■ TSH, free T_4 ■ CT of chest, abdomen, and pelvis ■ Brain MRI with contrast, if neurologic symptoms ■ Bone scan and other scans as clinically indicated
MEDICATIONS	■ Supportive therapy: acetaminophen (650 mg q4h), Indomethacin (50–75 mg q8h), ranitidine (50 mg, q8h), or H_2 blocker for up to 24 hours after discontinuing IL-2 ■ Diuretics as needed	
OUTCOMES	■ VS return to normal ■ Laboratory values normalize without intervention ■ Weight returns to baseline ■ Neurologic status returns to baseline ■ Verbalizes post IL-2 precautions and symptoms that require notification of health care team ■ On day of discharge, states return date for next cycle of treatment	*Long-term follow-up: Every 3 months × 3 years Every 6 months for 2 years, then annually

Source: Reprinted with permission. Mavroukakis, S.A., Muehlbauer, P.M., Schwartzentruber, D.J., and White, R.L. 2001. Clinical pathways for managing patients receiving Interleukin-2. *CJON* 5(5):210–212.

of ischemia; ventricular arrhythmias; sustained sinus tachycardia that persists after correcting hypotension, fever, and hypoxemia; diarrhea greater than 1 liter per 8 hours; vomiting unresponsive to medication; O_2 saturation < 94% despite oxygen therapy; sustained oliguria; and disorientation or hallucinations (Schwartzentruber 2000; Schwartzentruber 2001; Mavroukakis *et al.* 2001; Schwartz *et al.* 2002; Dutcher *et al.* 2001). These side effects generally reverse within 24 hours after stopping IL-2 therapy. However, because neurologic toxicities can worsen after therapy is completed, it is imperative to closely observe patients experiencing any symptoms of neurologic alterations.

Patients who receive LD IL-2 have less severe toxicities. Some reasons that a patient on LD IL-2 may delay or stop therapy include a rise in creatinine to > 2.5 mg/dl, shortness of breath, or constitutional symptoms that are not controlled with prophylactic medications. Major toxicities, including those similar to the HD IL-2 regimen, would warrant a discontinuation of therapy (Schwartzentruber 2001; Mavroukakis *et al.* 2001).

Retreatment with IL-2

Patients may undergo a second course of IL-2 therapy if they exhibit some evidence of either stable disease or tumor regression. Retreatment cycles

TABLE 4.5 Clinical Pathway for Patients Receiving Subcutaneous Interleukin-2
(Reprinted with permission from Mavroukakis *et al.* 2001, p 213–214.)

DATE	Pre-Treatment Evaluation (DATE:)
SITE	Clinic
ASSESSMENT & INTERVENTIONS	■ History and physical, noting exact size and location of lesions ■ Complete baseline assessment of all systems ■ Obtain informed consent if patient is participating in an investigational study
LABS	Metabolic panel: (incl. as minimum): 　■ electrolytes 　■ creatinine 　■ BUN 　■ glucose 　■ AST/SGOT 　■ ALT/SGPT 　■ total bilirubin 　■ CK 　■ calcium 　■ phosphorus 　■ magnesium 　■ albumen ■ CBC, differential ■ PT/PTT ■ Urinalysis ■ TSH, free T_4 ■ HIV antibody ■ Hepatitis screen: Hb_sAg, anti-HCV ■ Beta HCG pregnancy test for women of childbearing age
DIAGNOSTIC TESTS	■ Chest x-ray ■ EKG ■ Baseline scans within 6 weeks of starting therapy: 　■ Brain MRI with contrast, 　■ CT of chest, abdomen, and pelvis 　■ Bone scan if indicated
TEACHING	■ Assess for social work needs ■ Meet with reimbursement personnel ■ Teaching: including no steroids, IL-2 side effects and management ■ Advise regarding the availability of spiritual support
OUTCOMES	■ Able to describe the purpose of treatment and potential side effects ■ Able to discuss measures to alleviate side effects and prevent complications

(Continued)

TABLE 4.5 (Continued)

(DATE) Approximate Day of Cycle (Course/Cycle)	(DATES) Day 1–5 (Day 6–7 Rest) Day 8–12 (Day 13–14 Rest) [Repeated on weeks 3 through 6] Course ☐ /Cycle ☐	2 weeks after the conclusion of the 6th week of therapy evaluate for retreatment and long-term follow-up*
SITE	Outpatient/At home once competent in self-injection	Outpatient
ASSESSMENT & INTERVEN- TIONS	■ Nursing assessment ■ Weight and height for baseline ■ Vital signs and pulse oximetery for baseline ■ Patient to weigh daily, take temperature daily, document self-injection, and signs and symptoms in diary	■ History and physical examination. Measurement of evaluable lesions with physical examination

LABS	Metabolic panel (incl. as minimum): Initially, then once a week while at home:
	  ■ electrolytes
	  ■ creatinine
	  ■ BUN
	  ■ glucose
	  ■ AST/SGOT
	  ■ ALT/SGPT
	  ■ total bilirubin
	  ■ CK
	  ■ calcium
	  ■ phosphorus
	  ■ magnesium
	  ■ albumen
	■ CBC
		Metabolic panel: (incl. as minimum):
		  ■ electrolytes
		  ■ creatinine
		  ■ BUN
		  ■ glucose
		  ■ AST/SGOT
		  ■ ALT/SGPT
		  ■ total bilirubin
		  ■ CK
		  ■ calcium
		  ■ phosphorus
		  ■ magnesium
		  ■ albumen
		■ CBC, differential
		■ Urinalysis and TSH, free T_4

MEDICATIONS	■ 250,000 IU/kg SQ for 5 days (followed by a 2 day rest) then 125,000 IU/kg SQ for each 5 day cycle thereafter (followed by a 2 day rest) ■ Initiate supportive therapy immediately upon starting IL-2: acetaminophen (650 mg q4h), Indomethacin (50–75 mg prn), ranitidine (150 mg, bid, p.o.) or H_2 blocker ■ Other medications prescribed in response to patient complaints of signs and symptoms	
DIAGNOSTIC TESTS		■ CT of chest, abdomen, and pelvis ■ Brain MRI with contrast, if patient develops neurologic symptoms ■ Bone scan and other scans as clinically indicated
TEACHING	■ Initial assessment of needs and family support ■ Teach patient or reliable significant other to perform subcutaneous administration of IL-2	

(Continued)

TABLE 4.5. (Continued)		
SITE	Outpatient/At home once competent in self-injection	Outpatient

OUTCOMES	■ Teach patient what to monitor, side effects to report and interventions to treat side effects, use of diary, blood work requirements
	■ Demonstrates competent self-administration of IL-2
	■ Verbalizes daily activities to perform, how to treat side effects and symptoms that require notification of health care team
	■ At home:
	  ■ Documents self-injection, weight, and temperature, and signs and symptoms daily
	  ■ Performs daily activities, treats side effects, and reports significant symptoms to the health care team
		*Long-term follow-up:
		Every 3 months × 3 years
		Every 6 months for 2 years, then annually

are administered in the same fashion as the initial cycle, although patients receiving HD IL-2 usually do not tolerate the same number of doses. Major responses after two unsuccessful courses of IL-2 are thought to be rare, although clinical trials to investigate this possibility have not been reported in the literature. Patients who respond are offered additional courses of therapy. If a patient has a complete response, defined as a disappearance of all clinical evidence of disease, two additional cycles are administered in an attempt to consolidate that response. Retreatment is begun 4–6 weeks after the last course (Proleukin prescribing information 2000; Mavroukakis *et al.* 2001).

Discharge Teaching

Persistent side effects are commonly noted at the time of discharge. Appropriate discharge instructions are important and are delineated in Table 4.6. For patients receiving SC IL-2, self-administration of the SC IL-2 is taught with return demonstrations until the patient is comfortable. Patients keep a diary of their daily weights and temperatures, documentation of self-administration of the IL-2 injection, and any side effects that occur during treatment (Mavroukakis *et al.* 2001).

Follow-Up Evaluation

Routine response evaluation of the patient receiving IL-2, including blood work and imaging scans outlined in the clinical pathways, should be performed 3–6 weeks after each course of therapy to determine retreatment options. Once treatment is concluded, follow-up allows assessment of overall survival and disease-free survival and provides the patient with a significant support system. Patients with recurrent or progressive disease may benefit from other treatment interventions or may elect to pursue palliative care (Mavroukakis *et al.* 2001).

Summary

IL-2–based treatments are among the biologic therapies in this emerging field. Knowledge of the indications, toxicity assessment and management, and dosing regimens can support the clinician in providing safe and competent care.

TABLE 4.6 Discharge Instructions for Patients Receiving IL-2

- Gradually increase their food intake. Push fluids, about 12 or more 8-ounce glasses a day.
- Nutrition tips can be found in the NCI's "Eating Hints for Cancer Patients: Before, During and After Treatment" booklet (http://www.cancer.gov/cancerinfo/eatinghints). These tips will also assist with any lingering GI side effects.
- Gradually increase exercise and take frequent rest breaks during the day.
- Sleep disturbances and unusual dreams may continue for 2 to 3 weeks after therapy.
- Use a strong sunblock with an SPF of 15 or greater even if it is cloudy or overcast.
- Wear hats with broad brims, long sleeves, and pants for extra protection against the sun.
- Skin side effects may last for 6 weeks. Continue using the creams, oils, and lotions used while in the hospital.
- Continue to use mild soaps and try to avoid swimming in chlorinated or salt water. If you do swim, rinse off immediately and use lotions or creams on your skin.
- Do not drive for 1 week after therapy.
- Do **NOT** use any products containing **steroids** or **cortisone**. Many over-the-counter products including moisturizers contain these ingredients. Check with the health care team **BEFORE** using *any* medications, creams, or ointments.

Symptoms to Report to the Health care Team
- Nausea, vomiting, or diarrhea, which lasts for more than 48 hours
- Any new onset of nausea, vomiting, or diarrhea
- Trouble with breathing
- Temperature greater than 100.8°F
- Chest pain
- Any new onset of pain including headaches

Hints to Help Fight Cancer-Related Fatigue
- Do not spend all your time in bed. This only worsens fatigue.
- Treat energy levels as a bank with "deposits" and "withdrawals".
- Drinking up to 2 liters of fluid daily can help decrease feelings of fatigue.
- Short walks and other activity can help increase energy. Try to increase activity to 30 minutes continuously.
- *Remember:* There are many contributing factors to fatigue such as the disease, cancer treatments, stress, nutrition, and emotional state.

The Interferons

Interferons (IFN) are a group of naturally occurring antiviral cytokines first described by Issacs and Lindenman, which, when induced, can inhibit the replication of other viruses (Williams 2000; Cuaron and Thompson 2001; Skalla 1996). They are named interferons because of their ability to "interfere" with viral replication. Interferons were the first identified cytokines. There are three main interferons with clinical indications: alpha (α), beta (β), and gamma (γ). Two other interferons, tau and omega, are not approved for therapeutic use in humans. In the 1970s, IFN-α was derived from donated human blood (Cuaron and Thompson 2001; Williams 2000; Cantell *et al*. 1975). These early preparations were impure, but they provided a chance to test IFN as an anticancer therapy. As with IL-2, it was not until recombinant DNA technology was available that IFN could be produced in quantities sufficient enough to use in clinical trials (Skalla 1996; Cuaron and Thompson 2001; Williams 2000). The only IFN approved for use as cancer therapy is IFN-α.

Biologic Activity

When a stimulus such as a virus, bacteria, parasite, or cancer activates a cell, IFN is produced. IFNs are recognized by the body as foreign, thus stimulating an immune response. IFN binds to a cell surface receptor site and activates downstream signal transduction pathways. A signal is sent to the cell nucleus where it attaches to certain genes, which then regulate cell activities including inducing apoptosis (Clemens 2003; Cuaron and Thompson 2001; Williams 2000; Skalla 1996; Gantz et al. 1995; Baron et al. 1991). Once the signal is activated, there is significant interaction between the cytokine, hormone, and growth factor signaling pathways that block viral and possibly cellular RNA development (Interferon alfa 2004; Cuaron and Thompson 2001; Baron et al. 1991).

The major actions of IFNs are antiviral, immunomodulatory, and antiproliferative. However, each IFN has similar and distinct characteristics. For example, there is evidence that IFN-α has antiangiogenic properties when given in lower doses. Endogenous IFN, a regulator of angiogenesis, inhibits endothelial cell migration, basic fibroblast growth factor, and IL-8, which promote tumor angiogenesis (Cáceres and González 2003; Muehlbauer 2003; Krown et al. 2002; Cuaron and Thompson 2001; Kerbel et al. 2000; Singh and Fidler 1996; Baron et al. 1991). Table 4.7 summarizes the types, names, actions, clinical indications, and recommended dosages of each IFN. IFN-α is the only IFN discussed in detail in this chapter.

IFN-α: Indications for Use

The FDA-approved indications for use of IFN-α are outlined in Table 4.7. However, studies continue to examine the effectiveness of IFN-α alone or in combination with other agents for a variety of malignancies. This next section provides a brief synopsis of some of the research being conducted with IFN-α in a variety of malignancies.

Chronic Myeloid Leukemia (CML)

Until the recent launch of imatinib mesylate (Gleevec), IFN-α was the standard treatment for patients in the chronic phase of CML (Marin et al. 2003). Several studies are underway or completed comparing the effects of IFN-α with imatinib mesylate in patients with CML, a clonal myeloproliferative disorder of the myeloid stem cells. Hughes et al. (2003) report a randomized trial (n = 1106) comparing imatinib mesylate to IFN-α plus cytarabine in patients newly diagnosed with chronic-phase CML. CML creates a fusion gene, BCR-ABL, which expresses an activated tyrosine kinase leading to the pathogenesis of CML. They looked at the presence of molecular markers of BCR-ABL at baseline and after complete cytogenic remission was obtained. Complete cytogenic remission was defined as the complete absence of Philadelphia chromosome–positive cells in metaphase among a minimum of 20 cells in metaphase in a bone marrow aspirate. The Philadelphia chromosome is a malignant clonal disorder in CML (Hughes et al. 2003; Cuaron and Thompson 2001). Patients were allowed to cross over from the IFN-α plus cytarabine group to the imatinib mesylate group. Overall, the authors found that the rates of hematologic and cytogenetic responses in newly diagnosed patients with chronic-phase CML were higher in the imatinib mesylate group versus patients treated with IFN-α plus cytarabine.

Hehlmann et al. (2003) report the results of combination IFN-α plus hydroxyurea versus hydroxyurea alone in newly diagnosed patients with CML in chronic phase receiving no prior therapy (n = 340). This study was conducted by the German CML Study Group in 1991, prior to the approval of imatinib mesylate. Duration of chronic phase in the IFN-α plus hydroxyurea group was 55 months versus 41 months for hydroxyurea alone (P < 0.0001). There was a survival advantage for the combination group over the monotherapy group (64 months vs 53 months, respectively; P = 0.0063). The authors concluded that combination IFN-α plus hydroxyurea should be considered standard therapy of CML and that this regimen should be used in comparison studies of new drugs and treatment modalities.

Interferon	Actions	Trade Names	FDA-Approved Indications	Dose
Alpha (α)	Antiviral Inhibits growth of normal and malignant cells Enhances NK cell activity Enhances class I MHC expression Influences differentiation of cells Induces apoptosis Antiangiogenic properties	INTRON A (IFN-alfa-2b) (Schering)	Hairy cell leukemia	2 MIU/m^2 IM or SC 3 × week for up to 6 months
			Malignant melanoma	**Induction regimen:** 20 MIU/m^2 IV daily for 5 consecutive days for 4 weeks **Maintenance regimen:** 10 MIU/m^2 SC 3 × week for 48 weeks
			Follicular lymphoma	5 MIU SC 3 × week for up to 18 months with anthracycline-containing chemotherapy
			Condylomata acuminata	1 MIU injected into each lesion 3 × week for 3 weeks
			AIDS-related Kaposi's sarcoma	30 MIU/m^2 SC or IM 3 × week
			Chronic hepatitis C	3 MIU SC or IM 3 × week
			Chronic hepatitis B	30–35 MIU SC or IM weekly for 16 weeks
		Roferon (IFN-alfa-2a) (Roche Laboratories)	Chronic hepatitis C	3 MIU SC or IM 3 × week for 12 months
			Hairy cell leukemia	**Induction:** 3 MIU QD for 16–24 weeks given SC or IM **Maintenance:** 3 MIU SC or IM
			CML	9 MIU QD given SC or IM
			AIDS-related Kaposi's sarcoma	**Induction:** 36 MIU QD for 10–12 weeks given SC or IM **Maintenance:** 36 MIU SC or IM given 3 × week
		Alferon N Injection (IFN-alfa-n3) (Hemispherx)	Intralesional treatment for condylomata acuminata	0.05 ml (250,000 IU) per wart, twice weekly for up to 8 weeks
		Infergen (IFN alfacon-1) (InterMune)	Chronic hepatitis C virus infection	9 μcg given SC 3 × week for 24 weeks
Beta (β)	Antiviral Enhances NK cell activity Enhances class I MHC expression Induces apoptosis	Avonex (IFN-beta-1a) (Biogen Neurology)	Multiple sclerosis	30 μcg IM once weekly
		Betseron (IFN-beta-1b) (Berlex)	Multiple sclerosis	0.25 mg SC QOD

(Continued)

Table 4.7 (Continued)

Interferon	Actions	Trade Names	FDA-Approved Indications	Dose
		Rebif (IFN-beta-1a) (Pfizer)	Multiple sclerosis	44 μcg SC 3 × week
Gamma (γ)	Antiviral Inhibits growth of normal and malignant cells Enhances macrophage activity Enhances class I and II MHC expression Generates secretion of other cytokines Impacts differentiation of cells Enhances immunoglobulin synthesis with other cytokines Induces apoptosis	Actimmune (IFN-gamma-1b) (InterMune)	Chronic granulomatous disease Osteoporosis	**For both diseases:** 50 μg/m^2 (1 MIU/ m^2) for patients with BSA > 0.5 m^2 and 1.5 μcg/kg/dose for patients with BSA ≤ 0.5 m^2

NK, natural killer; MHC, major histocompatibility complex; IFN, interferon; IM, intramuscular; SC, subcutaneous; IV, intravenous; QD, every day; BSA, body-surface area

O'Brien *et al.* (2003) combined IFN-α, cytarabine (ARA-C), and homoharringtonine (HHT) in a clinical trial for patients with a diagnosis of Philadelphia chromosome–positive CML in early chronic phase (n = 90). When imatinib mesylate became available, 78 patients had their therapy changed to imatinib mesylate. The authors found that the sequence of IFN-α, Ara-C, and HHT followed by imatinib mesylate resulted in an estimated 5-year survival rate of 88%, and the incidence of blastic phase was 9%. They postulated that the triple-agent regimen has different mechanisms of action in CML. Imatinib mesylate may reduce the incidence of imatinib mesylate–resistant mutant CML clones, resulting in reduced rates of disease transformation. They concluded that imatinib in combination with other agents may overcome CML resistance based on the responses obtained with combination IFN-α, ARA-C, and HHT followed by imatinib mesylate.

Follicular Non-Hodgkin's Lymphoma (NHL)

A meta-analysis of 25 articles, abstracts, and unpublished manuscripts describing separate study populations for NHL was conducted by Allen *et al.* (2001). Two types of IFN-α were used in the analyzed clinical trials including IFN-α-2b (INTRON A) and IFN-α-2a (Roferon). Progression-free survival (PFS) and overall survival (OS) were the primary outcomes of interest; the studies varied considerably regarding the definition of PFS and OS. Results indicate that, in previously untreated patients with high–tumor burden follicular NHL, IFN-α therapy significantly increased 5-year OS and PFS rates at 3 and 5 years compared with control arms of individual studies. The best advantages were shown in patients receiving anthracycline-containing induction regimens along with IFN-α as either induction or maintenance therapy. Progression free survival in this group was

20% greater than in control arms, but this group had a somewhat smaller survival advantage. Allen *et al.* (2001) suggest that the results of their review indicate a significant benefit for IFN-α, but these findings must be viewed with caution because of the uneven quality of study designs, methods, and results in the analyzed clinical trials.

Kaposi's Sarcoma (KS)

The AIDS Clinical Trials Group studied the efficacy and safety of a low and intermediate daily dose of IFN-α-2b with didanosine, an antiretroviral agent, in patients with AIDS-related KS (Krown *et al.* 2002). Sixty-eight eligible patients were randomized to receive either 1 MIU IFN-α-2b (low dose) or 10 MIU IFN-α-2b once daily with twice daily doses of didanosine. Response, toxicity, changes in CD4 counts, and survival were evaluated. Patients on the intermediate dose of IFN-α-2b had a higher rate of treatment discontinuation because of toxicities, including grade 3/4 neutropenia (21% in intermediate dose vs 3% in low dose), grade 3 constitutional and central nervous system toxicities, elevations in AST, and thrombocytopenia. There was no statistically significant difference in the complete or partial response rates of the two dosage groups (0.40 for low dose vs 0.55 for intermediate dose). The authors concluded that a low, minimally toxic daily dose of IFN-α-2b combined with antiretroviral therapy induced KS regression.

Hepatocellular Carcinoma (HCC)

IFN-α is effective in treating patients infected with hepatitis B virus (HBV) and hepatitis C virus (HCV). Lin *et al.* (2003) state that IFN-α improves the prognosis of patients with chronic liver disease, reduces cirrhosis, and delays the development of HCC. Studies have indicated that IFN-α is effective in preventing HCV-related HCC recurrence after tumor resection and preventing HBV-related HCC recurrence. Patients treated with IFN-α for 6 to 12 months showed lower rates of HCC than untreated patients (Lin *et al.* 2003; Oon and Chen 2003; Yao and Terrault 2001).

Superficial Bladder Cancer (SBC)

Intravesical instillation of IFN-α has been studied for treatment of SBC as both a monotherapy and combined with other therapies. SBCs are defined as stages Ta or Tcis (tumors confined to the mucosa) or stage T1 (tumors invading the lamina propria) and account for 80% of primary bladder tumors (Santhanam *et al.* 2002). Clinical studies imply that intravesical IFN-α has antiproliferative activity against SBC via several mechanisms including increasing production of IFN-γ and increasing the cytotoxic activity of T cells and natural killer cells by increasing the infiltration of these cells into the bladder wall (Ziotta and Schulman 2000; Santhanam *et al.* 2002).

IFN-α was not as effective as BCG in several trials as first-line therapy. Studies indicate that IFN-α has potential as a second-line therapy for patients not responding to prior intravesical chemotherapy or BCG. Efficacy of intravesical IFN-α in SBC appears to be greater with higher doses such as 100 MIU (Ziotta and Schulman 2000; Santhanam *et al.* 2002). Ziotta and Schulman (2000) report that BCG and IFN-α are biocompatible and may be used in combination intravesically as a single mixture that would produce or enhance the therapeutic response versus BCG alone. Clinical trials are underway to investigate this combination and other combinations with chemotherapy (Ziotta and Schulman 2000; Santhanam *et al.* 2002).

Melanoma

Since FDA approval was obtained for HD IFN-α-2b (HDI) as adjuvant treatment for patients with melanoma at high risk of recurrence (American Joint Committee on Cancer [AJCC] stage IIB or IIC [thick lesions 2.01–4.0 mm and > 4.0 mm] or stage III [lymph node positive]) in the mid-1990s, several trials in the United States and abroad evaluated the efficacy of IFN-α on overall survival (OS) and relapse-free survival (RFS) (Moschos *et al.* 2004; Masci and Borden 2002). The reason for continuing studies is that the impact of HDI on long-term survival has been under scrutiny because of cost and toxicity of the regimen as well as the absence of survival benefit. In a separate trial (E1690), the Eastern Oncology Cooperative Group was pivotal in getting HDI FDA approved for this patient population (Moschos *et al.* 2004). Moschos *et al.* (2004) report that, in Europe, the Association of Dermatologic Oncologists in Germany, the Italian Melanoma Intergroup, and the Hellenic Oncology Group in Greece have studied HDI only recently. These organizations evaluate the efficacy of lower doses of IFN-α-2b. Study results demonstrate that lower doses of IFN-α-2b show no survival benefit (Moschos *et al.* 2004; Hancock *et al.* 2004; Schuchter 2004; Eggermont and Punt 2003; Decatris *et al.* 2002). An overview of current clinical trials can be found in Moschos *et al.* (2004).

Renal Cell Carcinoma (RCC)

IFN-α has a roughly 10% to 20% response rate when used alone to treat RCC. Igarahsi *et al.* (1999) studied the effects of IFN-α combined with 5-fluorouracil (5-FU). Patients received IFN-α 3 MIU SC three times a week for 12 weeks and 600 mg/m^2 of 5-FU as a continuous infusion for the first 5 days followed by 600 mg/m^2 weekly from weeks 3 to 12. The overall response rate was 20% which was no better than IFN alone. The authors concluded that this regimen has limited value for treatment of patients with advanced RCC.

Another combination studied thalidomide, an antiangiogenic agent, with IFN-α. Investigators at Helsinki University Central Hospital hypothesized that IFN-α combined with thalidomide may enhance the antiangiogenic effects. Patients were given 0.9 MIU IFN-α SC three times a day for 1 month and then 1.2 MIU IFN-α three times a day. The thalidomide dose was escalated from 100 mg/day for the first week to 300 mg/day thereafter. Investigators measured serum vascular endothelial growth factor (VEGF), which is a potent stimulator of tumor angiogenesis. Serum VEGF levels decreased in the patients who responded to therapy compared with patients with stable or progressive disease. However, all responses were partial responses, and the biomarkers did not correlate with significant clinical benefit (Hernberg *et al.* 2003).

Other combinations have been tried with IFN-α in the treatment of RCC, including combining IFN-α with retinoids. Efficacy in two clinical trials was minimal in terms of response rate or overall survival. IFN-α has been combined separately with vinblastine, aspirin, histamine, and IFN-γ with overall mixed results. IFN-α as a monotherapy has modest activity in metastatic RCC. Response to IFN-α correlates with characteristics such as good performance status, few metastatic sites, prior nephrectomy, and low erythrocyte sedimentation rate (Decatris *et al.* 2002).

PEG-Intron

Pegylation of therapeutic proteins involves the addition of polyethylene glycol (PEG) to the therapeutic agent to allow for slower release of the agent. Pegylation has been done with a variety of therapeutic agents including adenosine deaminase, L-asparginase, IL-2, granulocyte colony-stimulating factor, tumor necrosis factor alpha, and human growth hormone (Bukowski *et al.* 2002; Neulasta [pegfilgrastim] prescribing information 2002). PEG-Intron is a conjugate of recombinant IFN-α with a single straight-chain molecule of polyethylene glycol and demonstrates similar biologic activity compared with IFN-α-2b (Bukowski *et al.* 2002; Hussar 2002). The impetus in pegylating IFN-α-2b was to delay clearance of IFN-α-2b, thus sustaining the duration of activity of IFN-α-2b and allowing for a once-weekly injection. PEG-Intron is FDA approved for hepatitis C virus (HCV) infection as a monotherapy and in combination with ribavirin (Rebetol) (Bukowski *et al.* 2002; Hussar 2002). It has been investigated in patients with CML and solid tumors including melanoma and RCC. The toxicity profile has been similar for patients with CML and HCV, whereas fatigue has been reported as a dose-limiting toxicity in patients with solid tumors. Further studies are needed to determine the optimal dose and to establish whether PEG-Intron can achieve dose intensification and improve efficacy (Michallet *et al.* 2004; Bukowski *et al.* 2002; Hussar 2002).

IFN-α: Side Effects and Medical and Nursing Management

Side effects with IFN-α are not insignificant. Nursing interventions are key in helping patients tolerate what is generally extended therapy. Knowledge of these side effects and how to manage them will be crucial when caring for the patient receiving IFN-α. Consideration should be given to adjustment of dose or schedule of administration if the patient is experiencing unremitting toxicities.

The most common side effects reported with IFN-α include fatigue, flu-like symptoms (fever, chills, myalgias, headaches, and malaise), neutropenia, anorexia, nausea/vomiting, increased liver function tests, depression, diarrhea, alopecia, and altered taste sensation (Interferon alfa 2004; Cuaron and Thompson 2001; Battiato and Wheeler 2000; Tretter *et al.* 2000; Donnelly 1998; Kiley and Gale 1998; Skalla 1996; Sandstrom 1996; Baron *et al.* 1991). Management of these reactions may necessitate a multidisciplinary approach. An overview of the more common side effects with suggested nursing management strategies is provided in Table 4.8.

Fatigue

Fatigue, the most frequently reported symptom experienced by patients with cancer, was reported in 96% of patients receiving IFN-α-2b for treatment of high-risk melanoma (INTRON-A 2002; Portenoy and Itri 1999; Kirkwood *et al.* 1996; Dean *et al.* 1995). Fatigue is common in all treatment regimens of IFN-α but more pronounced in patients receiving doses of 10 MIU/m^2 or greater (Cuaron and Thompson 2001). It is one of the most persistent and pervasive symptoms, can be difficult to manage, and can lead to dose alterations (Dean *et al.* 1995; Kirkwood *et al.* 1996; Dean 2001; Kiley and Gale 1998). Cancer-related fatigue is a complex, multifactorial disorder with

physical, mental, and psychological dimensions and is affiliated with diminished quality of life (Curt 2000; Portenoy and Itri 1999). Quesada *et al.* (1986) and Adams *et al.* (1984) speculate that IFN-induced fatigue, appetite changes, and cognitive-emotional disorders may be the consequence of central nervous system toxicity or frontal lobe neurotoxicity. IFN potentially has a direct effect on the frontal lobe or on deeper brain structures. Central and peripheral mechanisms could be a contributory factor by releasing cytokines (i.e., immunomodulators) that alter fatigue sensations (Quesada *et al.* 1986; Adams *et al.* 1984; Skalla and Rieger 1995; Kiley and Gale 1998). Other causes of fatigue in the patient receiving IFN-α include depression, anorexia, sleep disturbances, anemia, hypovolemia, hypoglycemia, and thyroid dysfunction. Mental fatigue is affiliated with cognitive dysfunction and may persist throughout therapy. Contributing factors include the disease itself, chronic pain, fever, and dehydration (Cella *et al.* 2002; Cuaron and Thompson 2001; Dean 2001; Aistairs 1987). It is important to understand all the underlying causes of fatigue and to be able to distinguish between fatigue and depression when assisting patients in managing their fatigue.

Flu-Like or Constitutional Symptoms

Flu-like symptoms (FLS) include fevers, chills, headaches, myalgias, and malaise. These side effects develop during the first week of treatment but lessen over time because of tachyphylaxis (decreasing symptoms with increasing exposure to drug). Fevers may reach 39–40°C 2 to 4 hours after IFN-α administration and last 4 to 8 hours (Kiley and Gale 1998; Shelton 2001; Kirkwood 2000; Baron *et al.* 1991).

Body temperature is controlled by a thermoregulatory set point. The anterior hypothalamic brain centers sense deviations from a set temperature range of 36.4–37.3°C and regulate thermal balance by either heat production, causing vasoconstriction and shivering, or by heat loss, causing vasodilation and sweating. The basis of

TABLE 4.8 Interferon-Alfa: Toxicities and Management Strategies (Dean 2001; Kiley and Gale 1998; Battiato and Wheeler 2000; Donnelly 1998; Skalla and Rieger 1995; Skalla 1996; Sandstrom 1996; Winningham 1991; Piper 1991; Aistars 1987)

Side Effect	Nursing Interventions
Flu-like symptoms	Premedicate with antipyretics and NSAIDS such as acetaminophen and indomethacin ■ These help alleviate fever/mylagias/headaches Increase fluid intake Administer IFN before bedtime or at dinner time (about 6 pm) Layer warm blankets for chills
Fatigue	Evaluate periods of rest with activity ■ Promote adequate balance of rest with activity Promote moderate daily exercise, such as walking Use distraction techniques, such as reading, watching movies, meditation, biofeedback Assist patient with time management Ensure adequate nutrition and hydration ■ Enlist registered dietician (RD) to assist ■ Ask patient to keep food diary for a period of time for evaluation by RD ■ Suggest patient drink 2 to 3 liters of fluid/day Suggest patient keep a diary of activity to help identify factors contributing to fatigue ■ Schedule activities important to patient during time of least fatigue ■ Help patient modify activities that promote fatigue Differentiate fatigue from depression
Neurologic	Evaluate psychiatric history at baseline Evaluate patient on ongoing basis for symptoms of depression Encourage support group participation Include family in education and encourage communication for signs of behavior changes Referral, as indicated, to psychiatrist and other support systems Patient may need medically prescribed antidepressants in some cases Use nonpharmacologic interventions such as relaxation therapy and guided imagery
Anorexia and weight loss	Monitor weight Promote small, frequent meals Encourage use of premade meals to conserve energy Cafeteria-style restaurants allow patients to eat what they want when they want Enlist RD Medicate with antiemetics as needed Assess patient for symptoms of fluid and electrolyte imbalance
Dermatologic	Assess for history of dermatologic problems (i.e., psoriasis) Assess skin at start of therapy and throughout therapy Instruct patient to use mild soaps and cleansers without a lot of fragrance Instruct patient to use fragrance-free lotions, creams, and emollients Instruct patient to use sunscreen with SPF 15 or greater every day Instruct patient to wear broad-brimmed hats and to cover exposed areas Consult with dermatologist if needed MD may prescribe histamine blockers for urticaria and rash

IFN fevers may be a result of the release of pyrogenic factors induced by cytokine administration including the stimulation of IL-1, IL-6, and tumor necrosis factor. These cytokines act on thermal brain centers via prostaglandin release, creating a higher body temperature set point, thus increasing body temperature (Shelton 2001; Battiato and Wheeler 2000; Sandstrom 1996). Chills and rigors precede a rise in fever and manifest as muscle contractions. This increased muscle activity generates heat to change the body temperature when the thermoregulatory set point rises. Chills, rigors, myalgias, and headaches may occur 1 hour before the onset of fever (Kiley and Gale 1998; Battiato and Wheeler 2000; Shelton 2001). Myalgias are characterized by general muscle aches and weakness unrelieved by rest. These effects can last after other FLS abate in part because of the muscle exertion generated when a patient has chills and rigors. Rigors and chills require a large consumption of energy and oxygen. Coupled with vasoconstriction, unnecessary demands are placed on myocardial tissue, so rigors and chills need to be controlled to avoid unnecessary cardiac stress (Cuaron and Thompson 2001; Shelton 2001; Battiato and Wheeler 2000).

Administration of antipyretics and non-steroidal anti-inflammatory agents prior to IFN-α is beneficial (Shelton 2001; Tretter et al. 2000; Kiley and Gale 1998; Sandstrom 1996; Skalla 1996). Giving IFN-α at bedtime may be helpful to some patients, allowing them to sleep through side effects; however, it may disrupt sleeping patterns for others (Donnelly 1998; Baron et al. 1991). A better time to administer IFN-α for these patients would be dinner time (around 6 pm) because this allows for the worst of the initial side effects to subside prior to bedtime. If fevers persist for more than 8 hours and are unrelieved by antipyretics, the presence of infection needs to be evaluated (Kiley and Gale 1998).

Cutaneous Reactions

Although flu-like symptoms are some of the most common side effects, cutaneous reactions of varying degrees have also been associated with IFN-α therapy. Alopecia, pruritus, rash, skin dryness and itching, erythema, exacerbations of herpes labialis, cutaneous vascular lesions, xerostomia, and injection site reactions have all been reported (Stafford-Fox and Guindon 2000; Asnis and Gaspari 1995; Toyofuku et al. 1994; Quesada et al. 1986). Asnis and Gaspari (1995) indicate that psoriasis can be exacerbated with IFN-α therapy. Treatment varies depending on the severity but may include observation or administration of topical, oral, or parenteral medication. Patients should be taught how to rotate injection sites to avoid injection site necrosis and either warm or cold compresses can be applied depending on which feels better to the patient. Diphenhydramine may be helpful in reducing itching, but the sedating effects must be considered (Stafford-Fox and Guindon 2000).

Systemic steroids, such as prednisone, have been shown to block some antiviral activity of IFN. Therefore systemic steroids should be avoided for patients on IFN-α. IFN-α therapy may cause severe cutaneous reactions in some instances, necessitating holding therapy (Stafford-Fox and Guindon 2000; Tretter et al. 2000).

Other strategies are similar to those suggested for IL-2 including using mild soaps; using lotions, creams, or ointments frequently; and encouraging adequate oral hydration. It is imperative that patients use a strong sunscreen with a SPF 15 or greater, wear hats with broad brims, and cover exposed skin because photosensitivity has been reported (Stafford-Fox and Guindon 2000; Donnelly 1998; Sandstrom 1996; Skalla 1996).

Periodic assessment of injection sites and administration techniques may be useful. Smaller gauge needles, room temperature solution, and slow injection of drug help alleviate injection site reactions. Other nursing considerations include ensuring that the injections are SC and not intradermal and that the correct dose and volume are being administered (Stafford-Fox and Guindon 2000).

Anorexia and Altered Taste Sensations

Weight loss from anorexia is not uncommon because of the duration of therapy. Anorexia occurs in 43% to 69% of patients receiving higher doses of IFN-α (Cuaron and Thompson 2001). IFN induces secondary cytokines, such as TNF-α, which may be a factor in anorexia because cytokines are known to alter protein, carbohydrate, and lipid metabolism. TNF-α is also a cachetin responsible for increased muscle catabolism and lipolysis (Cuaron and Thompson 2001).

Depression impacts appetite and nutritional status and is a common symptom in patients with cancer, and depression has been reported to occur in up to 40% of patients on IFN-α-2b. Some symptoms of depression include decrease in appetite and weight loss (Cuaron and Thompson 2001).

Taste alterations range from decreased taste to salty, bitter, or metallic taste to intolerance of sweets (Sandstrom 1996). Patients report that certain foods or beverages they enjoyed prior to IFN-α therapy are no longer appealing during therapy. A registered dietician (RD) is helpful in assisting patients to ingest adequate calories. Interventions include small, frequent meals, premade meals, exercise prior to eating, and eating at cafeteria-style restaurants where patients can choose what they are hungry for at that moment. A food diary assists the RD in evaluation of caloric intake and a breakdown of those calories. Evaluation of adequate calories from protein, carbohydrates, and fat allow the RD to make suggestions to maximize calories and maintain weight (Stafford-Fox and Guindon 2000; Donnelly 1998; Kiley and Gale 1998; Sandstrom 1996; Skalla 1996).

Neurologic Symptoms

The most common neurologic symptoms reported with IFN-α include mental fatigue, confusion, lack of concentration, memory problems, and depression. Patients also complain of lack of motivation, anxiety, sleep disturbances, and decreased libido. With higher doses, there are pronounced toxicities that occur including lethargy, somnolence, behavior changes, irritability, and confusion (Cuaron and Thompson 2001; Kiley and Gale 1998; Sandstrom 1996).

Several mechanisms help explain these neurologic toxicities. Potential contributory causes result from IFN-α, secondary cytokines, or both acting directly on the brain, inducing alterations in mood and cognition. Cytokine administration alters the production of neuroendocrine hormones, resulting in increased levels of cortisol, adrenocorticotrophic hormone (ACTH), and β-endorphin. IFNs are structurally similar to ACTH and β-endorphin and share a common signaling pathway. IFNs induce the production of other cytokines, such as IL-1 and TNF, which cross the blood-brain barrier and mimic neurologic changes seen in patients in septic shock (Cuaron and Thompson 2001; Atkins et al. 1986).

Close observation of patients' behavior, mood, and mental status is imperative. IFN-α has been associated with depression and suicidal behavior including suicidal ideation, suicide attempts, and suicide (INTRON-A 2002). Education of the family and patient help identify mental status changes early so that interventions are not delayed. Interventions include the use of antidepressants, dose delays or reduction, and referral to a psychiatrist. Other interventions include short-term administration of antianxiety agents such as lorazepam, the use of guided imagery, relaxation techniques, and participation in support groups (Kiley and Gale 1998; Donnelly 1998; Cuaron and Thompson 2001).

Supportive Care: Hematopoietic Growth Factors

Hematopoietic growth factors (HGF) are biologic agents used for supportive care with myelosuppressive chemotherapy or bone marrow transplantation in cancer. They are not primary anticancer treatments. Chemotherapy agents induce neutropenia, thrombocytopenia, and anemia, which can adversely affect quality of life. The myelosuppressive nature of chemotherapy can negatively affect patient outcomes by causing dose reductions, interruptions of treatment regimens, life-threatening sequelae, and problematic side effects. HGFs accelerate engraftment after autologous bone marrow transplant (BMT) and are used for patients with delayed engraftment following allogeneic BMT. HGFs mobilize the release of bone marrow stem cells into peripheral circulation where they are collected without difficulty (Battiato and Wheeler 2000; Wujcik 2001; Ozer 2001). Current FDA-approved HGFs, indications, and side effects can be found in Table 4.9.

Hematopoiesis

Hematopoiesis (Figure 4.1) or blood cell production occurs primarily in the bone marrow of the flat and long bones of the skeleton. The development of hematopoietic cells begins with the pleuripotent stem cell and terminates with mature cells that enter the circulation and tissue to perform their distinctive function. A single stem cell has the unique ability to self-replicate and differentiate into any of the hematopoietic cells. These activities occur in response to the need for certain cells to maintain homeostasis. Each cell line includes a variety of steps involving production of a series of immature cells prior to the functional mature cell (Naeim 1998; Emerson 1998; Wujcik 2001).

There are two major cell lineages that the stem cell designates: myeloid and lymphoid. The myeloid linage creates two categories of white blood cells (WBC), the granulocytes and agranulocytes, and the red blood cells (erythrocytes) and platelets (megakaryocytes). The lymphoid linage creates the B and T lymphocytes and megakaryocytes (Battiato and Wheeler 2000; Wujcik 2001).

The granulocytes (neutrophils, eosinophils, and basophils) provide the main defense against bacterial infection and have a life span of only a few hours. Neutrophils are mature WBCs and comprise 50% to 70% of the total WBC count. Because there are about three times as many neutrophils in the bone marrow as there are circulating

neutrophils, a stash of neutrophils is always available as bands. These immature cells are seen in the circulation in small quantities unless the demand is increased, at which point a high band count may be seen as the marrow works to meet the demand. Neutrophils are the first cells on the scene of any injury (Naeim 1998; Emerson 1998; Wujcik 2001).

Another granulocyte, eosinophils, constitutes 4% of the total WBC count. These cells ingest bacteria and release chemicals that modify the inflammatory response. Eosinophils are usually elevated in patients with parasitic infections and patients experiencing allergic reactions.

Basophils, the third granulocyte, release substances such as histamine and heparin in response to a stimulating factor, thus contributing to hypersensitivity reactions. Basophils comprise 0.05% of the WBC count and increase in patients with asthma, allergies, and some cancers (Naeim 1998; Wujcik 2001).

Two additional cells produced from the myeloid precursor are erythrocytes, or red blood cells (RBCs), and the megakaryocytes, or platelets. Erythrocytes transport oxygen via the hemoglobin molecule to the tissues and move carbon dioxide from tissue to the lungs. The immature erythrocyte, the reticulocyte, is circulating in small quantitites as the production of erythrocytes is managed by the bone marrow. However, when there is an increased need for RBCs by the body (e.g., hemorrhage) the production of reticulocytes increases to meet the demand for additional erythrocytes to reestablish homeostasis. The megakaryocytes are the mature cells that have the ability to release platelets into the circulation. Platelets aid the body in clotting. This clotting action is the first-line defense in tissue damage and is necessary to stop bleeding and allow the clotting cascade to complete the process of clot development and healing (Naeim 1998).

The agranulocytes include the monocytes and macrophages. When monocytes are mature, they are released into the blood stream and circulate for 1 to 3 days. Once monocytes enter tissues, they

TABLE 4.9 FDA-Approved Hematopoietic Growth Factors

Growth Factor (Generic/ Trade Name)	Indications and Route	Side Effects	Nursing Implications
G-CSF, Filgrastim (Neupogen; Amgen, Inc.)	■ Decrease the incidence of infection in patients receiving myelosuppressive chemotherapy with nonmyeloid malignancies ■ After induction or consolidation chemotherapy to decrease time of neutophil recovery in adult patients with AML ■ Reduce neutropenia and neutropenia-related side effects in nonmyeloid malignancies after myelosuppressive chemotherapy and BMT ■ Mobilization of hematopoietic progenitor cells for collection via leukapheresis ■ Chronic administration to reduce incidence and duration of neutropenia sequelae in symptomatic patients with congenital neutropenia, cyclic neutropenia, or idiopathic neutropenia **Route of administration:** SC, IV	■ Mild to moderate bone pain in areas with high bone marrow reserve, usually 2 to 3 days after initiation of therapy and prior to neutrophil recovery ■ Transient increases in liver function tests ■ Occasionally, pain at injection site ■ Rarely, allergic reactions including rash, urticaria, facial edema, dyspnea, hypotension, tachycardia ■ Nausea and vomiting ■ Pain during injection ■ Rarely, splenic rupture	■ Administer nonnarcotic analgesics as needed ■ Prior to injection, warm medication to room temperature and inject slowly to minimize pain with injection ■ CBC with differential and platelet counts at baseline and at regular intervals during therapy with filgrastim ■ Instruct patient regarding side effects ■ Assess for complaints of left upper abdominal or shoulder tip pain because this could be a sign of splenomegaly or splenic rupture ■ Teach patient self-injection technique and proper disposal of needles if to be self-administered
GM-CSF, Sargramostim (Leukine; Berlex)	■ After induction chemotherapy in older adults with AML	■ Bone pain ■ Flu-like symptoms including flushing, rigors,	■ Instruct patient regarding side effects ■ Monitor CBC with differential and platelets, reticulocyte count at baseline, then twice weekly

- Mobilization of hematopoietic progenitor cells into peripheral circulation for collection via leukapheresis
- Accelerate bone marrow recovery after BMT
- Delayed or failed engraftment after BMT
- **Route of administration:** SC, IV

- myalgias, arthalgias
- Dose-related fluid retention
- "First dose reaction" with first IV administration includes flushing, hypotension, transient hypoxia, and tachycardia
- Dyspnea

- Monitor liver enzymes, bilirubin, and creatinine in patients with preexisting renal dysfunction and/or hepatic dysfunction
- Use with caution in patients with preexisting fluid retention, pulmonary infiltrates, or CHF
- Assess for presence of pleural and/or pericardial effusions; fluid retention may worsen these conditions
- Reduce rate of infusion by half if patient experiences dyspnea; stop infusion if respiratory symptoms worsen
- Assess for preexisting cardiac condition
- Teach patient self-injection technique and proper disposal of needles if to be self-administered

Pegfilgrastim (Neulasta; Amgen, Inc.)

- Decrease incidence of febrile neutropenia and infection in patients with nonmyeloid malignancies receiving myelosuppressive chemotherapy
- **Route of administration:** SC

- Bone pain
- Fatigue
- Alopecia
- Diarrhea
- Nausea and vomiting
- Constipation
- Reversible elevations in LDH, alkaline phosphatase, and uric acid
- Splenic rupture has been reported with parent compound, filgrastim

- Administer nonnarcotic analgesics as needed
- Baseline CBC with differential and platelet count and at regular intervals
- Instruct patient regarding side effects
- Assess for complaints of left upper abdominal or shoulder tip pain because this could be a sign of splenomegaly or splenic rupture
- Do not administer between 14 days before and 24 hours after chemotherapy because of the possibility of increased sensitivity of rapidly dividing myeloid cells to cytotoxic chemotherapy
- Teach patient self-injection technique and proper disposal of needles if to be self-administered

Epoetin alfa (Procrit, Ortho Biotech, Inc.; Epogen, Amgen, Inc.)

- Anemia in patients with chronic renal failure
- Anemia related to zidovudine therapy in HIV-infected persons
- Anemia related to chemotherapy in patients with nonmyeloid malignancies
- Anemic patients scheduled for elective, noncardiac,

- Pain at injection site
- Fever
- Diarrhea
- Nausea
- Vomiting
- Edema
- Asthenia
- Fatigue
- Dyspnea
- Headache
- Arthalgias

- Instruct patient regarding side effects including signs/ symptoms of hypertension
- Teach patient self-injection technique and proper disposal of needles if to be self-administered

Baseline Assessment
- Obtain CBC
- Obtain iron deficiency test
- Evaluate for source of blood loss or other causes of anemia such as infection, underlying hematologic disease, and hemolysis

(Continued)

TABLE 4.9 (Continued)

Growth Factor (Generic/Trade Name)	Indications and Route	Side Effects	Nursing Implications
	nonvascular surgery to minimize need for blood transfusions **Route of administration:** SC, IV	■ Hypertension ■ Thrombotic events ■ Seizures (rare) **Contraindications:** ■ Uncontrolled hypertension ■ Hypersensitivity to mammalian cell-derived products ■ Hypersensitivity to human albumin	■ Vital signs including BP ■ QOL assessment **Assessment During Therapy** ■ Obtain weekly CBC, reticulocyte count ■ Monitor BP ■ Assess for injection site reaction ■ Assess for changes in QOL ■ Assess for other causes of anemia if no response to treatment after 6 weeks of treatment
Darbepoetin alfa (Aranesp; Amgen, Inc.)	■ Chemotherapy-induced anemia in patients with nonmyeloid malignancies ■ Anemia in patients with chronic renal failure **Route of administration:** SC, IV	■ Fatigue ■ Edema ■ Fever ■ Dizziness ■ Headache ■ Diarrhea ■ Constipation ■ Arthalgias ■ Hypertension ■ Injection site pain ■ Seizures (rare) **Contraindications:** ■ Uncontrolled hypertension ■ Hypersensitivity to epoetin alfa	■ Obtain baseline CBC ■ Obtain weekly hemoglobin levels until hemoglobin has stabilized, then obtain at regular intervals ■ Assess iron levels at baseline and periodically ■ Obtain baseline VS including BP, then monitor weekly BP ■ Assess baseline QOL and QOL as hemoglobin rises ■ Evaluate for source of blood loss or other causes of anemia such as infection, underlying hematologic disease and hemolysis ■ Instruct patient regarding side effects including signs/symptoms of hypertension ■ Teach patient self-injection technique and proper disposal of needles if to be self-administered ■ Assess for other causes of anemia if no response to treatment after 6 weeks of treatment

| Interleukin-11 Oprelvekin (Neumega; Wyeth Pharmaceuticals) | Prevention of severe thrombocytopenia and reduced need for platelet transfusions in patients with nonmyeloid malignancies after myelosuppressive chemotherapy

Route of administration: SC | Edema
Dyspnea
Tachycardia
Conjunctival redness/blurry vision
Palpitations
Pleural effusion
Atrial fibrillation/flutter
Decreased hemoglobin | Obtain baseline CBC with platelet count and then at regular intervals
Monitor platelet counts through expected nadir until adequate platelet recovery has occurred
Assess for risk factors including:
  History of atrial arrhythmias
  Cardiovascular disease
  Advanced age
  Diabetes mellitus
  Hypertension
Monitor for fluid retention including lungs for crackles and for peripheral edema
Instruct patient to weigh self weekly and report a 2-kg weight gain
Give diuretics as needed
Monitor fluid and electrolyte status with diuretics
Instruct patient to report shortness of breath and swelling in extremities
Monitor cardiac status
Instruct patient to report rapid heartbeat, chest discomfort, palpitations
Assess patient for signs/symptoms of anemia including fatigue
Assess for eye irritation or discomfort
Instruct patient to report eye redness and dryness
Use for need of artificial tears
Teach patient self-injection technique and proper disposal of needles if to be self-administered |

AML, acute myeloid leukemia; CBC, complete blood cell count; BMT, bone marrow transplantation; CHF, congestive heart failure; BP, blood pressure; QOL, quality of life; VS, vital signs

Sources: Neupogen (filgrastim) prescribing information 2002; Leukine (sargramostim) prescribing information 2002; Neulasta (pegfilgrastim) prescribing information 2002; EPOGEN (epoetin alfa) prescribing information 2003; Procrit (epoetin alfa) prescribing information 2002; Aranesp (darbepoetin alfa) prescribing information, 2002; Neumega (oprelvekin) prescribing information 2003; Rust *et al.* 1999; Battiato and Wheeler 2000; Wujcik 2001; Rieger and Haeuber 1995.

become macrophages providing nonspecific immunity against foreign invaders such as parasites, protozoa, and fungus. Monocyte levels make up 6% to 8% of the total WBC count. Macrophages reside in all body tissues such as the Kupffer cells in the liver and histiocytes in connective tissues (Wujcik 2001; Hyde 1992).

The second linage of cells is the lymphoid B and T lymphocytes and megakaryocytes (Battiato and Wheeler 2000; Wujcik 2001). Lymphocytes comprise 30% to 35% of the total WBC count. The pleuripotent stem cell gives rise to the lymphoid stem cell and differentiates into either T lymphocyte or B lymphocyte. T lymphocytes provide cellular immunity and produce cytokines that mediate a specific immune reaction in response to stimulation by specific antigens. T lymphocytes are comprised of subsets of T-helper cells, T-cytotoxic cells, T-memory cells, and T-suppressor cells, and each has its own function. B lymphocytes provide humoral immunity, responding to antigen-antibody binding on the cell surface membrane. B cells mature into either plasma cells or memory B cells. When stimulated, B lymphocytes secrete antibodies in response to antigen stimulation. Although B cells produce antibodies, the majority of production is by the plasma cell. Humoral and cell-mediated responses work together to fight pathogenic organisms (Wujcik 2001; Hyde 1992).

Hematopoiesis and HGFs

Hematopoiesis is regulated by HGFs via a complex feedback system. Stem cells die without differentiating if maintained in a nutritive environment only. To support the process of renewal, stem cells must be maintained closely with non-hematopoietic mesenchymal cells, which are called stromal cells. Stromal cells line the surfaces in the bone marrow cavity. Stromal cells consist of fibroblasts, endothelial cells, osteoblasts, and adipocytes. These cells provide HGF and membrane-bound attachment molecules that are required for hematopoietic cell regulation and differentiation (Emerson 1998; Wujcik 2001).

Hematopoietic progenitor cells, or stem cells, respond to growth factors. Hematopoietic stem cell division and differentiation is influenced by several growth factors. These growth factors are a class of glycoproteins that are produced in sequence. Initially, certain colony-stimulating factors (CSF) are produced by small amounts of granulocyte-macrophage colony-stimulating factor (GM-CSF), stem cell factor (SCF), IL-6, and Flt-3 ligand produced by the stromal cells in response to plasma protein stimulation. It is this adaptive production of these CSFs that maintains blood counts in the normal range. For example, CSFs have the ability to repopulate the bone marrow after myelosuppressive therapy and maintain hematopoiesis. CSF secretion is greatly increased in response to infection. Bacterial and viral products activate monocytes, which secrete IL-1, tumor necrosis factor alpha (TNF-α), granulocyte colony-stimulating factor (G-CSF), and macrophage colony-stimulating factor (M-CSF). Therefore, HGFs stimulate cell division and maturation in an organized fashion. Some HGFs affect cell differentiation and proliferation at the progenitor level, whereas other HGFs influence specifically the precursor and mature cells (Emerson 1998; Naeim 1998; Wujcik 2001).

FDA-Approved Growth Factors in Clinical Use

Granulocyte Colony-Stimulating Factor (G-CSF): Filgrastim (Neupogen; Neulasta)

G-CSF is a potent regulator of neutrophil recovery in the bone marrow. G-CSF is a single lineage HGF promoting the differentiation, proliferation, and activation of mature neutrophils from the PSC. G-CSF increases the neutrophils' ability to fight infection (Battiato and Wheeler 2000; Ozer and Tfayli 2002).

Filgrastim (Neupogen), a recombinant form of G-CSF, was approved to treat patients with non-myeloid malignances receiving myelosuppressive chemotherapy to enhance neutrophil recovery and prophylaxis against febrile neutropenia. It has

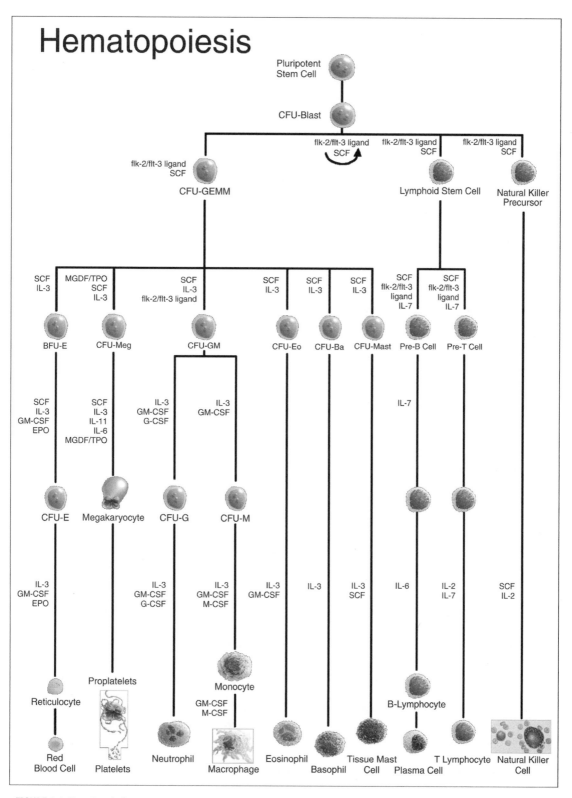

FIGURE 4.1 Hematopoiesis.

Source: Reprinted with permission from Amgen, Inc., copyright 2000, Thousand Oaks, CA.

been shown to shorten the duration of neutropenia, decrease the incidence of febrile neutropenia, and decrease the number of hospital days for patients receiving chemotherapy. The American Society of Clinical Oncology (ASCO) published evidence-based practice guidelines for the use of G-CSF (Ozer *et al*. 2000). ASCO recommends that primary administration of CSFs be reserved for patients receiving myelosuppressive chemotherapy, in whom the expected incidence of febrile neutropenia is $\geq$ 40%. ASCO cites special circumstances where patients receiving less myelosuppressive chemotherapy may benefit from CSF administration if they are at risk of developing chemotherapy-induced infectious complications. Some of these special populations include patients with preexisting neutropenia from disease, extensive prior chemotherapy, previous irradiation to the pelvis or other high bone marrow–containing areas, or a history of recurrent febrile neutropenia while receiving previous chemotherapy (Ozer *et al*. 2000).

Crawford *et al*. (2004) report that CSF is not as effective in preventing infectious complications in afebrile neutropenic patients as it is when used for prophylaxis. This is in concurrence with ASCO guidelines (Ozer *et al*. 2000). Crawford *et al*. (2004) cite a retrospective analysis showing a widespread practice of CSF administration initiation 5 days or more after the patient started chemotherapy. Additionally, CSF was not started until days 1 to 14, the expected time of ANC nadir, in 32% of patients.

Another FDA-approved indication for G-CSF includes mobilization of peripheral-blood stem cells (PBSC) in patients undergoing bone marrow transplant (BMT) both to increase the amount of PBSC collected via leukapheresis for use in PBSC transplantation and to hasten neutrophil recovery after transplantation. G-CSF is approved for adult patients undergoing induction or consolidation chemotherapy who have acute myelogenous leukemia (AML). Use of G-CSF has not been associated with increased leukemic growth or with a negative impact on remission rate or survival in adults with AML (Sylvester 2002; Battiato and Wheeler 2000; Ozer *et al*. 2000; Neupogen [filgrastim] prescribing information 2002). G-CSF is also approved for use in patients with congenital, cyclic, and idiopathic neutropenia. The most common side effect is mild to moderate bone pain, which is caused when the WBC proliferate (Battiato and Wheeler 2000; Wujcik 2001; Neupogen [filgrastim] prescribing information 2002).

The recommended time to start filgrastim is 24 hours after chemotherapy is initiated, and treatment should continue daily for up to 2 weeks until the ANC reaches 10,000/μl after the expected chemotherapy-induced neutrophil nadir. The ASCO recommended dose for G-CSF is 5 μg/kg/day in adults for all clinical settings other than PBSC stimulation. The recommended dose for PBSC stimulation is 10 μg/kg/day. G-CSF is administered either SC or IV (Neupogen [filgrastim] prescribing information 2002; Ozer *et al*. 2000).

A new form of G-CSF, Pegfilgrastim, is the pegylated form of filgrastim that has recently become available. Pegfilgrastim (Neulasta), a long-acting form of filgrastim, consists of a 20-kD polyethylene glycol (PEG) molecule attached to one end of the filgrastim protein. The pegylated form extends the half-life of filgrastim, decreasing the need for frequent injections. A single 6-mg SC injection of pegfilgrastim given once per cycle of chemotherapy is sufficient to prevent chemotherapy-induced neutropenia in adults (Neulasta [pegfilgrastim] prescribing information 2002). Pegfilgrastim reduces renal clearance and self-regulates for neutrophil-mediated clearance, allowing the drug to remain in the blood throughout the neutropenic period and then be cleared rapidly when neutrophils recover toward normal levels. As the ANC rises, pegfilgrastim clears the body (Holmes *et al*. 2002; Neulasta [pegfilgrastim] prescribing information 2002). The most common side effect is mild-to-moderate medullary bone pain similar to that experienced with filgrastim (Neulasta [pegfilgrastim] prescribing information 2002).

Granulocyte-Macrophage Colony-Stimulating Factor (GM-CSF): Sargramostim (Leukine)

GM-CSF is a multilineage growth factor affecting neutrophils, eosinophils, macrophages, and occasionally lymphocytes (Ozer and Tfayli 2002; Battiato and Wheeler 2000; Emerson 1998). Additionally, GM-CSF affects the immune system by enhancing effector cell activity in antigen presentation and cell-mediated immunity (Battiato and Wheeler 2000).

Sargramostim was initially FDA approved in 1991 for use in patients with non-Hodgkin's lymphoma, acute lymphoblastic leukemia, and Hodgkin's disease undergoing autologous BMT to accelerate myeloid engraftment. It has since received approval for the following indications: allogeneic or autologous BMT when engraftment is delayed or has failed; in older adults with AML after induction chemotherapy to reduce time of neutrophil recovery and in the incidence of severe/life-threatening infections; to accelerate myeloid recovery in patients undergoing allogeneic BMT from human-leukocyte antigen (HLA)–matched related donors; and to mobilize hematopoietic progenitor cells into peripheral circulation for collection via leukapheresis for PBSC transplant or BMT (Battiato and Wheeler 2000; Wujcik 2001; Sylvester 2002). Both sargramostim and filgrastim are accepted therapies for AIDs-associated neutropenia, drug-induced neutropenia, and myelodysplastic syndromes (MDS) complicated by infection (Sylvester 2002).

Side effects include fever, lethargy, myalgias, bone pain, anorexia, injection site redness, dose-related fluid retention, and rash. A reaction with the first dose may be seen and includes flushing, tachycardia, hypotension, dyspnea, nausea, and vomiting. Sargramostim is administered either SC or IV (Wujcik 2001; Battiato and Wheeler 2000; Leukine [sargramostim] prescribing information 2002).

Erythropoietin (Epogen, Procrit, Aranesp)

Erythropoietin is the major regulator of erythropoiesis or red blood cell production. Erythropoietin is a hormone synthesized primarily by peritubular cells in the kidney, and its production increases with hypoxia. Endogenous erythropoietin may be suppressed in patients with cancer for a variety of reasons including as a result of inflammatory cytokines, such as IL-1, IFN-γ, and TNF, that may suppress erythropoiesis and erythropoietin production. The suppression of erythropoietin production, cancer chemotherapy, and the inhibitory effects of cancer and cytokines on erythropoiesis contribute to cancer-related anemia (Crawford 2002a; Libretto et al. 2001; Battiato and Wheeler 2000).

Administration of recombinant erythropoietin relieves anemia and is produced by both Amgen (Epogen) and Ortho Biotech (Procrit). It is FDA approved for treatment of anemia caused by myelosuppressive chemotherapy in patients with non-myeloid malignancies, for anemia associated with chronic renal failure, for zidovudine (AZT)-induced anemia in HIV-infected persons, and for anemia in surgical patients to reduce the need for allogeneic transfusions. Recombinant erythropoietin increases hemoglobin levels and reduces the need for transfusions in patients receiving chemotherapy. ASCO published evidence-based guidelines for use of recombinant erythropoietin, recommending it when the hemoglobin concentration declines to ≤ 10 g/dl. The ASCO guidelines suggest that recombinant erythropoietin be administered in patients with declining hemoglobin levels of < 12 but > 10 g/dl based on clinical circumstances (Rizzo et al. 2002). Recombinant erythropoietin is not indicated in patients whose anemia is caused by other etiologies such as folate or iron deficiency, hemolysis, or gastrointestinal bleeding; therefore, other sources for anemia need to be ruled out prior to initiating this therapy (Crawford 2002a; Rizzo et al. 2002; Battiato and Wheeler 2000; Wujcik 2001).

The FDA-recommended dose of recombinant erythropoietin is 150 IU/kg SC three times per week for cancer patients receiving chemotherapy. It is usually administered IV in patients on dialysis. If the hematocrit does not increase by 5% or

6% after 4 weeks of therapy and iron levels are adequate, the dose is increased to 300 IU/kg. For hematocrit increases of more than 4% in a 2-week period or if the hematocrit is approaching 36%, the frequency of administration is decreased to twice weekly (Wujcik 2001; efacts Drug Comparison 2004). ASCO guidelines recommend hemoglobin levels be increased to close to 12 g/dl, and then recombinant erythropoietin should be titrated to maintain that level (Rizzo et al. 2002). Side effects include hypertension, flu-like symptoms, and injection site reactions (Wujcik 2001; efacts Drug Comparison 2004).

A new long-acting form of recombinant erythropoietin is darbepoetin alfa (Aranesp). The increased in vivo activity of darbepoetin alfa compared with epoetin alfa can be attributed to two additional N-linked carbohydrate chains. Darbepoetin alfa binds to the same receptor as recombinant erythropoietin and stimulates erythropoiesis by the same mechanism as endogenous erythropoietin. The increased sialic acid–containing carbohydrate content of darbepoetin alfa results in a longer serum half-life of approximately threefold. For this reason, it can be administered less frequently than the original forms of recombinant erythropoietin (Aranesp [darbepoetin alfa] prescribing information 2002; Joy 2002).

Darbepoetin alfa is indicated for treatment of anemia associated with chronic renal failure and in cancer patients with nonmyeloid malignancies with chemotherapy-induced anemia. The recommended starting dose for cancer patients receiving chemotherapy is 2.25 μg/kg SC weekly. If the increase in hemoglobin is less than 1.0 g/dl after 6 weeks of therapy, darbepoetin alfa should be increased to 4.5 μg/kg. If hemoglobin increases by more than 1.0 g/dl in 2 weeks or if the hemoglobin is greater than 12 g/dl, the dose should be reduced by 25% (Aranesp [darbepoetin alfa] prescribing information 2002; Joy 2002). An alternative regimen is described by the US Oncology Network and is based on a multicenter review of medical records of patients who were either on recombinant erythropoietin and switched to darbepoietin alfa or who had not recently been treated with recombinant erythropoietin but were started with darbepoietin alfa. The US Oncology Network concluded that a starting dose of 200 μg SC given every 2 weeks is effective in treating chemotherapy-induced anemia (Thames et al. 2004).

The positive effect of recombinant erythropoietin on quality of life (QOL) is well documented. Crawford (2002b) and Itri (2002) reviewed the results of three trials with a combined database of more than 7,000 patients. These trials defined the impact of hemoglobin level on QOL. All patients received recombinant erythropoietin and reported significant improvements in symptoms of energy, activities of daily living, and overall QOL when the hemoglobin improved to > 2 g/dl or reached ≥ 12 g/dl. Iconomou et al. (2003) conducted a prospective, single-center, randomized trial of erythropoietin versus placebo in cancer patients with solid tumors (n = 122). The primary end point was QOL. Hemoglobin levels were significantly increased in the recombinant erythropoietin arm at week 12. The authors concluded that patients treated with recombinant erythropoietin reported statistically significant improvements in levels of fatigue, higher energy levels, and an enhanced overall sense of well-being. This trial showed a positive and statistically significant association between the magnitude of the increase of hemoglobin levels and the extent of improvement in QOL. These results correlate with the results from the three previously mentioned studies. To add to the clinical trial knowledge, a series of 12 case studies reported by Libretto et al. (2001) describe QOL in patients with solid tumors and hematologic malignancies receiving epoetin alfa. Of particular interest in this series was the impact of anemia on levels of fatigue. Patients universally described feelings of fatigue, lethargy, and being "washed out." They reported that they lacked motivation for social activities and activities of daily living, leading to frustration, irritability, and depression. As patients' hemoglobin levels increased to clinically acceptable levels while receiving recombinant erythropoietin, patients reported feelings of less fatigue and renewed energy.

Oprelvekin (IL-11; Neumega)

Oprelvekin, or IL-11, is a thrombopoietic growth factor that stimulates megakaryocyte progenitor cells, inducing megakaryocyte maturation that results in increased platelet production. IL-11 is indicated for prevention of severe thrombocytopenia and reduced need for platelet transfusions after myelosuppressive chemotherapy in adults with nonmyeloid malignancies who are at a high risk of developing severe thrombocytopenia. In clinical studies, IL-11 showed no effect on platelet function, including platelet aggregation and platelet reactivity. IL-11 was not associated with significant changes in prothrombin time or partial thromboplastin time (Reynolds 2000).

The recommended dose of oprelvekin is 50 μg/kg/day SC 6 to 24 hours after completion of chemotherapy. It is recommended that dosing should be continued until the postnadir platelet count is $\geq 50,000/\mu l$. When reconstituted, oprelvekin should be used within 3 hours. Complete blood counts, including platelet counts, should be evaluated prior to starting chemotherapy and then periodically throughout the expected nadir (Neumega [oprelvekin] prescribing information 2003; Wujcik 2001; Reynolds 2000; Rust et al. 1999). To date it is the only available platelet growth factor on the market (Reynolds 2000).

The most common side effects with IL-11 include edema, dyspnea, tachycardia, and conjunctival redness. Other side effects include atrial arrhythmias, palpitations, and pleural effusions. These are mostly mild to moderate in severity and related to fluid retention. The fluid retention is not affiliated with capillary leak syndrome, as are other biologics such as IL-2. Rather, it is related to an increase in plasma volume secondary to sodium retention. Patients may experience fatigue while taking IL-11, and transient anemia has been observed because of plasma volume shift. Prior to starting oprelvekin, patients should be evaluated for cardiovascular disease, a history of atrial arrhythmias, advanced age, diabetes, and hypertension. Patients should be monitored for fluid retention during therapy (Rust et al. 1999; Reynolds 2000).

Use of Growth Factors in the Elderly

As our aging population increases, so does the risk of cancer. About 80% of all cancers occur in persons over 60 years of age. Multiple genetic mutations occur over many years, changing normal cells into malignant cells. Several factors contribute to this transformation, including increased exposures to carcinogens and the deterioration of host defenses with age. The most common dose-limiting toxicity with systemic chemotherapy is myelosuppression, and this is of particular importance with older persons because the functional reserve of bone marrow and other organs diminishes with age. For these reasons and others, older patients are often undertreated with chemotherapy. Growth factor support can reduce the risk of infectious complications from chemotherapy in older adults (Lyman et al. 2003; Balducci and Carreca 2002; Repetto et al. 2003; Hood 2003).

Balducci and Carreca (2002) and Repetto et al. (2003) report that better outcomes in elderly patients can be achieved when chemotherapy dose-intensity is maintained. However, older patients are at a greater risk of chemotherapy-related toxicities, particularly hematologic toxicities and mucositis, than younger patients. Comorbid conditions, such as diabetes, hypertension, and coronary artery disease, also contribute to the impact of chemotherapy-induced toxicities. The risk of febrile neutropenia increases with age and may be greatest during the first cycle of chemotherapy. Febrile neutropenia in the elderly leads to serious complications including sepsis and death (Lyman et al. 2003; Balducci and Carreca 2002; Repetto et al. 2003; Hood 2003).

The prophylactic use of filgrastim or pegfilgrastim in elderly cancer patients is recommended starting with the first cycle of chemotherapy to reduce the risk of febrile neutropenia, infection, and complications of infection associated with chemotherapy. This recommendation is substantiated by studies of patients with non-Hodgkin's lymphoma, a common malignancy in patients > 65 years of age, who were treated with G-CSF during the first cycle of chemotherapy. The incidence, severity, and duration of neutropenia were decreased in these patients. Additionally, elderly patients, particularly those ≥ 70 years, fall into the "special circumstances" category of the ASCO guidelines for using HGF because these patients are at a greater risk of developing neutropenia (Lyman *et al.* 2003; Balducci and Carreca 2002; Repetto *et al.* 2003; Hood 2003; Ozer *et al.* 2000; Ozer 2001).

The risk of neutropenic infection and death in older individuals is highest during the first cycle of chemotherapy. Chemotherapy dose-intensity can be maintained with use of prophylactic G-CSF, and maintenance of dose-intensity is affiliated with better clinical outcomes in older patients. Cost benefits from using growth factors in elderly patients include prevention of hospitalization for neutropenic infection and complications (Lyman *et al.* 2003; Balducci and Carreca 2002; Repetto *et al.* 2003; Hood 2003).

Experimental Therapies

The field of biologic therapy changes rapidly. New experimental agents enter clinical trials on a regular basis. This next section provides an overview of two promising experimental therapies: cancer vaccines and the adoptive transfer of cells.

Cancer Vaccines

Vaccination is the administration of an agent that stimulates the immune system to react against the foreign substances of the vaccine. These foreign substances are known as antigens. The expectation is that the immunized person will develop immunity so subsequent exposures to the antigen will cause the immune system to destroy the antigen. Examples of successful vaccines include polio and smallpox vaccines (Muehlbauer and Schwartzentruber 2003; Siemens and Ratliff 2001; Kinzler and Brown 2001; Restifo 2000).

Cancer vaccines differ from traditional or preventive vaccines in that they are considered therapeutic but not preventive. An argument can be made that preventive cancer vaccines do exist, but these are vaccines that are already in use to prevent the carcinogen. Vaccines that can be considered prophylactic include vaccination against human papilloma virus, which has been linked to cervical cancer, and vaccination against hepatitis, which can lead to liver cancer (King 2004; Muehlbauer and Schwartzentruber 2003; Restifo 2000; Mitchell 2002; Lowy and Schiller 1998; Matzku and Zoller 2001).

The goal of cancer vaccines is to mobilize the immune system into attacking existing cancer cells. This is done by targeting tumor-associated antigens (TAA). TAAs are structures that are present on tumor cells but absent or only minimally present on normal cells. These TAAs can be proteins, enzymes, or carbohydrates, and they provide a target for immune system recognition and destruction (Siemens and Ratliff 2001; Kinzler and Brown 2001; Matzku and Zoller 2001; Schreiber 1999). TAAs are divided into different categories, which are outlined in Table 4.10.

Melanoma has served as the prototype for many subsequent tumor vaccines because the most comprehensive model for TAA has been established in malignant melanoma (Mitchell 2002; Muehlbauer and Schwartzentruber 2003; Boon and Van den Eynde 2000; Nestle *et al.* 1999). The most common melanoma-associated antigens are also expressed on normal melanocytes and include MART-1/Melan A, tyrosinase, and gp100. Other examples of TAAs that are found on normal cells include the human melanoma-associated ganglioside GD2, which is normally expressed on neural tissues, and the cancer testis antigens, such as melanoma-associated antigen (MAGE). MAGE is expressed in the testis and placenta and is not perceived as foreign by the immune system (Kinzler and Brown 2001; Dermime *et al.* 2002; Muehlbauer and Schwartzentruber 2003; Schreiber 1999).

The primary goal of cancer vaccines is to generate an immune response leading to recognition and destruction of the tumor cell. Specific antitumor T-cell immunity must occur so that the immune response can produce a clinical response. The immune system must recognize the TAA as foreign and respond with the proliferation of T cells that have the ability to recognize this specific antigen once the cancer vaccine containing the TAA is administered. These T cells circulate, find the tumor expressing the same antigen, and orchestrate its destruction. Two major obstacles in developing adequate cancer vaccines include the identification of suitable antigens to target and generating a sufficiently strong immune response against the tumor antigens (Siemens and Ratliff 2001; Kinzler and Brown 2001; Borello and Sotomayor 2002; Muehlbauer and Schwartzentruber 2003).

Major Histocompatability Complex (MHC)

For vaccines to work, T cells must be stimulated to distinguish self from nonself. T cells cannot distinguish self-antigens from nonself-antigens unless the antigens are presented to them in association with MHC molecules (Siemens and Ratliff 2001; Kinzler and Brown 2001; Schreiber 1999). MHC molecules are unique to each person, are present on most cells in the body, and are known as human leukocyte antigens (HLA). The T-cell receptor (TCR) on the surface of the T cell specifically interacts with a peptide/MHC complex on the tumor cell surface. If a peptide is not presented for immune recognition in the form of a peptide/MHC complex, then the desired immune response will not occur. This process is known as MHC restriction.

There are three classes of MHC in humans, but only classes I and II actively participate in antigen presentation. MHC class I molecules are found on nearly all nucleated cells and platelets. They restrict antigen presentation to cytotoxic T cells via interaction with the CD8$^+$ molecule. MHC class II molecules are found on subsets of antigen-presenting cells such as dendritic cells, macrophages, monocytes, and B cells. MHC class II molecules restrict

antigen presentation to T-helper cells via interaction with the CD4$^+$ molecule (Hyde 1992).

Immunoadjuvants

The goal of cancer vaccines is to mount an effective T-cell reaction against the tumor. Tumor cells do not produce the necessary proinflammatory cytokines and chemokines, or danger signals, necessary for the immune system to mount an adequate immune response. Cytokines are crucial in mediating T-cell activation and proliferation. Chemokines are a group of cytokines that act as chemo attractants. They are produced locally by tissues, usually when a pathogen is present, and act on leukocytes to induce immune-cell activation. By adding cytokines, chemokines, or other costimulatory molecules to vaccines, the necessary warning signals can be generated. These molecules are known as immunoadjuvants (Muehlbauer and Schwartzentruber 2003; Kinzler and Brown 2001; Restifo 2000).

The role of immunoadjuvants is to promote, expedite, or lengthen the immune response to a vaccine (Salgaller 2000). Immunoadjuvants recruit antigen-presenting cells, activate nonspecific immune responses, initiate the reticuloendothelial system, and stimulate recruitment of innate immune responses. The interaction of the T cells and tumor cells in this type of environment enhances the chances of inducing cell kill by the tumor vaccine. The responses are nonspecific to cytokines and chemokines because those responses are broad. The overall immune effect is intensified by stimulating macrophages, natural killer cells, and T cells (Muehlbauer and Schwartzentruber 2003; Kinzler and Brown 2001; Restifo 2000; Akporiaye and Hersh 1995).

Various adjuvants are under clinical investigation. Adjuvants can be of bacterial origin (i.e., BCG), cytokines, such as IL-12, that activate natural killer cells and T cells, growth factors such as GM-CSF, or gel-type adjuvants, such as aluminum hydroxide, that enhance the humoral response. Another adjuvant is incomplete Freund's adjuvant, which is an emulsifier with mineral oil that allows for slow

TABLE 4.10 Prospective Targets for Cancer Vaccines (Muehlbauer and Schwartzentruber 2003; Dermime *et al.* 2002; Bremers and Parmiani 2000)

Antigen Type	Description	Antigen (Ag)	Neoplasia
Tissue-specific antigen/differentiation antigens	■ Found on the tissue of origin of the tumor ■ Examples include retina of the eye and melanocytes (MART)	Prostate-specific Ag Prostate-specific membrane Ag Tyrosinase MART-1, Gp100 α-fetoprotein CEA	Prostate cancer Prostate cancer Melanoma Melanoma Liver cancer Colon, breast, pancreas cancers
Cancer testis antigen	■ Expressed in the testis but not in other normal tissues ■ MAGE, or melanoma-associated antigen, is expressed in placenta and is not perceived as foreign by the immune system	MAGE-1, MAGE-3, MAGE-12, BAGE, GAGE NY-ESO-1	Melanoma, lung, gastric, head and neck, bladder cancers Melanoma, breast, lung cancers
Tumor-specific antigen	■ These are unique antigens for individual tumors ■ They represent normal proteins containing mutations or gene fusions that result in the generation of unique proteins	Immunoglobin idiotype TCR BCR/ABL Mutant p53	B-cell NHL, myeloma T-cell NHL CML Lung, colorectal, head and neck, bladder cancers

Overexpressed antigens	■ Antigens shared by normal tissues but overexpressed or altered on tumor cells ■ These mutations cause altered protein sequences in cancer cells making them recognizable by the immune system as foreign	Mutated *Ras* Her2/neu MUC-1 CEA Normal p53	Pancreas Breast, ovarian, lung cancers Pancreatic, lung, breast, colorectal cancers Colorectal Breast, colon, other cancers
Viral antigens	■ Certain malignancies are strongly correlated with viruses ■ Viral antigens expressed on tumor cells can serve as specific targets for immune destruction ■ Potentially, these can be considered prophylactic cancer vaccines	Human papilloma virus Hepatitis B virus Epstein-Barr virus Hepatitis C virus	Cervical cancer Hepatocellular cancer Burkitt's lymphoma Hepatocellular cancer

CEA, carcinoembryonic antigen; CML, chronic myeloid leukemia; NHL, non-Hodgkin's lymphoma antigen release and extended exposure of antigens to cells and immunogenic proteins, such as keyhole limpet hemocyanin, which induces CD4$^+$ responses and boosts natural killer cell activity (Muehlbauer and Schwartzentruber 2003; Kinzler and Brown 2001; Salgaller 2000).

Cancer Vaccine Strategies

A number of cancer vaccine clinical trials using various strategies exist. Multiple trials have been conducted in patients with melanoma, but several clinical trials have been conducted or are underway to test vaccination in patients with cancers of the lung, colon, stomach, and prostate and hematologic malignancies (Muehlbauer and Scwhartzentruber 2003). This is a rapidly evolving field, so no specific clinical trials will be mentioned in this chapter. An up-to-date summary can be found at http://www.cancer.gov.

The manner in which TAA is supplied or expressed by the cancer vaccine to be presented to the APC can be classified into one of several major categories. The first category includes peptide vaccines, which are taken up by empty MHC molecules on the surface of the APC for presentation. The second category consists of preparations of TAA that are internalized by the APC, processed, and presented in conjunction with an MHC molecule. Vaccines in this category include tumor cells, tumor lysates, and whole tumor bodies. The third category is genetic material that is used to transduce host cells, leading to endogenous expression of the TAA. Examples include recombinant viruses, bacteria, and naked nucleic acid molecules. A fourth category includes the administration of the APC itself expressing the appropriate TAA. Examples of this approach include dendritic cells that have been pulsed with peptides or transduced with a gene encoding the TAA (Muehlbauer and Schwartzentruber 2003; Siemens and Ratliff 2001; Kinzler and Brown 2001; Matzku and Zoller 2001; Bremers and Parmiani 2000). A further overview of various cancer vaccine strategies, including advantages and limitations, is summarized in Table 4.11.

Nursing Management

Nursing management varies by route of administration. Prophylactic analgesia may be necessary for vaccines administered intradermally. Frequent injections are given over time, so the sites of injections need to be monitored for redness, swelling, ulceration, tenderness, induration, and any site-specific symptoms. Some vaccines administered IV require pretreatment with antipyretics because patients can develop fever and chills, although constitutional symptoms are generally minimal. Patients should be assessed for systemic effects regardless of the route of injection. Patients are monitored in the clinical setting for at least 15 minutes after vaccination in the event of an allergic reaction. Educating patients about side effects and what to report is necessary to monitor vaccine reactions and treat accordingly (Muehlbauer and Schwartzentruber 2003; Kinzler and Brown 2001).

Current Status and Future Directions

No cancer vaccines have been FDA approved for cancer treatment as of press time. The search for therapeutic cancer vaccines remains a major area of research. Cancer vaccines are increasingly incorporated as part of multimodality regimens including combinations with surgery, other biologic agents, chemotherapy, radiation therapy, and stem-cell transplantation (Kinzler and Brown 2001; Kwak 1998). Patients with intact immune systems and a small volume of disease may be the best candidates for cancer vaccine trials. Efficacy of the vaccine will be established when clinical end points, such as tumor shrinkage, delay in time to disease progression, and improvement in survival, are measured rather than immunologic end points. However immunologic end points may be helpful in directing efforts to optimize a vaccine strategy and its delivery (Simon *et al.* 2001).

Although innate cytotoxic T lymphocytes (CTL) can be generated against vaccines, there is frequently no correlation with clinical regression of disease. Investigators are left wondering why the CTL activity does not overcome the targeted

TABLE 4.11 Vaccine Approaches

Vaccine Approach	Description	Advantages	Limitations	Diseases Targeted/ Clinical Studies
Peptide / Protein (Disis 2002; Dermime *et al.* 2002; Parmiani *et al.* 2002; Salit *et al.* 2002; Kinzler and Brown 2001; Rosenberg 2000b)	▪ Peptides provide the minimal target required for T-cell recognition, and vaccines using peptides can elicit T-cell–mediated immunity ▪ Evidence shows that T-cell immunity is augmented when peptide vaccines are given with adjuvants ▪ The immunogenicity of peptide vaccines may be improved by modifying amino acid sequences, thus potentiating the interaction with HLA or with the specific T-cell receptor (TCR)	▪ Immune response is directed mainly against tumor cells and not normal tissues ▪ Low toxicity profile ▪ Inexpensive to manufacture	▪ Peptides may not be processed naturally by APCs, leading to the possibility of generating an unimportant peptide-specific response ▪ Low clinical response rates reported and possibly a result of previous chemotherapy or radiation therapy ▪ Advanced disease stage of many participants ▪ Immune escape of tumors	▪ The first peptide vaccines used in clinical studies were in patients with metastatic melanoma ▪ Attempts are underway to develop peptide vaccines for common epithelial tumors such as those with mutations in the *ras* oncogene (pancreas, colon, and lung cancer), HER-2/*neu* oncogene (breast, ovary, and colorectal cancer), and prostate specificantigen (PSA) ▪ Peptide vaccine trials directed against viruses such as human papilloma virus (HPV) are also in progress
Recombinant viral (poxvirus and adenovirus)/bacterial (Dermime *et al.* 2002; Kinzler and Brown 2001; Roberts 2000; Schlom and Panicali 2000; Bremers and Parmiani, 2000)	▪ Recombinant techniques allow tumor antigen genes to be introduced into viruses (poxvirus or adenovirus) that attract APCs and maximize antigen presentation to the immune system ▪ This strong immune response is generated by a viral infection that is foreign to the host and produces a significant inflammatory response	▪ Recombinant gene products tend to be more immunogenic ▪ Poxviruses have a large capacity available within their genomes to insert foreign DNA and multiple genes ▪ Poxvirus-based vaccines are stable for long periods of time, safe, easy to administer, and cost-effective	▪ Require available cloned antigens ▪ Neutralizing antibodies may recognize the viral vector, especially with adenovirus	▪ Clinical studies with poxviruses include those directed against cancers overexpressing CEA, HPV, MART, gp100, and PSA ▪ Trials using adenoviral vectors have been performed in patients with melanoma, breast cancer, and neuroblastoma

(Continued)

TABLE 4.11 (Continued)

Vaccine Approach	Description	Advantages	Limitations	Diseases Targeted/ Clinical Studies
	■ Several modalities can be used for generating viral cancer vaccines including: 1. Tumor cells may be used as the source of antigens, and adenovirus and poxvirus vectors deliver the immunomodulatory genes to the tumor cells 2. One or more TAA genes can be inserted into a virus and administered as a traditional vaccine or intravenously 3. Viral vaccines can be delivered by infecting dendritic cells *in vitro* with either recombinant poxvirus or adenoviral vectors containing tumor antigen genes or costimulatory genes	■ Possible continuous supply of tumor antigen–derived peptides for immune presentation ■ Accurate replication		
Dendritic Cell (DC) Vaccines (Dermime *et al.* 2002; Morse 2002; Kinzler and Brown 2001; Dallal *et al.* 2000; Bremers and Parmiani 2000; Kugler *et al.* 2000)	■ Dendritic cells are the most potent APC and are found throughout the body, principally in areas that are entry sites for infectious organisms ■ DC capture, process, and uptake antigens from tissues, and transport the antigens from	■ Hypothesized that using DC may lead to prolonged tumor response by efficient activation of specific T cells ■ Generally well tolerated with few toxicities	■ Generating DC is labor intensive, requiring large facilities to generate sufficient DC preparation	■ Several phase I and II clinical trials have been performed using DC-based vaccine therapy in an attempt to treat multiple cancers including melanoma, B-cell lymphoma, renal cell carcinoma, and neuroendocrine, brain, lung, and prostate

- peripheral to primary and secondary lymphoid sites
- The DC express high levels of MHC class I and II molecules and high levels of costimulatory molecules necessary to signal T-cell activation
- Primary tumors with histologic evidence of infiltration with DC have been associated with prolonged patient survival and decreased metastatic disease in patients with cancers of the bladder, lung, esophagus, and nasopharynx
- Conversely, a poorer prognosis has been observed in patients with tumors containing little infiltration of DC
- A variety of methods have been explored to load the MHC molecules of DC with appropriate TAA including pulsing with peptides, protein, and cell lysates, transfection with viral vectors, and fusing with whole tumor cells
- DC vaccines have been administered via a variety of routes including subcutaneous,

cancers.
- Improving early results of DC therapy may lie in understanding the best possible routes of administration, methods to load DC, and the role of concomitant cytokine therapy

(Continued)

TABLE 4.11 (Continued)

Vaccine Approach	Description	Advantages	Limitations	Diseases Targeted/ Clinical Studies
	intravenous, intradermal, intranodal, intralymphatic, and directly into the tumor ■ Optimization of DC-based therapies may be obtained by adding cytokines, such as IL-2, IL-12, IL-7, IL-15, IFN-α, or Flt-3 ligand, thus increasing the immune response.			
Cellular Vaccines (Whole cell and tumor lysate) (Dermime *et al.* 2002; Mocellini *et al.* 2002; Weber 2002; Belli *et al.* 2002; Sondak *et al.* 2002; Matzku and Zoller 2001; Sivanandham *et al.* 2000; Kugler *et al.* 2000; Harris *et al.* 2000; Bremers and Parmiani 2000)	■ Cellular vaccines use whole tumor cells that are either irradiated or lysed by viral infection ■ With autologous tumor cell vaccines, tumor tissue is isolated from various sites on the patient to prepare the vaccine ■ Allogeneic tumor cells have been used to prepare tumor cell vaccines to overcome some of the disadvantages of autologous preparations ■ Allogeneic tumor cell lines need to be screened for the highest expression of TAAs to induce immune responses in the recipient ■ More recent clinical stud-	**Autologous vaccines:** ■ Lack of allogeneic tissue-specific antigens that may induce unwanted immune responses in patients receiving vaccine **Allogeneic tumor cell vaccines:** ■ Use multiple established tumor cell lines with no requirement for defined tumor antigen, reducing the chance of antigen selection and tumor escape	**Autologous vaccines:** ■ During the early stage of patient's disease, no tumor cells may be available ■ Many laborious steps are necessary to prepare and standardize this type of vaccine **Allogeneic tumor cell vaccines:** ■ Moderate potency ■ Changes of tumor cell lines in culture may result in lack of consistent antigen expression and hence stability and reproducibility of vaccine	■ Clinical trials have been conducted for melanoma (i.e., Melacine and CancerVax vaccines), breast, colorectal, glioblastoma, lung (i.e., GVAX), pancreas (i.e., GVAX), leukemia, sarcoma, renal, and ovarian cancers with modest results ■ Some clinical trials use cell extracts or semipurified proteins, instead of whole cells, called heat shock proteins (HSP); HSP are naturally occurring intracellular substances that

accompany a large variety of antigenic proteins present in the cell and channel these into MHC class I and II pathways
- HSP are also able to elicit the necessary warning signals to trigger DC-mediated antigen presentation
- The use of DC to augment cellular vaccines is under investigation

ies have used modified tumor cells (autologous or allogeneic or both) and genetically manipulated them to express immunostimulatory cytokines such as IL-2, granulocyte-macrophage colony-stimulating factor or IFN-γ.
- This diminishes the toxicities from systemic administration of these cytokines while providing the vaccine with the modulatory activity of cytokines

DNA Vaccines
(Dermime et al. 2002; Sundaram et al. 2002; Morse et al. 2002; Matzku and Zoller 2001; White and Conry 2000)
- Interest in developing DNA vaccines comes from the observation that when naked DNA is injected into muscle, a powerful response is generated including cellular and humoral immunity
- These vaccines may induce long-lasting immune responses by the continuous expression of the tumor antigen from the DNA-infected cell

- Easy access to DNA
- Easy handling
- Low cost of production

- No good responses in humans reported
- Potentially, DNA-encoding self-tumor antigens could integrate into the host genome, causing them to be at a high risk for cellular transformation
- Potential exists to elicit anti-DNA autoantibodies, resulting in the induction or exacerbation of systemic autoimmune disease

- Cancer clinical trials have included those directed against AIDS, hepatitis B, colon cancer, B-cell lymphoma, non-Hodgkinis lymphoma, melanoma, and cutaneous T-cell lymphoma

APC, antigen-presenting cell; HLA, human leukocyte antigen; TAA, tumor-associated antigens; MHC, major histocompatability complex tumors, raising the possibility that tumors resist immunotherapy because of an insufficient immune response. It is also possible that tumors adapt to the immune pressure and switch to less immunogenic phenotypes (Marincola 2000).

The optimal vaccine, route, and immunization schedule remain to be determined. The most advantageous strategies for presenting antigens to the immune effector cells continue to be elucidated. Progress in the ability to monitor immune response allows for greater understanding of how vaccines work and how tumors escape immune recognition (Dermime *et al.* 2002; Mocellin *et al.* 2002; Disis and Schiffman 2001; Marincola 2000).

Adoptive Cellular Transfer

Dr. Steven A. Rosenberg of the National Cancer Institute (NCI) has been a pioneer in the study of adoptive cell transfer as a cancer therapy. He describes this therapy as the "transfer of immune cells with antitumor activity that can mediate, directly or indirectly, antitumor effects in the tumor-bearing host [person]" (Rosenberg 2000a, p 322). The success of this treatment depends on a number of factors, including lymphocyte subtype, presence of the target antigen on the tumor cell for which the lymphocytes are reactive, and the ability of the transferred lymphocytes to overcome suppressive factors that might be present in the patient's immune system or at the tumor site that would prevent the transferred cells from reacting with the tumor. Other factors include how well the lymphocytes recognize the target antigens and the ability of lymphocytes to traffic to tumor locations (Rosenberg 2000a).

As mentioned in the vaccine section, melanoma is highly immunogenic, and much work has been done in identifying and characterizing melanoma antigens. Hence, cell transfer studies have primarily been done in persons with melanoma. Various cell types have been used for this therapy including tumor-infiltrating lymphocytes (TIL), peripheral lymphocytes sensitized *in vitro* to tumor antigens, and lymphocytes obtained from sites of tumor vaccinations. Recently, other studies have been reported using cell transfer therapy for malignancies such as nasopharyngeal carcinoma, renal cell carcinoma, and colorectal cancer (Dillman *et al.* 2003; Comoli *et al.* 2004). These studies remain experimental, but Rosenberg (2000a), Rosenberg and Dudley (2004), Dudley and Rosenberg (2003), Dillman *et al.* (2003), Comoli *et al.* (2004), and Kawai *et al.* (2003) report antitumor effects in patients treated with adoptive cell transfer.

Tumor-infiltrating lymphocytes (TILs) from melanoma patients exhibit an extensive variety of melanoma-associated antigens (i.e., MART-1, gp100, and tyrosinase) as well as antigens that are expressed on other cancers, such as the cancer testes antigen. Each of these antigens is recognized by TIL in an MHC-restricted manner (Rosenberg 2000b). Attempts at immunization against these target antigens with cancer vaccines have only rarely induced cancer regression, despite the evidence that antitumor T cells recognize tumor antigens. The generation of antitumor T cells via immunization does not appear adequate to induce regression of metastatic disease. Theoretically, the use of cell transfer therapy may overcome some of the limitations of immunization. Cell transfer therapy allows for administration of large numbers of selected cells with high affinity for recognition of tumor antigens. Reasons that make this a potentially superior therapy include the ability for the cells to be manipulated *ex vivo* so that they demonstrate antitumor effector function. A major bonus of cell transfer therapy is that the regulatory lymphocytes, those that compete with the transferred cells, can be eliminated or manipulated prior to reinfusion (Rosenberg and Dudley 2004).

The culture and growth of these TIL cells is a long, complex process taking about 5 to 8 weeks from harvest of the cells to infusion into the patient (M.E. Dudley, personal communication, October 1, 2004). The cells are collected either via peripheral blood or by harvesting tumor. Dudley (2000) states that, after immune effector cells are collected, they are cultured *ex vivo* to elude normal immune regulatory and suppressive effects. Cellular characteristics that make this therapy viable can be enhanced in cell culture. The methods applied may not be possible *in vivo* because the agents used to achieve the desirable cellular characteristics may be toxic or could compromise the patient's health. Once the cells have been activated and expanded, they are infused back into the autologous patient (Dudley 2000). IL-2 is generally given after infusion of adoptive TIL cells. The reason is that IL-2 causes *in vivo* proliferation and prolonged survival of cells. The efficacy of IL-2 has shown to be enhanced when given in conjunction with cellular therapy (Belldegrun *et al.* 2000).

Dr. Rosenberg and his colleagues at the NCI arguably have some of the most extensive experience with adoptive transfer of autologous cells. The NCI experience with adoptive cell transfer has been primarily in patients with metastatic melanoma and has evolved throughout the years. Initially, nonspecific, activated lymphocytes, such as lymphokine-activated killer (LAK) cells, were tested. The response rates using LAK cells with IL-2 versus IL-2 alone in patients with metastatic melanoma or renal cell carcinoma were not statistically significant. These early studies indicated that tumor antigen–specific lymphocytes were necessary for successful cell transfer cancer therapy (Dudley and Rosenberg 2003; Rosenberg and Dudley 2004).

TIL cells provide more antigen-specific lymphocytes, and several approaches have been studied. The adoptive transfer of cloned T cells (CD4$^+$ and CD8$^+$) was attempted because efficacy was seen in clinical trials using this approach for viral prophylaxis with anticytomegalovirus clones. However, no objective tumor regression was seen in patients with transferred clone cells with or without IL-2 administration. Immunologic studies showed that these cloned cells disappeared rapidly from the patient's circulation. Dudley and Rosenberg (2003) concluded that, although highly avid recognition of tumor antigens by the transferred lymphocytes is necessary, it is not enough to induce significant clinical responses.

Currently, trials are underway that combine a lymphocyte-depleting chemotherapy preparatory regimen (cyclophosphamide 60 mg/kg for 2 days then fludarabine 25 mg/m^2 for 5 days) followed by TIL cell infusion and administration of high-dose IL-2 (720,000 IU/kg). The elimination of the patient's lymphocytes makes room in the lymphocyte compartment for the TIL cells and provides an environment for the adoptively transferred lymphocytes to survive and proliferate. Theories have been put forth that innate CD4$^+$ T lymphocytes may suppress the antitumor effects of TIL. The elimination of CD4$^+$ CD25$^+$ regulatory T cells with the lymphodepletive chemotherapy regimen may improve adoptive immunotherapy (Dudley and Rosenberg 2003; Shimizu *et al.* 1999). The chemotherapy preparative regimen has no known effects on melanoma, and the sole use is to eliminate innate T lymphocytes prior to cell transfer. These ongoing trials so far have shown the ability for transferred cells to survive and grow in patients for several months after adoptive transfer. Rosenberg and Dudley (2004) also report that 6 of 13 patients showed an objective response and four additional patients had mixed responses.

Dillman *et al.* (2003) report the use of autologous activated lymphocytes (AAL) for use in autolymphocyte therapy (ALT) in 47 patients with a variety of malignancies including colorectal cancer; renal cell carcinoma; breast, lung, pancreas, prostate, endocrine, and gastric cancers; and sarcoma and melanoma. They describe ALT as therapy involving helper T lymphocytes but not cytotoxic T lymphocytes. Instead of using a tumor as a source of lymphocytes, the lymphocytes were obtained from peripheral-blood mononuclear cells (PBMC) via leukapheresis procedures. The initial leukapheresis procedure was done to obtain mononuclear cell products enriched for PBMC enriched for lymphocytes. The cells were then washed, and some were suspended in medium. These autologus lymphokine (ALK) cells had significant measurements of TNF-α, IL-1β, IFN-γ, and IL-6 but no IL-2. Patients then underwent up to 6 monthly leukapheresis procedures to collect PBMC for AAL. These cells were cultured in the ALK cells and resulted in increased T lymphocytes, decreased natural killer cells, decreased suppressor T cells, and increased helper T cells. The final product for IV infusion of AAL was placed in a 50-ml bag of 25% human albumin.

In the study by Dillman *et al.* (2003), patients received 600 mg of the histamine type 2 blocker cimetidine orally every 6 hours prior to infusion of AAL and then daily until the end of treatment. Treatments were given monthly for 6 months or until disease progression in the outpatient setting. Patients did not receive IL-2 in this study. A variety of support medications were given if the patient experienced side effects such as fever or chills. The authors report objective tumor responses in patients with renal cell carcinoma and colorectal cancer (Dillman *et al.* 2003).

In conclusion, adoptive cell transfer is evolving as more is learned about the role of the host immune environment on tumor therapy (Dudley and Rosenberg 2003; Gardini *et al.* 2004; Shi *et al.* 2004). Researchers are looking at alternative methods for obtaining potent cells for adoptive transfer by first priming the patient with autologous tumor vaccination then expanding activated T cells *in vivo* that will be reinfused (Chan *et al.* 2003). Concurrent vaccination and after T-cell transfer has potential for improving adoptive cell transfer therapy (Dudley and Rosenberg 2003). Other methods for advancing cell transfer include genetically modifying lymphocytes to increase antitumor effects by introducing genes encoded with cytokines, T-cell receptors, or antiapoptotic molecules (Rosenberg and Dudley 2004).

References

Adams, F., Quesada, J., and Gutterman, J. 1984. Neuropsychiatric manifestations of human leukocyte interferon therapy in patients with cancer. *Journal of the American Medical Association* 151:938–941.

Aistars, J. 1987. Fatigue in the cancer patient: A conceptual approach to a clinical problem. *Oncology Nursing Forum* 14(6):25–30.

Akporiaye, E., and Hersh, E. 1995. Cancer vaccines: Clinical applications. Immune Adjuvants. In V.T. DeVita, S. Hellman, and S.A. Rosenberg (Eds): *Biologic Therapy of Cancer* (ed 2). Philadelphia: JB Lippincott, pp 635–647.

Allen, I.E., Ross, S.D., Borden, S.P., Monroe, M.W., Kupelnick, B., Connelly, J.E., and Ozer, H. 2001. Meta-analysis to assess the efficacy of interferon-α in patients with follicular non-Hodgkin's lymphoma. *Journal of Immunotherapy* 24(1):58–65.

Aranesp (darbepoetin alfa): Prescribing information. 2002. Thousand Oaks, CA: Amgen.

ASHP. 1999. ASHP therapeutic guidelines on the pharmacologic management of nausea and vomiting in adult and pediatric patients receiving chemotherapy or radiation therapy or undergoing surgery. *American Journal of Health-System Pharmacy* 56:729–764.

Asnis, L.A., and Gaspari, A.A. 1995. Cutaneous reactions to recombinant cytokine therapy. *Journal of American Academy of Dermatology* 33:393–412.

Atkins, M., Gould, J., Allegretta, M., *et al.* 1986. Phase I evaluation of recombinant interleukin 2 in patients with advanced malignant disease. *Journal of Clinical Oncology* 4:1380–1391.

Atkins, M.B., Sparano, J., Fisher, R.I., *et al.* 1993. Randomized phase II trial of high-dose interleukin-2 either alone or in combination with interferon alpha-2b in advanced renal cell carcinoma. *Journal of Clinical Oncology* 11:661–670.

Atzpodien, J., Hänninen, E.L., Kirchner, H., *et al.* 1995. Multi-institutional home-therapy trial of recombinant interleukin-2 and interferon-alfa in progressive metastatic renal cell carcinoma. *Journal of Clinical Oncology* 13:497–501.

Balducci, L., and Carreca, I. 2002. The role of myelopoietic growth factors in managing cancer in the elderly. *Drugs* 62(Suppl 1):47–63.

Baron, S., Tyring, S.K., Fleischmann, W.R., Coppenhaver, D.H., Niesel, D.W., Klimpel, G.R., Stanton, J., and Hughes, T.K. 1991. The interferons: Mechanism of action and clinical applications. *Journal of the American Medical Association* 266(10):1375–1383.

Battiato, L.A., and Wheeler, V.S. 2000. Biotherapy. In C.H. Yarbro, M.H. Frogge, M. Goodman, and S.L. Groenwald (Eds): *Cancer Nursing Principles and Practice* (ed 5). Sudbury, MA: Jones & Bartlett, pp 543–579.

Belldegrun, A.S., Figlin, R.A., and Patel, B. 2000. Cell transfer therapy: Clinical applications, renal cell carcinoma. In S.A. Rosenberg (Ed): *Principles and Practice of the Biologic Therapy of Cancer* (ed 3). Philadelphia: Lippincott Williams & Wilkins, pp 333–345.

Belli, F., Testori, A., Rivoltini, L., *et al.* 2002. Vaccination of metastatic melanoma patients with autologous tumor-derived heat shock protein gp96-peptide complexes: Clinical and immunologic findings. *Journal of Clinical Oncology* 20:4169–4180.

Bindon, C., Czerniecki, M., Ruell, P., *et al.* 1983. Clearance rates and systemic effects of intravenously administered interleukin-2 (IL2) containing preparations in human subjects. *British Journal of Cancer* 47:123–133.

Boon, T., and Van den Eynde, B. 2000. Cancer vaccines: Cancer antigens: Shared tumor-specific antigens. In S.A. Rosenberg (Ed): *Principles and Practice of the Biologic Therapy of Cancer* (ed 3). Philadelphia: Lippincott Williams & Wilkins, pp 493–504.

Borrello, I.M., and Sotomayor, E.M. 2002. Cancer vaccines for hematologic malignancies. *Cancer Control* 9:138–151.

Bremers, A.J., and Parmiani, G. 2000. Immunology and immunotherapy of human cancer: Present concepts and clinical developments. *Critical Reviews in Oncology/Hematology* 34:1–25.

Bukowski, R.M., Tendler, C., Cutler, D., Rose, E., Laughlin, M.M., and Statkevich, P. 2002. Treating cancer with PEG Intron. *Cancer* 95(2):389–396.

Buzaid, A.C. 2002. Biochemotherapy for advanced melanoma. *Critical Reviews in Oncology/Hematology* 44:103–108.

Cáceres, W., and González, S. 2003. Angiogenesis and cancer: Recent advances. *Puerto Rico Health Sciences Journal* 22(2):149–151.

Cantell, K., Hervonen, S., Cavalletto, L., *et al.* 1975. Human leukocyte interferon production, purification and animal experiments. In C. Waymouth (Ed): *In vitro.* Baltimore: Baltimore Tissue Culture Association, pp 35–38.

Cella, D., Lai, J.S., Chang, C.H., Peterman, A., and Slavin, M. 2002. Fatigue in cancer patients compared with fatigue in the general United States population. *Cancer* 94(2):528–538.

Chan, B., Lee, W., Hu, C.X.L., Ng, P., Li, K.W., Lo, G., Ho, G., Yeung, D.W., and Woo, D. 2003. Adoptive cellular immunotherapy for non-small cell lung cancer: A pilot study. *Cytotherapy* 5(1):46–54.

Chiron Corporation. 2000. Proleukin (aldesleukin for injection): Package insert. Emeryville, CA: Chiron Therapeutics.

Choyke, P.L., Miller, D.L., Lotze, M.T., Whiteis, J.M., Ebbit, B., and Rosenberg, S.A. 1992. Delayed reactions to contrast media after interleukin-2 immunotherapy. *Radiology* 183:111–114.

Clemens, M.J. 2003. Interferons and apoptosis. *Journal of Interferon and Cytokine Research* 23:277–292.

Coffe, R.J., Richards, J.S., Remmert, C.S., LeRoy, S.S., Schoville, R.R., and Baldwin, P.J. 1992. An introduction to critical pathways. *Quality Management in Health Care* 1:45–54.

Coley, W.B. 1898. The treatment of inoperable sarcoma with the mixed toxins of erysipelas and *Bacillus prodigiosus. Journal of the American Medical Association* 31:389–395.

Coley, W.B. 1911. A report of recent cases of inoperable sarcoma successfully treated with mixed toxins of erysipelas and *Bacillus prodigious. Surgical Gynecology and Obstetrics* 13:174–190.

Comoli, P., De Palma, R., Siena, S., Nocera, A., Basso, S., Del Galdo, F., Schiavo, R., Carminati, O., Tagliamacco, A., Abbate, G.F., Locatelli, F., Maccario, R., and Pedrazzoli, P. 2004. Adoptive transfer of allogeneic Epstein-Barr virus (EBV)-specific cytotoxic T cells with *in vitro* antitumor activity boosts LMP2-specific immune response in a patient with EBV-related nasopharyngeal carcinoma. *Annals of Oncology* 15:113–117.

Conrad, A. 2003. Interleukin-2: Where are we going? *Journal of the Association of Nurses in AIDS Care* 14(6):83–88.

Crawford, J. 2002a. Recombinant human erythropoietin in cancer-related anemia: Review of clinical evidence. *Oncology* September(Suppl):41–53.

Crawford, J. 2002b. Clinical uses of pegylated pharmaceuticals in oncology. *Cancer Treatment Reviews* 28(Suppl A):7–11.

Crawford, H., Dale, D.C., and Lyman, G.H. 2004. Chemotherapy-induced neutropenia: Risks, consequences and new directions for its management. *Cancer* 100(2):228–237.

Cuaron, L., and Thompson, J. 2001. The interferons. In P. Rieger (Ed): *Biotherapy: A Comprehensive Overview* (ed 2). Sudbury, MA: Jones and Bartlett, pp 125–194.

Curt, G.A. 2000. The impact of fatigue on patients with cancer: Overview of FATIGUE 1 and 2. *The Oncologist* 5(Suppl 2):9–12.

Dallal, R.M., Mailliard, R ., and Lotze, M.T. 2000. Cancer vaccines: Clinical applications: Dendritic cell vaccines. In S.A. Rosenberg (Ed): *Principles and Practice of the Biologic Therapy of Cancer* (ed 3). Philadelphia: Lippincott Williams & Wilkins, pp 705–721.

Darrow, T.L., Abdel-Wahab, Z., and Seigler, H.F. 1995. Immunotherapy of human melanoma with gene-modified tumor cell vaccines. *Cancer Control* 2: 415–423.

Davey, R.T., Chaitt, D.G., Piscitelli, S.C., Wells, M., Kovacs, J.A., Walker, R.E., Falloon, J., Polis, M.A., Metcalf, J.A., Masur, H., Fyfe, G., and Lane, H.C. 1997. Subcutaneous administration of interleukin-2 in human immunodeficiency virus type-1 infected persons. *The Journal of Infectious Diseases* 175:781–789.

Dean, G.E. 2001. Fatigue. In P.T. Rieger (Ed): *Biotherapy: A Comprehensive Overview* (ed 2). Boston: Jones and Bartlett, pp 547–575.

Dean, G.E., Spears, L., Ferrell, B.R., Quan, W.D., Groshon, S., and Mitchell, M.S. 1995. Fatigue in patients with cancer receiving interferon alpha. *Cancer Practice* 3(3):164–172.

Decatris, M., Santhanam, S., and O'Byrne, K. 2002. Potential of interferon-α in solid tumours: Part 1. *Biodrugs* 16 (4):261–281.

Dermime, S., Armstrong, A., Hawkins, R.E., and Stern, P.L. 2002. Cancer vaccines and immunotherapy. *British Medical Bulletin* 62:149–162.

Dillman, R.O., Soori, G., DePriest, C., Nayak, S.K., Beutel, L.D., Schiltz, P.M., de Leon, C., and O'Connor, A.A. 2003. Treatment of human solid malignancies with autologous activated lymphocytes and cimetidine: A phase II trial of the cancer biotherapy research group. *Cancer Biotherapy and Radiopharmaceuticals* 18(5):727–733.

Disis, M.L. 2002. Introduction and overview. Therapeutic cancer vaccines: Targeting the future of cancer treatment. http://www.medscape.com.

Disis, M.L., and Schiffman, K. 2001. Issues on clinical applications of cancer vaccines. *Journal of Immunotherapy* 24:104–105.

Donnelly, S. 1998. Patient management strategies for interferon alfa-2b as adjuvant therapy of high-risk melanoma. *Oncology Nursing Forum* 25(5):921–927.

Dudley, M.E. 2000. Cell transfer therapy: Basic principles and preclinical studies. In S.A. Rosenberg (Ed): *Principles and Practice of the Biologic Therapy of Cancer* (ed 3). Philadelphia: Lippincott Williams & Wilkins, pp 305–321.

Dudley, M.E., and Rosenberg, S.A. 2003. Adoptive-cell-transfer therapy for the treatment of patients with cancer. *Nature* 3:666–675.

Dutcher, J. 2002. Current status of interleukin-2 therapy for metastatic renal cell carcinoma and metastatic melanoma. *Oncology* 16(Suppl):4–10.

Dutcher, J., Atkins, M.B., Margolin, K., Weiss, G., Clark, J., Sosman, J., Logan, T., Aronson, R., and Mier, J. 2001. Kidney cancer: The cytokine working group experience (1986–2001). *Medical Oncology* 18(3):209–219.

Eggermont, A.M.M., and Punt, C.J.A. 2003. Does adjuvant systemic therapy with interferon-α for stage II-III melanoma prolong survival? *American Journal of Clinical Dermatology* 4(8):531–536.

Emerson, S.G. 1998. Hematopoiesis: The development of blood cells. In F.J. Schiffman (Ed): *Hematologic Pathophysiology*. Philadelphia: Lippincott-Raven, pp 1–24.

efacts Drug Comparison. Epoetin alfa, recombinant. 2004. http://www.efactsweb.com.

EPOGEN (epoetin alfa): Full prescribing information. Thousand Oaks, CA: Amgen, 2003.

Fisher, B., Keenan, A.M., Garra, B.S., Steinberg, S.M,. White, D.E., DiBisceglie, A.M., Hoofnagle, J.H., Yolles, P., Rosenberg, S.A., and Lotze, M.T. 1989. Interleukin-2 induces profound reversible cholestasis: A detailed analysis in treated cancer patients. *Journal of Clinical Oncology* 7:1852–1862.

Flaherty, L.E., Atkins, M., Sosman, J., Weiss, G., Margolin, K., Dutcher, J., Gordon, M.S., Lotze, M., Mier, J., Sorokin, P., Fisher, R.I., Appel, C., and Du, W. 2001. Outpatient biochemotherapy with inteleukin-2 and interferon alf-2b in patients with metastatic malignant melanoma: Results of two phase II Cytokine Working Group trials. *Journal of Clinical Oncology* 19(13):3194–3202.

Fyfe, G., Fisher, R.I., Rosenberg, S.A., Sznol, M., Parkinson, D.R., and Louie, A.C. 1995. Results of treatment of 255 patients with metastatic renal cell carcinoma who received high-dose recombinant interleukin-2 therapy. *Journal of Clinical Oncology* 13:688–696.

Gale, D., and Sorokin, P. 2001. The interleukins. In P. Rieger (Ed): *Biotherapy: A Comprehensive Overview* (ed 2). Sudbury, MA: Jones and Bartlett, pp 198–244.

Gallagher, J. 1995. Management of cutaneous symptoms. *Seminars in Oncology Nursing* 11:239–247.

Gantz, S., Tomaszewski, J.G., DeLaPena, L., Molenda, J., Bernato, D.L., and Kryk, J. 1995. Interferons. *Cancer Nursing* 18(6):479–494.

Gardini, A., Ercolani, G., Riccobon, A., Ravaioli, M., Ridolfi, L., Flamini, E., Ridolfi, R., Graze, G.L., Cavallari, A., and Amadori, D. 2004. Adjuvant, adoptive immunotherapy with tumor infiltrating lymphocytes plus interleukin-2 after radical hepatic resection for colorectal liver metastases: 5-year analysis. *Journal of Surgical Oncology* 87(1):46–52.

Ghezzi, S., Vicenzi, L., Tambussi, G., Murone, M., Lazzarin, A., and Poli, G. 1997. Experiences in immune reconstitution. The rationale for interleukin-2 administration to HIV-infected individuals. *Journal of Biological Regulators and Homeostatic Agents* 11:74–78.

Guleria, A.S., Yang, J.C., Topalian, S.L., Weber, J.S., Parkinson, D.R., MacFarlane, M.P., White, R.L., Steinberg, S.M., White, D.E., Einhorn, J.H., Seipp, C.A., Austin, H.A., Rosenberg, S.A., and Schwartzentruber, D.J. 1994. Renal dysfunction associated with the administration of high-dose interleukin-2 in 199 consecutive patients with metastatic melanoma or renal carcinoma. *Journal of Clinical Oncology* 12:2714–2722.

Hancock, B.W., Wheatley, K., Harris, S., Ives, N., Harrison, G., Horsman, J.M., Middleton, M.R., Thatcher, N., Lorigan, P.C., Marsden, J.R., Burrows, L., and Gore, M. 2004.

Adjuvant interferon in high-risk melanoma: The AIM HIGH study—United Kingdom Coordinating Committee on Cancer Research randomized study of adjuvant low-dose extended duration interferon alfa-2a in high-risk resected malignant melanoma. *Journal of Clinical Oncology* 22(1):53–61.

Harris, J.E., Ryan, L., Hoover, H.C., Jr., *et al.* 2000. Adjuvant active specific immunotherapy for stage II and III colon cancer with an autologous tumor cell vaccine: Eastern Cooperative Oncology Group Study E5283. *Journal of Clinical Oncology* 18:148–157.

Hauschild, A., Weichenthal, M., Balda, B.-R., Becker, J.C., Wolff, H.H., Tilgen, W., Schulte, K.-W., Ring, J., Schadendorf, D., Lischner, S., Burg, G., and Dummer, R. 2003. Prospective randomized trial of interferon - alfa-2b and interleukin-2 as adjuvant treatment for resected intermediate and high risk primary melanoma without clinically defectable node metastasis. *Journal of Clinical Oncology* 21(15):2883–2888.

Hehlmann, R., Berger, U., Pfirrmann, M., Hochhaus, A., Metzgeroth, G., Maywald, O., *et al.* 2003. Randomized comparison of interferon alpha and hydroxyurea with hydroxyurea monotherapy in chronic myeloid leukemia (CML study II): Prolongation of survival by the combination of interferon α and hydroxyurea. *Leukemia* 17:1529–1537.

Hernberg, M., Virkkunen, P., Bono, P., Maenpaa, H., and Joensuu, H. 2003. Interferon alfa-2b three times daily and thalidomide in the treatment of metastatic renal cell carcinoma. *Journal of Clinical Oncology* 21(20): 3770–3776.

Holmes, F.A., Jones, S.E., O'Shaughnessey, J., *et al.* 2002. Comparable efficacy and safety profiles of once-per-cycle pegfilgrastim and daily injection filgrastim in chemotherapy-induced neutropenia: A multicenter dose-finding study in women with breast cancer. *Annals of Oncology* 13:903–909.

Hood, L.E. 2003. Chemotherapy in the elderly: Supportive measures for chemotherapy-induced myelotoxicity. *Clinical Journal of Oncology Nursing* 7(2):185–190.

Hughes, T.P., Kaeda, J., Branford, S., Rudzki, Z., Hochhaus, A., Hensley, M.L., Gathmann, I., Bolton, A.E., van Hoomissen, I.C., Goldman, J.M., and Radich, J.P. 2003. Frequency of major molecular responses to imatinib or interferon alfa plus cytarabine in newly diagnosed chronic myeloid leukemia. *New England Journal of Medicine* 349(15):1423–1432.

Hussar, D.A. 2002. New drugs 2002. *Nursing* 32(4):56–62.

Hyde, R.M. 1992. *The national medical series for independent study: Immunology* (ed 2). Philadelphia: Harwal Publishing.

Iconomou, G., Koutras, A., Rigopoulos, A., Vagenakis, A.G., and Kalofonos, H.P. 2003. Effect of recombinant human erythropoietin on quality of life in cancer patients receiving chemotherapy: Results of a randomized, controlled trial. *Journal of Pain and Symptom Management* 25(6):512–518.

Igarashi, T., Marumo, K., Onishi, T., Kobayashi, M., Aiba, K., Tsushima, T., Ozono, S., Tomita, Y., Terachi, T., Satomi, Y., Kawamura, J., and the Japanese Study Group Against Renal Cancer. 1999. Interferon-alpha and 5-Fluorouracil therapy in patients with metastatic renal cell cancer: An open multicenter trial. *Urology* 53:53–59.

Interferon alfa. 2004. *Martindale: The complete drug reference*. http://micromedex.com.

INTRON-A for injection. 2002. *Physician's Desk Reference*. http://micromedex.com.

Itri, L.M. 2002. The use of epoetin alfa in chemotherapy patients: A consistent profile of efficacy and safety. *Seminars in Oncology* 29(3):81–87.

Joy, M.S. 2002. Darbepoetin alfa: A novel erythropoiesis-stimulating protein. *The Annals of Pharmacology* 36:1183–1191.

Kammula, U.S., White, D.E., and Rosenberg, S.A. 1998. Trends is the safety of high dose bolus interleukin-2 administration in patients with metastatic cancer. *Cancer* 83(4):797–805.

Katterhagen, G. 1996. Physician compliance with outcome-based guidelines and clinical pathways in oncology. *Oncology* 10(Suppl):113–121.

Kawai, K., Saijo, K., Oikawa, T., Morishita, Y., Noguchi, M., Ohno, T., and Akaza, H. 2003. Clinical course and immune response of a renal cell carcinoma patient to adoptive transfer of autologous cytotoxic T lymphocytes. *Clinical and Experimental Immunology* 134:264–269.

Keilholz, U., Stoter, G., Punt, C.J.A., Scheibenbogen, C., Lejeune, F., and Eggermont, A.M.M. 1997. Recombinant interleukin-2-based treatments for advanced melanoma: The Experience of the European Organization for Research and Treatment of Cancer Melanoma Cooperative Group. *The Cancer Journal from Scientific American* 3:S22–S28.

Kerbel, R.S., Viloria-Petit, A., Klement, G., and Rak, J. 2000. 'Accidental' anti-angiogenic drugs: Anti-oncogene directed signal transduction inhibitors and conventional chemotherapeutic agents as examples. *European Journal of Cancer* 26:1248–1257.

Kiley, K.E., and Gale, D.E. 1998. Nursing management of patients with malignant melanoma receiving adjuvant alpha interferon-2b. *Clinical Journal of Oncology Nursing* 2(1):11–16.

King, S.E. 2004. Therapeutic cancer vaccines: An emerging treatment option. *Clinical Journal of Oncology Nursing* 8(3):271–278.

Kinzler, D., and Brown, C. 2001. Cancer vaccines. In P. Rieger (Ed): *Biotherapy: A Comprehensive Overview* (ed 2). Sudbury, MA: Jones & Bartlett, pp 357–382.

Kirkwood, J.M. 2000. Interferon-α and -β: Clinical applications: Melanoma. In S.A. Rosenberg (Ed): *Principles and Practice of the Biologic Therapy of Cancer* (ed 3). Philadelphia: Lippincott Williams & Wilkins, pp 224–251.

Kirkwood, J.M., Strawderman, M.H., Ernstoff, M.S., Smith, T.J., Bordern, E.C., and Blum, R.H. 1996. Interferon alfa-2b adjuvant therapy of high-risk resected cutaneous melanoma: The Eastern Cooperative Oncology Group trial EST 1684. *Journal of Clinical Oncology* 14(1):7–17.

Kragel, A.H., Travis, W.D., Steis, R.G., Rosenberg, S.A., and Roberts, W.C. 1990. Myocarditis or acute myocardial infarction associated with interleukin-2 therapy for cancer. *Cancer* 66:1513–1516.

Krown, S.E., Li, P., Von Roenn, J.H., Paredes, J., Huang, J., and Testa, M.A. 2002. Efficacy of low-dose interferon with antiretroviral therapy in Kaposi's sarcoma: A randomized phase II AIDS clinical trials group study. *Journal of Interferon and Cytokine Research* 22:295–303.

Kugler, A., Stuhler, G., Walden, P., *et al.* 2000. Regression of human metastatic renal cell carcinoma after vaccination with tumor cell-dendritic cell hybrids. *Nature Medicine* 6:332–336.

Kwak, L.W. 1998. Tumor vaccination strategies combined with autologous peripheral stem cell transplantation. *Annals of Oncology* 9(Suppl 1):S41–S46.

Lerner, D.M., Stoudemire, A., and Rosenstein, D.L. 1999. Neuropsychiatric toxicity associated with cytokine therapies. *Psychosomatics* 40:428–435.

Leukine (sargarmostim): Prescribing information. 2002. Richmond, CA: Berlex.

Libretto, S.E., Barrett-Lee, P.J., Branson, K., Gorst, D.W., Kaczmarski, R., McAdam, K.M., and Thomas, R. 2001. Improvement in quality of life of cancer patients treated with epoetin alfa. *European Journal of Cancer Care* 10:183–191.

Lin, S.M., Lin, C.J., Hsu, C.W., Tai, D.I., Sheen, I.S., Lin, D.Y., and Liaw, Y.F. 2003. Prospective randomized controlled study of interferon-alpha in preventing hepatocellular carcinoma recurrence after medical ablation therapy for primary tumors. *Cancer* 100(2):376–382.

Lokich, J. 1997. Spontaneous regression of metastatic renal cancer. *American Journal of Clinical Oncology* 20:416–418.

Lotze, M.T. 1995. Biology of cytokines: The intereleukins. In V.T. DeVita, S. Hellman, and S.A. Rosenberg (Eds): *Biologic Therapy of Cancer*. Philadelphia: JB Lippincott, pp 207–233.

Lowy, D.R., and Schiller, J.T. 1998. Papillomaviruses and cervical cancer: Pathogenesis and vaccine development. *Journal of National Cancer Institute Monographs* 23:27–30.

Lu, A.C., Jones, E.C., Chow, C., Miller, K.D., Herpin, B., Kress-Rock, D., Metcalf, J.A., Lance, H.C., and Kovacs, J.A. 2003. Increases in CD4[+] T lymphocytes occur without increases in thymic size in HIV-infected subjects receiving interleukin-2 therapy. *Journal of Acquired Immune Deficiency Syndrome* 34(3):299–303.

Lyman, G.H., Kuderer, N., Agboola, O., and Balducci, L. 2003. Evidence-based use of colony-stimulating factors in elderly cancer patients. *Cancer Control* 10(6):487–499.

MacFarlane, M.P., Yang, J.C., Guleria, A.S., White, R.L., Seipp, C.A., Einhorn, J.H., White, D.E., and Rosenberg, S.A. 1995. The hematologic toxicity of Interleukin-2 in patients with metastatic melanoma and renal cell carcinoma. *Cancer* 75:1030–1037.

Marin, D., Marktel, S., Szydlo, R., Klein, J.P., Bua, M., Foot, N., Olavarria, E., Shepherd, P., Kanfer, E., Goldman, J.M., and Apperley, J.F. 2003. Survival of patients with chronic-phase chronic myeloid leukaemia on imatinib after failure on interferon alfa. *The Lancet* 362:617–619.

Marincola, F.M. 2000. Cancer vaccines: Basic principles: Mechanisms of immune escape and immune tolerance. In S.A. Rosenberg (Ed): *Principles and Practice of the Biologic Therapy of Cancer* (ed 3). Philadelphia: Lippincott Williams & Wilkins, pp 601–617.

Masci, P., and Borden, E.C. 2002. Malignant melanoma: Treatments emerging, but early detection is still key. *Cleveland Clinic Journal of Medicine* 69(7):529–540.

Matzku, S., and Zoller, M. 2001. Specific immunotherapy of cancer in elderly patients. *Drugs Aging* 18:639–664.

Mavroukakis, S.A., Muehlbauer, P.M., White, R.L., and Schwartzentruber, D.J. 2001. Clinical pathways for managing patients receiving interleukin-2. *Clinical Journal of Oncology Nursing* 5(5):207–217.

McDermott, D., Flaherty, L., Clark, J., *et al.* 2001. A randomized phase III trial of high-dose interleukin-2 versus subcutaneous IL-2 plus interferon in patients with metastatic renal cell carcinoma. *Proceedings of the American Society of Clinical Oncology* 20(Abstr 685):172a.

Michallet, M., Maloisel, F., Delain, M., Hellmann, A., Rosas, A., Silver, R.T., and Tendler, C. 2004. Pegylated recombinant interferon alpha-2b vs. recombinant interferon alpha-2b for the initial treatment of chronic-phase chronic myelogenous leukemia: A phase III study. *Leukemia* 18:309–315.

Mier, J.W. 1993. Pathogenesis of the interleukin-2-induced vascular leak syndrome. In M.B. Atkins and J.W. Mier

(Eds): *Therapeutic Applications of Interleukin-2*. New York: Marcel Dekker, Inc, pp 363–379.

Mitchell, M.S. 2002. Cancer vaccines: A critical review—Part I. *Current Opinion in Investigational Drugs* 3:140–149.

Mitchell, M.S. 2003. Combinations of anticancer drugs and immunotherapy. *Cancer Immunology and Immunotherapy* 52:686–692.

Mocellin, S., Rossi, C.R., and Lise, M., *et al.* 2002. Adjuvant immunotherapy for solid tumors: From promise to clinical application. *Cancer Immunology and Immunotherapy* 51:583–595.

Morris, K. 1998. HAART and host: Balancing the response to HIV-1. *The Lancet* 352:1686.

Morse, M.A. 2002. Current status of dendritic cell vaccines. Therapeutic cancer vaccines: Targeting the future of cancer treatment. http://www.medscape.com.

Moschos, S., Kirkwood, J.M., and Konstantinopoulos, P.A. 2004. Present status and future prospects of adjuvant therapy of melanoma: Time to build upon the foundation of high-dose interferon alfa-2B. *Journal of Clinical Oncology* 22(1):11–14.

Muehlbauer, P.M. 2003. Antiangiogenesis in cancer therapy. *Seminars in Oncology Nursing* 19(3):180–192.

Muehlbauer, P.M., and Schwartzentruber, D.J. 2003. Cancer vaccines. *Seminars in Oncology Nursing* 19(3):206–216.

Naeim, F. 1998. *Pathology of Bone Marrow*. Baltimore: Williams & Wilkins.

Napolitano, L.A. 2003. Approaches to immune reconstitution in HIV infection. *Topics in HIV Medicine* 11(5):160–163.

Nestle, F.O., Burg, G., Dummer, R. 1999. New perspectives on immunobiology and immunotherapy of melanoma. *Immunology Today* 20:5–7.

Neulasta (pegfilgrastim): Prescribing information. 2002. Thousand Oaks, CA: Amgen.

Neumega (oprelvekin): Prescribing information. 2003. Cambridge, MA: Wyeth Pharmaceuticals.

Neupogen (filgrastim): Prescribing information. 2002. Thousand Oaks, CA: Amgen.

Noble, S., and Goa, K.L. 1997. Aldesleukin (recombinant interleukin-2): A review of its pharmacological properties, clinical efficacy and tolerability in patients with metastatic melanoma. *BioDrugs* 7(5):394–422.

O'Brien, S., Giles, F., Talpaz, M., Cortes, J., Rios, M.B., Shan, J., Thomas, D., Andreeff, M., Kornblau, S., Faderl, S., Garcia-Manero, G., White, K., Mallard, S., Freireich, E., and Kantarjian, H.M. 2003. Results of triple therapy with interferon-alpha, cytarabine, and homoharringtonine, and the impact of adding imatinib to the treatment sequence in patients with Philadelphia chromosome-positive chronic myelogenous leukemia in early chronic phase. *Cancer* 98(5):888–893.

Oon, C.J., and Chen, W.N. 2003. Lymphoblastoid alpha-interferon in the prevention of hepatocellular carcinoma (HCC) in high-risk HbsAg-positive resected cirrhotic HCC cases: A 14-year follow-up. *Cancer Invest* 21(3):394–399.

Ozer, H. 2001. Patients aged ≥ 70 are at high risk for neutropenic infection and should receive hemopoietic growth factors when treated with moderately toxic chemotherapy. *Journal of Clinical Oncology* 19(5):1583–1585.

Ozer, H., and Tfayli, A. 2002. Supportive care of cancer patients: Hematopoietic growth factors. http://www.medscape.com.

Ozer, H., Armitage, J.O., Bennett, C.L., Crawford, J., Demetri, G.D., Pizzo, P.A., *et al.* 2000. 2000 update of recommendations for the use of hematopoietic colony-stimulating factors: Evidence-based, clinical practice guidelines. *Journal of Clinical Oncology* 18(20): 3558–3585.

Parmiani, G., Castelli, C., Dalerba, P., *et al.* 2002. Cancer immunotherapy with peptide-based vaccines: What have we achieved? Where are we going? *Journal of the National Cancer Institute* 94:805–818.

Piper, B.F. 1991. Alteration in comfort: Fatigue. In J.C. McNally, E.T. Somerville, C. Misaskowski, and M. Rostad (Eds): *Guidelines for Oncology Nursing Practice*. Philadelphia: WB Saunders, pp 155–162.

Pockaj, B.A., Yang, J.C., Lotze, M.T., *et al.* 1994. A prospective randomized trial evaluating colloid versus crystalloid resuscitation in the treatment of the vascular leak syndrome associated with interleukin-2 therapy. *Journal of Immunotherapy* 15:22–28.

Portenoy, R.K., and Itri, L.M. 1999. Cancer-related fatigue: Guidelines for evaluation and management. *The Oncologist* 4:1–10.

Procrit (epoetin alfa): Full prescribing information. 2002. Raritan, NJ: Ortho Biotech.

Proleukin (interleukin 2): Prescribing information. 2000. Emeryville, CA: Chiron.

Quesada, J.R., Talpaz, M., Rios, A.L., Kurzrock, R., and Gutterman, J.U. 1986. Clinical toxicity of interferons in cancer patients: A review. *Journal of Clinical Oncology* 4:234–243.

Ravaud, A., Negrier, S., Cany, L., *et al.* 1994. Subcutaneous low-dose interleukin-2 and alpha-interferon in patients with metastatic renal cell carcinoma. *British Journal of Cancer* 69:1111–1114.

Repetto, L., Biganzoli, L., Koehne, C.H., Luebbe, A.S., Soubeyran, P., Tjan-Heijnen, V.C.G., and Aapro, M.S. 2003. EORTC cancer in the elderly task force guidelines for the use of colony-stimulating factors in elderly patients with cancer. *European Journal of Cancer* 39:2264–2272.

Repetto, L., Carreca, I., Maraninchi, D., Aapro, M., Calabresi, P., and Balducci, L. 2003. Use of growth factors in the elderly patient with cancer: A report from the Second International Society for Geriatric Oncology (SIOG) 2001 meeting. *Critical Reviews in Oncology/Hematology* 45:123–128.

Restifo, N.P. 2000. Cancer vaccines: Basic principles: General concepts and preclinical studies. In S.A. Rosenberg (Ed): *Principles and Practice of the Biologic Therapy of Cancer* (ed 3). Philadelphia: Lippincott Williams & Wilkins, pp 571–584.

Reynolds, C.H. 2000. Clinical efficacy of rhIL-11. *Oncology* 14(Suppl 8):32–40.

Rieger, P. 2001. Biotherapy: An overview. In P. Rieger (Ed): *Biotherapy: A Comprehensive Overview* (ed 2). Sudbury, MA: Jones and Bartlett, pp 3–37.

Rieger, P., and Haeuber, D. 1995. A new approach to managing chemotherapy-related anemia: Nursing implications of epoetin alfa. *Oncology Nursing Forum* 22:77–81.

Rizzo, D.J., Lichtin, A.E., Woolf, S.H., Seidenfeld, J., Bennett, C.L., Cella, D., *et al.* 2002. Use of epoetin in patients with cancer: Evidence-based clinical practice guidelines of the American Society of Clinical Oncology and the American Society of Hematology. *Journal of Clinical Oncology* 20(19):4083–4107.

Roberts, B. 2000. Cancer vaccines: Clinical applications: Adenovirus and other viral vaccines. In S.A. Rosenberg (Ed): *Principles and Practice of the Biologic Therapy of Cancer* (ed 3). Philadelphia: Lippincott Williams & Wilkins, pp 694–705.

Rosenberg, S.A., Lotze, M.T., Yang, J.C., Aebersold, P.M., Linehan, W.M., Seipp, C.A., and White, D.E. 1989. Experience with the use of high dose interleukin-2 in the treatment of b52 cancer patients. *Annals of Surgery* 210(4):474–484.

Rosenberg, S.A. 1997. Keynote Address: Perspectives on the use of interleukin-2 in cancer treatment. *The Cancer Journal from Scientific American* 3:S2–S6.

Rosenberg, S.A. 2000a. Cell transfer therapy: Clinical applications: Melanoma. In S.A. Rosenberg (Ed): *Principles and Practice of the Biologic Therapy of Cancer* (ed 3). Philadelphia: Lippincott Williams & Wilkins, pp 322–333.

Rosenberg, S.A. 2000b. Cancer vaccines: Clinical applications: Peptides and protein vaccines. In S.A. Rosenberg (Ed): *Principles and Practice of the Biologic Therapy of Cancer* (ed 3). Philadelphia: Lippincott Williams & Wilkins, pp 662–673.

Rosenberg, S.A., and Dudley, M.E. 2004. Cancer regression in patients with metastatic melanoma after the transfer of autologous antitumor lymphocytes. *Proceedings of the National Academy of Sciences of the United States of America.* 101(Suppl 2): 14639–14645.

Rosenberg, S.A., Yang, J.C., Topalian, S.L., Schwartzentruber, D.J., Weber, J.S., Parkinson, D.R., Seipp, C.A., Einhorn, J.H., and White, D.E. 1994. Treatment of 283 consecutive patients with metastatic melanoma or renal cell cancer using high-dose bolus interleukin 2. *Journal of the American Medical Association* 271:907–913.

Rosenberg, S.A., Yang, J.C., White, D.E., and Steinberg, S.M. 1998. Durability of complete responses in patients with metastatic cancer treated with high-dose interleukin-2: Identification of the antigens mediating response. *Annals of Surgery* 228:307–319.

Rust, D.M., Wood, L.S., and Battiato, L.A. 1999. Oprelvekin: An alternative treatment for thrombocytopenia. *Clinical Journal of Oncology Nursing* 3(2):57–62.

Salgaller, M.L. 2000. Cancer vaccines: Basic principles: Immune adjuvants. In S.A. Rosenberg (Ed): *Principles and Practice of the Biologic Therapy of Cancer* (ed 3). Philadelphia: Lippincott Williams & Wilkins, pp 584–601.

Salit, R.B., Kast, W.M., Velders, M.P. 2002. Ins and outs of clinical trials with peptide-based vaccines. *Frontiers in Bioscience* 7:e204–e213.

Sandstrom, K.S. 1996. Nursing management of patients receiving biological therapy. *Seminars in Oncology Nursing* 12:152–162.

Santhanam, S., Decatris, M., and O'Byrne, K. 2002. Potential of interferon-α in solid tumors: Part 2. *Biodrugs* 16(5):349–372.

Schlom, J., and Panicali, D. 2000. Cancer vaccines: Clinical applications: Recombinant poxvirus vaccines. In S.A. Rosenberg (Ed): *Principles and Practice of the Biologic Therapy of Cancer* (ed 3). Philadelphia: Lippincott Williams & Wilkins, pp 686–694.

Schreiber, H. 1999. Tumor Immunology. In W. Paul (Ed): *Fundamental Immunology* (ed 4). Philadelphia: Lippincott-Raven, pp 1237–1270.

Schuchter, L.M. 2004. Adjuvant interferon therapy for melanoma: High-dose, low-dose, no dose, which dose? *Journal of Clinical Oncology* 22(1):7–10.

Schwartz, R., Stover, L., and Dutcher, J. 2002. Managing toxicities of high-dose interleukin-2. *Oncology* 16 (Suppl):11–20.

Schwartzentruber, D.J. 2000. Chapter 3.1: Interleukin-2: Clinical applications. Principles of administration and management of side effects. In S.A. Rosenberg (Ed): *Principles and Practice of the Biologic Therapy of Cancer* (ed 3). Philadelphia: Lippincott Williams & Wilkins, pp 32–50.

Schwartzentruber, D.J. 2001. Guidelines for the safe administration of high-dose interleukin-2. *Journal of Immunotherapy* 24(4):287–293.

Shanahan, J.C., Moreland, L.W., and Carter, R.H. 2003. Upcoming biologic agents for the treatment of Rheumatic diseases. *Current Opinion Rheumatology* 15(3):226–236.

Sharp, E. 1995. The interleukins. In P.T. Reiger (Ed): *Biotherapy: A Comprehensive Overview*. Boston: Jones and Bartlett, pp 93–111.

Shelton, B.K. 2001. Flu-like syndrome. In P.T. Rieger (Ed): *Biotherapy: A Comprehensive Overview* (ed 2). Boston: Jones and Bartlett, pp 519–543.

Shi, M., Zhang, B., Tang, Z.R., Lie, Z.Y.L., Wang, H.F., Feng, Y.Y., Fan, Z.P., Xu, D.P., and Wang, F.S. 2004. Autologous cytokine-induced killer cell therapy in clinical trial phase I is safe in patients with primary hepatocellular carcinoma. *World Journal of Gastroenterology* 10(8):1146–1151.

Shimizu, J., Yamazaki, S., and Sakaguchi, S. 1999. Induction of tumor immunity by removing $CD25^+CD4^+$ T cells: A common basis between tumor immunity and autoimmunity. *Journal of Immunology* 163:5211–5218.

Siemens, D.R., and Ratliff, T.L. 2001. Vaccines in urologic malignancies. *Urology Research* 29:152–162.

Simon, R.M., Steinberg, S.M., Hamilton, M., et al. 2001. Clinical trial designs for the early clinical development of therapeutic cancer vaccines. *Journal of Clinical Oncology* 19:1848–1854.

Singh, R., and Fidler, I. 1996. *Current topics in microbiology and immunology*. Berlin: Spring-Verlag.

Sivanandham, M., Stavropoulos, C., and Wallack, M. 2000. Cancer vaccines: Clinical applications: Whole cell and lysate vaccines. In S.A. Rosenberg (Ed): *Principles and Practice of the Biologic Therapy of Cancer* (ed 3). Philadelphia: Lippincott Williams & Wilkins, pp 632–647.

Skalla, K. 1996. The interferons. *Seminars in Oncology Nursing* 12(2):97–105.

Skalla, K., and Rieger, P.T. 1995. Fatigue. In P.T. Rieger (Ed): *Biotherapy: A Comprehensive Overview*. Boston: Jones and Bartlett, pp 221–242.

Slavin, S., Morecki, S., Weiss, L., and Or, R. 2003. Immunotherapy of hematologic malignancies and metastatic solid tumors in experimental animals and man. *Critical Reviews in Oncology/Hematology* 46:139–163.

Smith, J.W. 2000. Tolerability and side effect profile of rhIL-11. *Oncology* 14(9 Suppl 8):41–47.

Sondak, V.K., Liu, P.Y., Tuthill, R.J., et al. 2002. Adjuvant immunotherapy of resected, intermediate-thickness, node-negative melanoma with an allogeneic tumor vaccine: Overall results of a randomized trial of the Southwest Oncology Group. *Journal of Clinical Oncology* 20:2058–2066.

Sparber, A.G., Biller-Sparber, K. 1993. Immunotherapy and neuropsychiatric toxicity: Nursing clinical management considerations. *Cancer Nursing* 16:188–192.

Stafford-Fox, V., and Guindon, K.M. 2000. Cutaneous reactions associated with alpha interferon therapy. *Clinical Journal of Oncology Nursing* 4(4):164–168.

Sundaram, R., Dakappagari, N.K., Kaumaya, P.T. 2002. Synthetic peptides as cancer vaccines. *Biopolymers* 66:200–216.

Sylvester, R.K. 2002. Clinical applications of colony stimulating factors: A historical perspective. *American Journal of Health-System Pharmacy* 59 (Suppl 2):s6–s12.

Thames, W.A., Smith, S.L., Scheifele, A.C., Yao, B., Giffin, S.A., and Alley, J.L. 2004. Evaluation of the US Oncology Network's recommended guidelines for substitution with darbepoetin alfa 200 mcg every 2 weeks in both naïve patients and patients switched from epoetin alfa. *Pharmacotherapy* 24(3):313–323.

Tomaszewski, J.G., DeLaPena, L., Molenda, J., Gantz, S., Bernato, D.L., and Folts, S. 1995. Programmed instruction: biotherapy module II. Overview of biotherapy. *Cancer Nursing* 18(5):397–414.

Tourani, J.M., Pfister, C., Tubiana, N., Ouldkaci, M., et al. 2003. Subcutaneous interleukin-2 and interferon-alfa administration in patients with metastatic renal cell carcinoma: Final results of SCAPP III, a large, multicenter, phase II, nonrandomized study with sequential analysis design—The Subcutaneous Administration Propeukin Program Cooperative Group. *Journal of Clinical Oncology* 21(21):3987–3994.

Toyofuku, K., Imayama, S., Yasumoto, S., Kiryu, H., and Hori, Y. 1994. Clinical and immunohistochemical studies of skin eruptions: Relationship to administration of interferon-alpha. *Journal of Dermatology* 21:732–737.

Tretter, C., Savage, P.D., Muss, H.B., and Ernstoff, M.D. 2000. Interferon-α and -β: Clinical applications: Renal cell cancer. In S.A. Rosenberg (Ed): *Principles and Practice of the Biologic Therapy of Cancer* (ed 3). Philadelphia: Lippincott Williams & Wilkins, pp 252–273.

Tushinski, R.J., and Mulé, J.J. 1995. Biology of cytokines: The intereleukins. In V.T. DeVita, S. Hellman, and S.A. Rosenberg (Eds): *Biologic Therapy of Cancer*. Philadelphia: JB Lippincott, pp 87–94.

Viele, C.S., and Moran, T.A. 1993. Nursing management of the nonhospitalized patient receiving recombinant interleukin-2. *Seminars in Oncology Nursing* 3:20–24.

Weber, J. 2002. Tumor-antigen vaccines for cancer. Therapeutics cancer vaccines: Targeting the future of cancer treatment. http://www.medscape.com.

Wheeler, V.S. 1996. Interleukins: The search for an anticancer therapy. *Seminars in Oncology Nursing* 12(2):106–114.

White, R.L., Schwartzentruber, D.J., Guleria, A., MacFarlane, M.P., White, D.E., Tucker, E., and Rosenberg, S.A. 1994. Cardiopulmonary toxicity of treatment with high dose interleukin-2 in 199 consecutive patients with metastatic melanoma or renal cell carcinoma. *Cancer* 74:3212–3222.

White, S., Conry, R. 2000. Cancer vaccines: Clinical applications: DNA vaccines. In S.A. Rosenberg (Ed): *Principles and Practice of the Biologic Therapy of Cancer* (ed 3). Philadelphia: Lippincott Williams & Wilkins, pp 674–686.

Wiemann, B., and Starnes, C.O. 1994. Coley's toxins, tumor necrosis factor and cancer research: A historical perspective. *Pharmacology Therapy* 64:529–564.

Williams, B.R.G. 2000. Interferon-α and -β: Basic principles and preclinical studies. In S.A. Rosenberg (Ed): *Principles and Practice of the Biologic Therapy of Cancer* (ed 3). Philadelphia: Lippincott Williams & Wilkins, pp 194–208.

Winningham, M.L. 1991. Walking program for people with cancer: Getting started. *Cancer Nursing* 14(5):270–276.

Wujcik, D. 2001. Hematopoietic growth factors. In P.T. Rieger (Ed): *Biotherapy: A Comprehensive Overview* (ed 2). Sudbury, MA: Jones and Bartlett, pp 245–282.

Yang, J.C., and Rosenberg, S.A. 1997. An ongoing prospective randomized comparison of interleukin-2 regimens for the treatment of metastatic renal cell cancer. *Cancer Journal from Scientific American* 3(Suppl 1):S79–84.

Yang, J.C., Sherry, R.M., Steinberg, S.M., Topalian, S.L., Schwartzentruber, D.J., Hwu, P., Seipp, C.A., Rogers-Freezer, L., Morton, K.E., White, D.E., Liewehr, D.J., Merino, M.J., and Rosenberg, S.A. 2003. Randomized study of high-dose and low-dose interleukin-2 in patients with metastatic renal cancer. *Journal of Clinical Oncology* 21(16):3127–3132.

Yao, F., and Terrault, N. 2001. Hepatitis C and hepatocellular carcinoma. *Current Treatment Options in Oncology* 2:473–483.

Ziotta, A.R., and Schulman, C.C. 2000. Biological response modifiers for the treatment of superficial bladder tumors. *European Urology* 37(Suppl 3):10–15.

Zukiwski, A.A., David, C.L., Coan, J., Wallace, S., Gutterman, J.U., Mavligit, G.M. 1990. Increased incidence of hypersensitivity to iodine-containing radiographic contrast media after interleukin-2 administration. *Cancer* 65:1521–1524.

Molecular Targeted Therapy

Gail M. Wilkes, M.S.N., R.N.C.

Introduction

For many years, cancer treatment has depended on eradication of malignant cells. Surgical removal of solid tumors resulted in cure for many patients with cancer, but for others, high risk for recurrence, perhaps because of disease involvement of regional lymph nodes, required adjuvant chemotherapy to eliminate micrometastatic disease. Chemotherapy is the use of cellular poisons to kill malignant cells; unfortunately, these poisons are not exclusively targeted to malignant cells, and normal cells that divide frequently are injured as well. Fortunately, normal cells have more effective repair mechanisms, and recovery occurs after a predictable interval. Patients are challenged by not only physiologic assaults on their body but by psychological threats as well, such as body image changes related to hair loss, changes in sexuality, and fatigue. The search for the "silver bullet," which would target malignant cells exclusively, is elusive.

As knowledge of the process of carcinogenesis and malignant transformation emerges, molecular flaws can be targeted, and "silver bullets" or targeted therapy can be developed to preferentially attack malignant cells, sparing normal cells. However, most agents identified to date are given along with chemotherapy or radiotherapy.

The 21st century has become the age of molecular targeted therapy, and as new and more sophisticated understanding of genetic mutations and their subsequent role in malignant transformation occurs, new agents are being developed in exponential numbers.

Andrew C. von Eschenbach, MD, director of the National Cancer Institute (NCI), has announced that the goal of the NCI is to eliminate suffering and death from cancer by the year 2015. He refers to this time in cancer care as the "era of molecular oncology." (It is known that cancer is a disease of the cell and, more importantly, a disease of sequential mutations that are not repaired and that then progress to malignant transformation.) To achieve this goal, von Eschenbach has identified major initiatives in seven areas of research and treatment (von Eschenbach 2003):

1. Molecular epidemiology (finding what causes specific mutations in the cell that then cause a specific cancer)
2. Integrated cancer biology (finding the steps in malignant transformation, invasion, metastases, and angiogenesis)
3. Strategic development of cancer interventions (such as partnering with the Food and Drug Administration to speed up approval of drugs and medical devices)
4. Early detection, prevention, and prediction
5. Integrated clinical trials (to find a better and faster way to do the testing)
6. Overcoming health disparities
7. Bioinformatics (using information technology and computers to make the tools needed to collect, share, and analyze biomedical data)

Because most people die from metatases and not from the primary tumor, von Eschenbach proposes that molecular targeted therapy can help keep the primary tumor small, at 1–3 mm so that cancer would become a chronic disease much like diabetes mellitus. Figure 5.1 shows the current disease trajectory of a cancer that is not cured (top line) compared with extended survival in cancer as a chronic disease (lower line).

Three major advances have brought this optimism to oncology:

1. Identification of molecular flaws leading to cancer and mechanisms to target these flaws, although this knowledge continues to grow
2. Identification of the almost 35,000 genes in the human genome
3. Gene and protein microarray technology, permitting genetic fingerprinting to diagnose cancers and the promise to be able to prescribe individualized, targeted treatment based on the genetic mutations

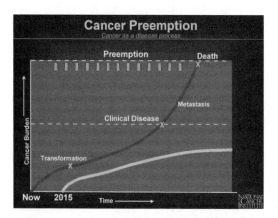

FIGURE 5.1 Goal of reduction of cancer deaths and suffering by 2015. The top line shows "now," as of 2003, the process of a cancer forming, getting large enough to be recognized as clinical disease, metastasizing, and leading to death, compared with the bottom line, where by 2015, the NCL goal is to keep the initial malignant tumor at a small size, so that cancer becomes a chronic disease, not causing death or suffering. The person is able to "live with cancer" as a chronic disease, much like diabetes or heart disease. Image reproduced from: http://www.cancer.gov/newscenter/benchmarks-vol3-issue2/Photo. Reproduced with permission.

Molecular Targets

Cancer is a disease of sequential mutations, as shown in Figure 5.2.

To understand how cancer is a disease of mutations, it is important to review deoxyribonucleic acid (DNA), mutations, how cells divide, and the process of malignant transformation. To begin with, let's think about ourselves. Genes are the blueprint for who we are and what we look like, such as whether we have brown or blue or hazel eyes or blonde or brown hair. The genes are found on two strands of DNA, which are twisted together in a double helix and stored in the chromosome. The chromosome is stored in the nucleus of the cell. Each strand of DNA is made up of four chemical bases, repeated millions of times and in many combinations. A chromosome is made up of DNA and contains many genes, which are specific segments of DNA. Not all genes are "turned on" or "expressed," and only those that are expressed are active, such as those for blue eyes in a blue-eyed person. "Expressed" also means that the gene portion of DNA is transcribed into messenger ribonucleic acid (mRNA) and then translated into protein, such as insulin in the latter example, or made into special types of RNA used to help in translation and synthesis of the protein (transfer and ribosomal RNA) (Genome Glossary 2004). The human cell has 23 pairs of chromosomes: 22 autosomal (somatic) and 1 sex (see Figures 5.3 to 5.6). Figure 5.7 depicts how the location of a gene on a chromosome is identified.

The sequence of the bases tells the message or the recipe for a specific protein that will do a task, which is later transcribed or copied by mRNA and taken outside of the cell nucleus to the ribosome in the surrounding cytoplasm, where it is translated. The translated message results in the production of a specific protein. The message or recipe is coded using four bases: adenine, thymine, guanine, and cytosine. Adenine always binds with thymine, and guanine binds with cytosine, forming *base pairs*. Proteins are responsible for body functions and are made up of a specific sequence

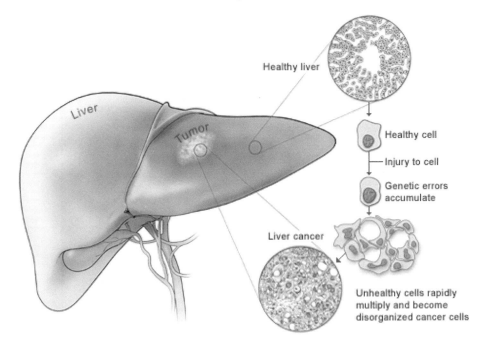

Healthy liver

Liver

Tumor

Healthy cell

Injury to cell

Genetic errors
accumulate

Liver cancer

Unhealthy cells rapidly
multiply and become
disorganized cancer cells

FIGURE 5.2 Cancer is a disease of mutations. The top right shows healthy liver cells, which undergo an environmental insult, causing injury to the cell and leading to genetic errors, which are allowed to accumulate in the cell's DNA. This leads to mutations in proto-oncogenes, tumor-suppressor genes, and DNA repair genes and permits malignant transformation. The lower right circle shows hepatoma cells. Image reproduced from: http://ghr.nlm.nih.gov/ghr/picture/cancer, accessed August 14, 2004. Reproduced with permission from Genetics Home Reference.

of amino acids. This process of the gene telling the body what proteins to make is called *gene expression* and involves *transcription* and *translation* (see Figure 5.8.). For example, let's say you just had lunch, and your body needs insulin to bring the glucose into the cells. Your pancreas cells have received a message from the body to make insulin. The genes coding for the protein insulin are copied by mRNA and move out of the nucleus to the ribosome, where they are translated, insulin is manufactured and then released into the blood.

In general, in the healthy individual, cell birth equals cell death. When the body needs new cells, cells that have the capacity to divide are stimulated by a growth factor or hormone, and a signal is sent to the cell's nucleus to start cell division, or proliferation. The body carefully regulates cell division or proliferation, which is promoted by proto-oncogenes. Cell division is balanced by halting forces (tumor-suppressor genes) that put the "brakes" on cell division and make sure there is a balance between cell division and cell death through apoptosis, or programmed cell death. When the prodivision force is stronger, the cell then prepares to divide and goes through specific phases of the cell cycle.

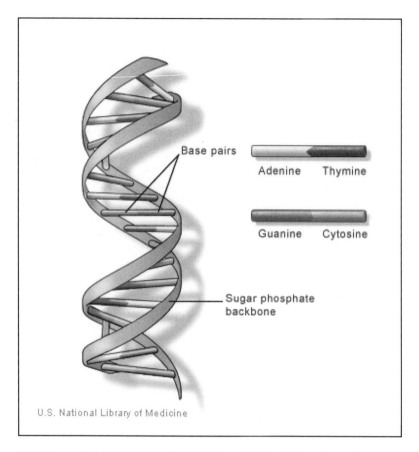

FIGURE 5.3 DNA double helix. The DNA helix is formed by the binding of base pairs (guanine with cytosine and adenine with thymine) attached to a sugar-phosphate backbone. Image reproduced from: http://ghr.nlm.nih.gov/info=basics/show/dna; jsessionid=8E1845BBD275FEB78F13E193E80C1193, accessed August 9, 2004. Reproduced with permission from Genetics Home Reference.

When originally studied, the cell cycle appeared to have "gaps" of time in the cycle, and G was used to identify them. G_0 is the resting phase, where cells rest until they need to divide and are recruited into the cell cycle. G_1 is the first phase, and it is during this time that the cell enlarges and begins to synthesize proteins to make DNA in the next phase, the synthesis phase. There is a restriction point near the end of the G_1 phase ("R") when the cell commits to cell division. Up until this time, the cell is following growth factor orders to divide. At the R_1 point, the cell takes over control and is no longer responding to growth factors. This is a crucial and irreversible step and is flawed in almost all malignant cells. Studies are continuing to help us understand the actual steps, but the retinoblastoma (Rb) protein, a tumor suppressor gene product, appears to play a major role. The Rb protein is the product of the tumor-suppressor retinoblastoma gene and is called the "master brakes" of the cell cycle. Once committed, the cell enters the synthesis phase, where the cell duplicates the DNA to be used for the daughter cell, and duplicates the chromosomes. Because the

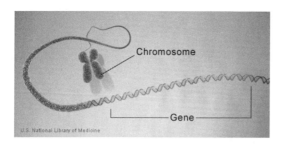

FIGURE 5.4 Genes are a segment of DNA. Genes are segments of DNA on a chromosome. Genes code for specific proteins that support all body processes. Each chromosome contains many genes. Image reproduced from: http://ghr.nlm.nih.gov/info=basics/show/gene; jsessionid=8E1845BBD275FEB78F13E193E80C1193, accessed August 9, 2004. Reproduced with permission from Genetics Home Reference.

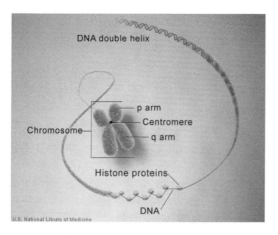

FIGURE 5.5 The human chromosome. The tightly wound DNA helix, along with histone proteins, make up the human chromosome. Image reproduced from: http://ghr.nlm.nih.gov/info=basics/show/chromosome; jsessionid=8E1845BBD275FEB78F13E193E80C1193, accessed August 9, 2004. Reproduced with permission from Genetics Home Reference.

entire strand of DNA needs to be copied exactly, there are many opportunities for mistakes, like mismatched base pairs, single base insertions, or deletions. Chapter 1 describes these genetic mutation possibilities in detail. Within this cycle is a DNA replication checkpoint where the DNA is closely examined to make sure that the DNA replication is completed. Throughout this process, p53

monitors the cell's health, especially the integrity of the DNA, making sure the cycles of the cell are completed correctly (Weinberg 1996), and also making sure that the DNA is only duplicated once, thus protecting against overexpression of certain genes. In certain breast cancers, genes, such as the *HER-2-neu* gene, are overexpressed. The cell then enters G_2 phase, where the cell makes the apparatus needed for mitosis, or cell division. Here, there is a third checkpoint called the G_2 DNA damage checkpoint, and the DNA is inspected to see whether there are any mutations or damage that needs to be repaired. Not unexpectedly, the genes responsible for repair are called mismatch repair genes, and their gene products closely compare the parental strand with the daughter strand. When they find a mistake, they unwind the DNA, degrade the flawed strand, and repair the error. Unfortunately, these genes may also be mutated, and then the flawed DNA is allowed to proceed through the rest of the cell cycle, with the genetic mutations being present in all subsequent cell divisions. In a normal cell, there continues to be mistakes or if the DNA is incorrectly replicated, the cell cannot progress to mitosis. The cell has time now to fix the mistakes or to complete the replication of DNA. Once the cell is certain that there are no mutations and that the DNA is correctly replicated, the cell moves into mitosis. Now, the chromosomes line up on the centromere of the mitotic spindle, the cell cytoplasm separates into two parts (cytokinesis), and two identical daughter cells are formed. See the phases in Figure 5.9. This figure also depicts the gene proteins (such as p21), cyclins, and CDCs (that control) progress through the cell cycle. Later in the chapter, this will be discussed in more detail because mutations in these factors can move cell division forward despite the presence of mutations that result in carcinogenesis.

Cells divide continually to replace cells that are used up through normal wear and tear, such as cells lining the intestinal microvilli, which are shed by the millions every minute during the digestion process. It is not surprising that given the

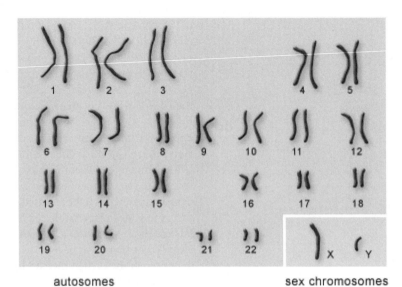

autosomes   sex chromosomes

FIGURE 5.6 Complement of human chromosomes. The human genome consists of 22 autosomes, which are numbered by size. The 23rd pair of chromosomes are the sex chromosomes, or X and Y chromosomes. Image reproduced from:http://ghr.nlm.nih.gov/info=basics/show/how_many_ chromosomes; jsessionid=8E1845BBD275FEB78F13E193E80C1193, accessed August 9, 2004. Reproduced with permission from Genetics Home Reference.

millions of cell divisions a minute and the billions of transcription and translation actions that occur, mutations are impossible to prevent. In addition, mutations can be caused by environmental mutagens, such as cigarette smoke in the bronchial tree, chemicals such as pesticides, *Helicobacter pylori* bacteria in the stomach, or human 185 papilloma virus (HPV) 16 and 18 viruses in the cervix of women. Mutations common in cancer are point mutations and insertion and deletion mutations (Gribbon and Loescher 2000). Point mutations are mutations involving the substitution of a single base, such as the substitution of thymine for guanine, and can be further classified as silent (does not change the message when the gene is transcribed), missense (mutation resulted in a change in the amino acid being copied, so it changes the protein product that is produced when the gene is transcribed), and nonsense (codes for a STOP codon so that the protein cannot be made and will be truncated), which are most commonly harmful.

Deletion or insertion mutations involve the loss or addition of one or more base pairs, so that the reading frame of the sequence of bases is shifted. If one or two base pairs are lost or added, it will result in a frameshift mutation; if three are lost, there will not be a frameshift because the code is in groups of three base pairs (Gribbon and Loescher 2000). Figure 5.10 illustrates a number of ways mutations can occur.

Translocations of genetic material involve large parts of the chromosome being moved from one chromosome to another nearby chromosome. Reciprocal translocations mean an exchange of genetic material from one chromosome to another and material from the second chromosome back to the first chromosome or to two places on the same chromosome. Often, this results in oncogene activation (changing a proto-oncogene to an

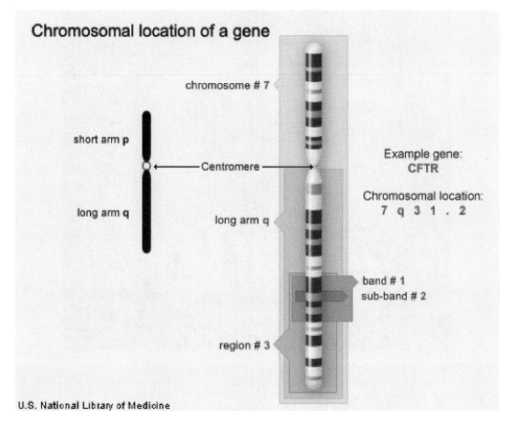

Chromosomal location of a gene

chromosome # 7

short arm p

Centromere

long arm q

long arm q

Example gene:
CFTR

Chromosomal location:
7 q 3 1 . 2

band # 1
sub-band # 2

region # 3

U.S. National Library of Medicine

FIGURE 5.7 Points of reference on a chromosome. The cystic fibrosis gene, *CFTR*, is located on the long arm (q) of chromosome 7, region 3, band 1, sub-band 2 (position 7q31.2). Image reproduced from:http://ghr.nlm.nih.gov/info=basics/show/gene_location; jsessionid=8E1845BBD275FEB78F13E193E80C1193, accessed 8.9.04. Reproduced with permission from Genetics Home Reference.

oncogene) through overexpression and fusion at areas where breaks commonly occur (breakpoint region) (Gribbon and Loescher 2000).

What is surprising is the fact that so few mutations become dangerous or lead to malignancy. This is because the cell has special DNA repair genes that attempt to repair the mutation (for example, in the base pairing). Once a cell is recruited into the G_1 phase, it undergoes close scrutiny to see whether the DNA is damaged in any way or mutated and, if so, whether the DNA can be repaired by the DNA repair genes. Figure 5.11 shows how effective DNA repair genes can circumvent malignant transformation. If they cannot, then the cell is destroyed through apoptosis,

or programmed cell death, as shown in Figures 5.12 to 5.14. The protein p53 is instrumental in orchestrating the destruction of cells in which the DNA mutations cannot be repaired by the DNA repair genes. Apoptosis is a process where the cells are broken apart and then engulfed by macrophages (National Cancer Institute 2004). That way, the integrity of the DNA is assured, and both daughter cells receive the full complement of intact DNA. However, if the mutations are in the DNA repair genes, then the protein made by these genes cannot repair the mutations. This allows mutations to accumulate and be passed on to the daughter cells if the genes responsible for cell death or apoptosis are also mutated, such as

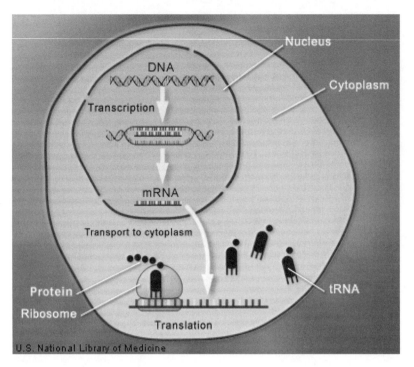

FIGURE 5.8 Transcribing a gene and translating it into a protein gene product. Through the processes of transcription and translation, the "recipe" from a gene is used to make a specific protein. The portion of DNA encoding for the gene is transcribed onto messenger RNA (mRNA) and then carried from the cell nucleus to the ribosome or protein factory in the cytoplasm. There transfer RNA brings amino acids to the ribosome where they are made into proteins using the recipe from the gene carried on mRNA. Image reproduced from: http://ghr.nlm.nih.gov/info=basics/show/making_protein; jsessionid= 8E1845BBD275FEB78F13E193E80C1193, accessed August 9, 2004. Reproduced with permission from Genetics Home Reference.

BCL-2 (a proto-oncogene). Unrepaired mutations in proto-oncogenes and tumor-suppressor genes lead to malignant transformation.

Mutations can occur in any part of the DNA. Not all mutations are harmful, but some can be harmful depending on whether the mutation allows the correct protein to still be made. For example, a mutation may just be an extra base pair and not be near an important gene, so the critical proteins can still be made. However, if the mutation is near a proto-oncogene or a tumor-suppressor gene, then it can be quite serious, as discussed later.

Let's look at the types of mutations that can occur. Germline mutations are mutations in the germ cells (ova or sperm) that are present at birth and represent the first mutation in the sequence of mutations that lead to malignant transformation. For example, when the baby is born, that particular mutation will occur in every cell of the body. An example is the *APC* germline mutation (adenomatous polyposis coli gene, a tumor-suppressor gene), where the child inherits the first mutation in the sequence leading to colon cancer (Fearon and Vogelstein 1990). There are two alleles, one from each parent, and here, one has the autosomal dominant mutation, which has 100% penetrance (the person who inherits the mutation will develop the disease). Having inherited a mutated gene usually does not confer a 100% risk

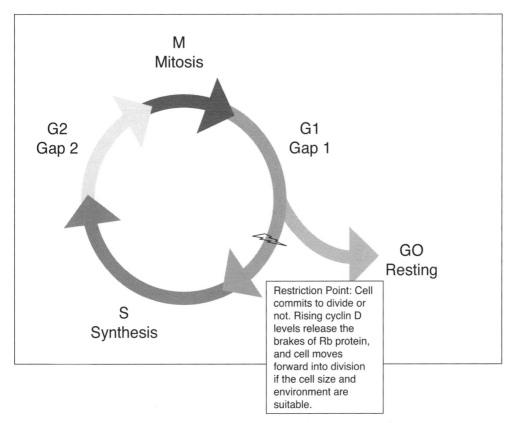

FIGURE 5.9a The cell cycle. The cell cycle is very tightly controlled to ensure that cells divide only when needed and that DNA in the chromosomes is intact so that daughter cells created have identical genes to the parent cell. G stands for GAP, and G_0 is the resting phase. G_1 is the phase where the cell decides whether to divide, and if so, the proteins necessary to replicate DNA are made. S is the synthesis phase, when DNA is copied and replicated, forming an identical double helix; G_2 is a time to ensure that the DNA is correctly replicated and to make the necessary apparatus for mitosis. M is the next phase, and the cell undergoes mitosis, forming two identical daughter cells, which usually go back to the G_0 phase. Mitosis is shown in Figure 5.9b. Proteins called *cyclins* regulate movement through the phases of the cell cycle once they are activated by binding to enzymes called *cyclin-dependent kinases*. There are three checkpoints during the cell cycle to ensure that cell division is going as planned, and the DNA is scrutinized to make sure it is not damaged: (1) before the cell enters the S phase at the G_1 checkpoint or restriction point shown by the lightning bolt in the figure; (2) during the S phase to make sure that the replicated DNA strands are correct; and (3) after the DNA has been replicated at the G_2 checkpoint, to make sure the replication is completed and DNA is undamaged. If the DNA is damaged, DNA repair gene products try to fix it, and if unsuccessful, the cell does not complete cell division, but undergoes programmed cell death or apoptosis. p53 gene product is very important in overseeing this process. Reproduced with permission. Yarbro, C. 2006. *Cancer Nursing Principles and Practice* (ed 6). Sudbury, MA: Jones and Bartlett Publishers.

of developing cancer because most mutations do not have 100% penetrance. A person inherits two copies of each gene, called alleles, one from each parent. Usually, the two alleles are not identical, so they are called heterozygous (homozygous means identical). If one is mutated

(e.g., inactivated tumor-suppressor function), then the other normal tumor-suppressor gene should provide normal function until it too is mutated. This loss of one of the alleles is called loss of heterozygosity (LOH) and is common in most malignant tumors that lose function of

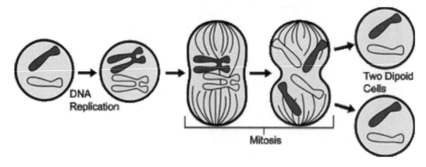

FIGURE 5.9b Mitosis. Image reproduced from: http://www.ncbi.nlm.nih.gov/About/primer/ genetics_cell.html, accessed August 9, 2004. Reproduced with permission from the National Center for Biotechnology Information, National Library of Medicine, The National Institute of Health.

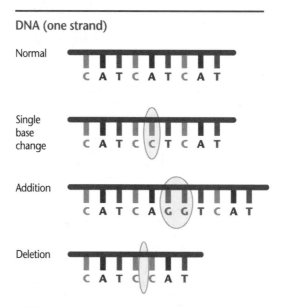

FIGURE 5.10 Types of mutations. Mutations in genes involve base pairs and can be simple, such as a change, either an addition or deletion of a single base, as shown above. The mutation may or may not affect whether the gene can make the correct protein when transcribed. However, bigger mistakes, like large segments of DNA which can be moved, deleted, or repeated, can occur with more damaging consequences. Image reproduced from: http://press2.nci.nih.gov/sciencebehind/cancer/cancer42.h tm, accessed August 9, 2004. Reproduced with permission.

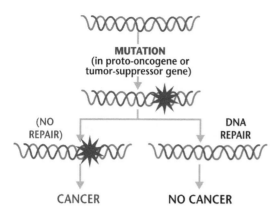

MUTATION
(in proto-oncogene or
tumor-suppressor gene)

(NO
REPAIR)

DNA
REPAIR

CANCER   NO CANCER

FIGURE 5.11 Effects of repair of mutations on carcinogenesis. Cancer appears related to mutations in proto-oncogenes, tumor-suppressor genes, and DNA repair genes. DNA repair genes code for proteins (gene products), which correct mutations that occur when the cell replicates its DNA before mitosis. If there is a mutation in the DNA repair gene, then the DNA mutation is not repaired, and mutations are allowed to accumulate in the cell's DNA along with mutations in tumor-suppressor genes and oncogenes. People with a hereditary type of colorectal cancer (hereditary nonpolyposis colon cancer or HNPCC) have defects in their DNA repair genes. Image reproduced from: http://press2.nci.nih.gov/sciencebehind/cancer/cancer51.htm. Reproduced with permission.

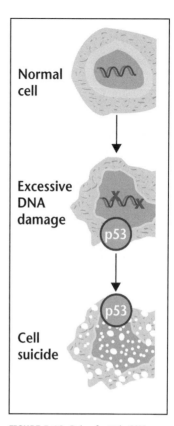

Normal cell

Excessive DNA damage

p53

p53

Cell suicide

FIGURE 5.12 Role of *p53* in DNA repair and apoptosis. The *p53* tumor-suppressor gene is the guardian of the cell cycle. If portions of DNA are mutated and cannot be repaired, the *p53* gene product, called p53 protein, stops cell growth and division and triggers "cell suicide," or apoptosis. This prevents the damaged cell from being copied, which would lead to more mutations. Image reproduced from: http://press2.nci.nih.gov/sciencebehind/cancer/cancer50.htm, accessed August 9, 2004. Reproduced with permission.

tumor-suppressor genes. When the second gene copy becomes mutated, the person can develop a malignancy. Rarely, such as in the case of familial adenomatous polyposis (FAP) (with the inherited *APC* mutation, a tumor-suppressor gene), the risk as the person approaches 40 years old is 100% because the genetic mutation is dominant and has 100% penetrance (eg., all individuals who inherit this gene mutation will develop the disease). A child of a person with FAP has a 50% chance of inheriting the mutated gene, assuming the other parent does not have the mutation. It is for this reason that genetic counseling is important to identify whether the child has the mutation, and if so, early screening or preventative surgery can be planned.

Most mutations are not inherited as germline mutations and are called somatic mutations. These occur in somatic cells, so the mutation happens during the course of one's life and is most commonly environmentally induced, such as the effect of cigarette smoking on the bronchial mucosal cells causing bronchogenic cancer. Other examples are human papilloma virus 16 and 18, which have been shown to cause the transformation to cervical cancer (Goldie *et al*. 2003). This can also be thought of as initiation, which is

Apoptosis

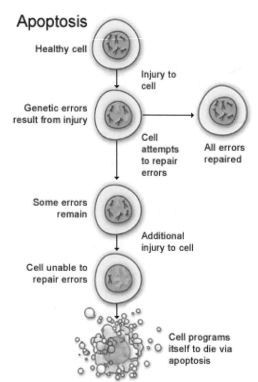

U.S. National Library of Medicine

FIGURE 5.13 Evaluation of success of repair of mutations. This figure shows the cell's evaluation process to see if the DNA mutation(s) have been successfully repaired, and if not, the cell undergoes programmed cell death or apoptosis. Image reproduced from: http://ghr.nlm.nih.gov/info=img%2Ccell_growth_and_division/show/apoptosis_process;jsessionid=8E1845BBD275FEB78F13E193E80C1193, accessed August 9, 2004. Reproduced with permission from Genetics Home Reference.

followed by a promotional mutation that leads to malignant transformation.

Location of the mutation is very important. For a malignant tumor to develop, there need to be mutations in the genes that control cell growth and division. Proto-oncogenes are genes that promote cell growth and division, as shown in Figure 5.15, and their action is finely balanced against that of tumor-suppressor genes, which make proteins that discourage cell growth and division. Thus, if the mutation occurs near or on the proto-oncogene, the gene can be mutated, forming

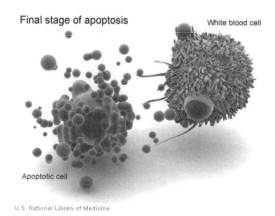

U.S. National Library of Medicine

FIGURE 5.14 Final stage of apoptosis: macrophage ready to engulf apoptotic cell. Image reproduced from: http://ghr.nlm.nih.gov/info=img,cell_growth_and_division/show/apoptosis_macrophage;jsessionid=8E1845BBD275FEB78F13E193E80C1193?js=1, accessed August 9, 2004. Reproduced with permission from Genetics Home Reference.

an oncogene, which leads to uncontrolled cell growth and division. For example, chronic myelogenous leukemia in patients with the Philadelphia chromosome involves the mutation of a proto-oncogene, forming an oncogene. Figures 5.16A and B describe the formation of this oncogene and compare a proto-oncogene to an oncogene. Figure 5.17 shows how an oncogene can lead to uncontrolled growth, and Figure 5.18 shows the formation of the Philadelphia chromosome, the gene mutation in chronic myogeneous leukemia. Chronic myleloid leukemia (CML) involves the reciprocal translocation of genetic material from the long arm (q) of chromosome 9 to the long arm of chromosome 22. This moves the *abl* proto-oncogene to be translocated to chromosome 22 at the breakpoint cluster region (Bcr), forming the *BCR-ABL* oncogene in a smaller Philadelphia chromosome. This mutation results in the production of a fused protein, Bcr-abl tyrosine kinase, which controls the overgrowth of primitive myeloid cells, causing CML. In certain types of B-cell leukemia and lymphoma, there is a mutation of a proto-oncogene, *BCL-2*, on chromosome 18, causing the *BCL-2* gene to be moved to chromosome 14, right next to a gene enhancer

Normal growth-control pathway

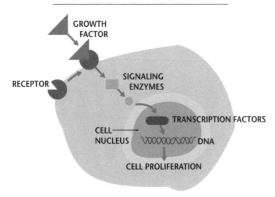

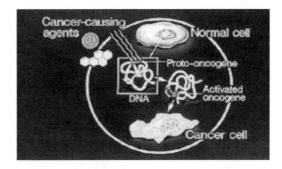

FIGURE 5.15 Normal control of cell growth. When the body needs new cells, a growth factor stimulates the cell surface receptor to divide. It sends signaling enzymes in a "bucket brigade"–like movement to the cell nucleus, where the message initiates transcription of specific genes. This causes proteins to be made that turn on cell division (e.g., move the cell through the cell cycle), so that a new cell is made that is identical to the original cell (e.g., two identical daughter cells). Image reproduced from: http://press2.nci.nih.gov/sciencebehind/cancer/cancer43.htm. Reproduced with permission.

FIGURE 5.16a Formation of an oncogene. Proto-oncogene codes for proteins involved in control of cell growth and division. When mutated, it is activated into an oncogene, that has the ability to turn on cell growth and division indefinitely through altered growth signaling pathways. Image reproduced from: http://press2.nci.nih.gov/sciencebehind/cioc/molecular/molecularframe.htm. Reproduced with permission.

for the antibody heavy-chain locus (DiBacco *et al.* 2000). A similar amount of DNA from chromosome 14 is placed on chromosome 18, forming a reciprocal translocation t(14;18). The *BCL-2* gene makes a gene product, the protein Bcl-2, which in sufficient amounts can prevent apoptosis, or programmed cell death. With the translocation, the *BCL-2* gene becomes an oncogene, not because it causes uncontrolled cell division but because it prevents cell death. The *BCL-2* gene turns on repeated transcription of its protein Bcl-2, which prevents apoptosis. By virtue of lying next to the gene that enhances the production of heavy-chain antibodies, huge quantities of the protein Bcl-2 are made along with the synthesized antibody. This mutation was identified in B-cell leukemias and some B-cell lymphomas, where the B-cell function is to make large amounts of antibody. Not only does this mutation result in immortal B-cell lymphocytes, which normally would die a few days after they

accomplish their tasks, but unfortunately, the high amounts of the protein Bcl-2 make these diseases difficult to treat. The cells are able to escape damage from chemotherapy and do not die. This will be further discussed later in this chapter.

Figure 5.19 depicts the function of a normal tumor-suppressor gene. If the tumor-suppressor gene is mutated, so that the protein that helps to put the brakes on cell division cannot be made, then cells can divide without control. The two copies of the genes a person has, one from each parent, are called alleles. If one of the tumor suppressor-gene alleles is mutated and the other is normal, then the normal one will prevail. If the normal allele becomes silenced, or is not expressed, again by some environmental insult or promotion, then there will be no production of the tumor-suppressor protein, such as p53 and cancer may result. p53 is mutated in more than 50% of solid malignancies (Rodrigues *et al.* 1990). Figure 5.20 shows a comparison between normal and mutated tumor-suppressor genes. Thus, malignant transformation occurs when there are mutations in proto-oncogenes, resulting in the activation of oncogenes; tumor-suppressor genes; and, finally, DNA repair genes, so the mutations are passed on to subsequent generations of cells.

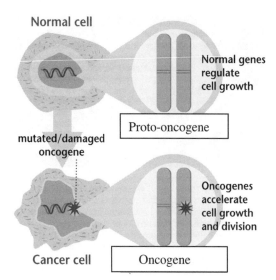

FIGURE 5.16b Comparison of proto-oncogene and oncogene. A proto-oncogene, shown in the top image, is responsible for making many of the proteins that bring about cell growth and division. Normally, proteins called growth factors bind to special receptors on the cell surface and activate the signal or message, which is sent to the cell nucleus via enzymes, where the signal activates transcription factors. The transcription factors "turn on" the genes that start cell growth or entry into the cell cycle for cell division. Many of these signaling enzymes, receptors, and transcription factors are made by proto-oncogenes, so if they are mutated to form oncogenes, cell growth and division is uncontrolled. Image reproduced from: http://press2.nci.nih.gov/sciencebehind/cancer/cancer45.htm. Reproduced with permission.

Figure 5.21 shows how mutations in proto-oncogenes and tumor-suppressor genes can lead to malignant transformation.

Now that the process of malignant transformation is better understood, let's look at specific targeting of the processes that result from malignant transformation.

Intracellular Malignant Flaws and Targets

The most promising molecular flaws to be targeted are acquired capabilities of cancer cells compared with normal cells: loss of tumor suppression and independence from growth signals, so that

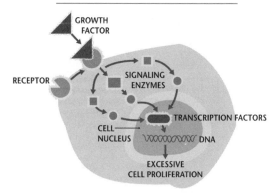

FIGURE 5.17 Oncogene leads to uncontrolled cell growth. Oncogenes produce abnormal or high quantities of proteins that control growth, so that the cell is turned on for cell growth and division, much like an accelerator stuck to the floor of a car. Image reproduced from: http://press2.nci.nih.gov/sciencebehind/cancer/cancer47.htm, accessed August 9, 2004. Reproduced with permission.

the stimulus to divide is always "on," metastatic potential, immortalization, angiogenesis, and resistance to programmed cell death or apoptosis. This section will review molecular flaws in the following areas: cell surface receptors, such as the epidermal growth factor receptor family, which allows uncontrolled cell division and growth; signal transduction, which carries the message for uncontrolled cell division and growth; proteasome function and inhibitors; angiogenesis; and the process of apoptosis, including Bcl-2 and oligonucleotide antisense agents, which can induce apoptosis.

Overexpression of Growth Factor Receptors and Mutations in Signaling Pathways

Many human cells have the capacity to divide, and when more cells are needed, growth factors or hormones, called ligands, attach to receptors on the cell surface and stimulate the cell to divide. As part of the malignant transformation process, these receptors may become overexpressed and essentially turn on the cell for continual cell

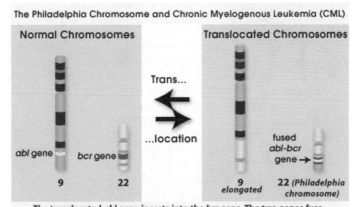

The Philadelphia Chromosome and Chronic Myelogenous Leukemia (CML)

The translocated *abl* gene inserts into the *bcr* gene. The two genes fuse.
The altered *abl* gene functions improperly, resulting in CML.

FIGURE 5.18 Philadelphia chromosome: mutation on a proto-oncogene, forming an activated oncogene. The *bcr* gene on chromosome 22 is translocated to chromosome 9, next to the *abl* gene, where the two genes fuse together forming the *bcr-abl* gene. It is a reciprocal translocation so that much of chromosome 22 translocates to chromosome 9, elongating it. The *bcr-abl* gene codes for a special tyrosine kinase that sends growth signals (signal transduction) to the cell nucleus, continually causing the cell to divide. This occurs in the hematopoietic stem cell, giving rise to chronic myelogenous leukemia (CML). Image reproduced from: http://gslc.genetics.utah.edu/units/disorders/karyotype/images/ philadelphia_cml.gif, accessed August 9, 2004. Reproduced with permission.

divisions. A cell can be turned on by a number of ways: the cell receptor for the epidermal growth factor (EGF) will dimerize (get together with another cell surface receptor), and together, they will initiate the message from outside the cell, which then passes into the cell, and the message is sent via a signaling cascade to the nucleus. If the two receptors are of the same type, like EGF-1, it is called homodimerization. If they are two different receptors from the same family, like EGF-1 and EGF-2, it is called heterodimerization and usually makes a stronger signal to the nucleus (Gribbon and Loescher 2000). Sometimes, the message is sent even when the receptors are not stimulated or there is no dimerization, which is called constituative signaling. Here, the receptor kinase is activated by phosphorylation, with the loss of a phosphate group, and initiates the message, so that cell division is continually in the "on"

position. When there are too many receptors (overexpressed), then many messages continue to be sent to the nucleus, and the cell proliferates without regard to body needs. Cell birth no longer equals cell death.

The EGF family of receptor tyrosine kinases are critical to everyday replacement of body cells. These include EGF-1 (ErbB1 or HER-1), EGF-2 (HER-2-neu or ErbB2), EGF-3 (ErbB3 or HER-3), and EGF-4 (ErbB4 or HER-4). The HER-2-neu receptor is very well known because of its role in breast cancer. Although HER-2-neu is only one receptor in this family of four, it appears to influence the function of EGF dimerization and is often found proximal to the EGF overexpressed receptors (Sundaresan *et al.* 1999).

Each receptor tyrosine kinase has three domains: (1) an extracellular domain that binds with a ligand (hormone or growth factor) and also

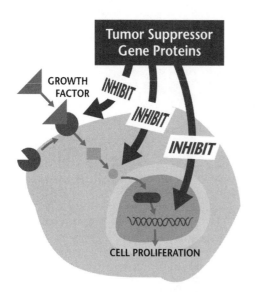

FIGURE 5.19 Tumor-suppressor genes. If oncogenes are the accelerator of a car, then tumor-suppressor genes are the brake pedal. Normally, tumor-suppressor genes help to balance the cell's growth and division signals. They are a large family of genes that make proteins (gene products) that restrain cell growth and division. If tumor-suppressor genes are mutated, they become silent and no longer oppose cell growth and division. Thus, in combination with oncogenes, there is uncontrolled cell growth and division. Image reproduced from: http://press2.nci.nih.gov/sciencebehind/cancer/cancer49.htm, accessed August 9, 2004. Reproduced with permission.

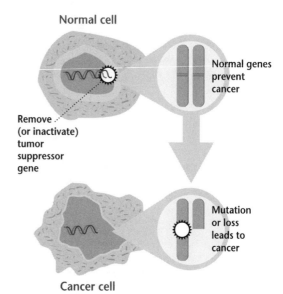

FIGURE 5.20 Comparison of a normal cell and a cell with a mutated tumor-suppressor gene. All genes come with two copies or alleles, one from each parent. To inactivate or silence a tumor-suppressor gene, both gene copies must be mutated. Thus, if a person is born with a mutated tumor-suppressor gene, the other copy is still functioning. However, if during the person's lifetime, the second allele is mutated, then the tumor-suppressor gene will be silenced, increasing the person's risk of developing cancer. Image reproduced from: http://press2.nci.nih.gov/sciencebehind/cancer/cancer48.htm, accessed August 9, 2004. Reproduced with permission.

dimerizes or pairs with another receptor close by; (2) a transmembrane domain; and (3) an inner cytoplasmic tyrosine kinase domain. When a ligand binds to the receptor, it causes the EGF receptor (EGFR) to dimerize with another receptor, either itself as a homodimer or another family member receptor (heterodimer). Dimerization activates the phosphorylation of the tyrosine kinase, which then autophosphorylates, giving up a phosphate group or energy for signaling. Once the receptor (protein) kinase is phosphorylated, docking or adaptor proteins bind to it to help send the signal along, such as the Ras protein or MAP kinases and cyclin D, a cell cyclin that operates the cell cycle. The phosphorylated receptor kinase can also modify another signaling protein and pass the message via phosphorylation, like a "bucket brigade." The

signal is transduced, or sent down (e.g., downstream), along the signaling pathway to the cell nucleus. This is called *signal transduction*. A variety of other pathways may be turned on as well, such as the Ras signaling cascade, which stimulates and turns on the ERK and JNK signaling pathways. Ultimately, the message reaches the nucleus and the chromosomes or DNA. Transcription factors are activated, such as c-fos, AP-1, and ELK-1, that begin the process of cell proliferation (Daly 1999). Other signaling pathways may be turned on as well. Cyclin D starts the cell cycle moving from G_0, or resting phase, to the G_1 phase. Cyclin D is produced or encoded by the gene *Bcl-1* and can be overexpressed when the *Bcl-1* gene is mutated, commonly by the t(11;14) translocation (Welzel *et al.* 2003). As can be imagined,

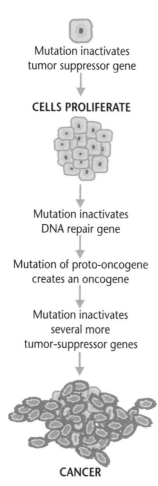

Mutation inactivates
tumor suppressor gene

CELLS PROLIFERATE

Mutation inactivates
DNA repair gene

Mutation of proto-oncogene
creates an oncogene

Mutation inactivates
several more
tumor-suppressor genes

CANCER

FIGURE 5.21 Malignant transformation resulting from mutations in proto-oncogenes, tumor-suppressor genes, and DNA repair genes. Image reproduced from: http://press2.nci.nih.gov/sciencebehind/cancer/cancer52.htm, accessed August 9, 2004. Reproduced with permission. Figure created by Susan Spangler.

overproduction of cyclin D continues to turn on the cell division mechanism so that the cell continues to divide. The cell cycle "clock" is turned on, and division starts with the increased levels of cyclin D and, later, by increased levels of cyclin E. The cyclins activate cyclin-dependent kinases (CDKs) which then transfer a phosphate group to a protein called pRB, which normally holds the cell cycle in the "off" position. Once pRB gets the phosphate group, it allows the cell cycle switch to be turned in the "on" position, and the cell divides (Weinberg 1996). These flaws are all potential molecular targets that are being explored.

In many solid tumors, EGF-1 is overexpressed. These tumors tend to be aggressive and metastasize. Many of these cells do not require ligand binding to activate the signaling cascade, but rather, they autophosphorylate continually. In addition, the cell takes on the following characteristics: the cell migrates, becomes invasive, secretes angiogenesis agents, such as vascular endothelial growth factor (VEGF), and ignores apoptotic signals. In breast cancer, EGFR-2 or HER-2-neu is overexpressed. Again, the prognosis for women with this overexpression is not as good as for women without this overexpression, and tumors are likely to be aggressive and metastasize. However, the good news is that there are drugs that interfere with this overexpression, such as trastuzumab (Herceptin). Figure 5.22 shows signal transduction.

Each of the signaling pathways may have a mutation, such as the ras pathway, which is a pathway that starts just inside the cell membrane when ras attaches to the activated protein kinase. When activated, ras sends a message to the nucleus, leading to transcription of genes and cell division. This pathway also controls many other effector pathways, such as protecting cells from apoptosis, by activating NF-kappa B (Downward 1998). The mitogen-activated protein kinase (MAPK) signaling pathway is normally stimulated by the ras molecules, but it is also stimulated by stress and inflammatory cytokines, which leads to growth, inflammation, or apoptosis. The MAPK pathway may be mutated, so scientists are working to develop drugs that will interfere with the malignant flaws in this and other pathways. For mutations in the Ras signaling, inhibitors, such as a farnesyltransferase inhibitor, that will stop the ras pathway from being automatically activated are being studied.

The greatest success so far has been with the EGFR inhibitors, including monoclonal 1) antibodies that block the extracellular domain and

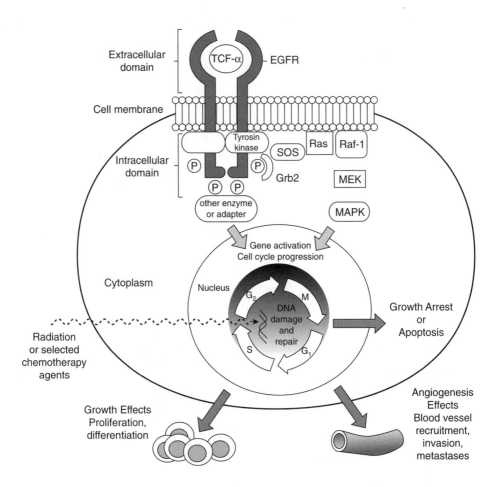

FIGURE 5.22 Growth factor stimulation and signal transduction. Two cell surface receptors dimerize, initiating the signal that is sent via a cascade effect or "bucket brigade" from the cell surface to the cell nucleus. Normally, this growth signal leads to cell growth and division, but with malignant transformation the cell is able to escape apoptosis, or programmed cell death, make vascular endothelial growth factor (VEGF) to make new blood vessels, become invasive, and metastasize. This figure shows potential targets from the inner cell membrane, along the signaling cascade, to the cell nucleus. Adapted from image http://www.novartisoncology.com/page/signal_transduction.jsp.

cause the receptor to be brought back into the cell so that it can no longer be stimulated, 2) the intracellular tyrosine kinase inhibitors, and 3) inhibitors of VEGF. Many exciting drugs are undergoing clinical investigation, such as drugs that block apoptosis and drugs that interfere with many intracellular or extracellular functions. Drugs that are able to block the overexpressed EGFR and prevent the message to divide from reaching the nucleus of the cell include cetuximab and trastuzumab, which are further described in Table 5.1.

Angiogenesis

Studies to find effective agents to stop angiogenesis have been loudly touted, beginning when endostatin and angiostatin were first announced by Judah Folkman in 1998 (Pistoi and Palmerini 2002). In the human body, there is balance between normal signals to grow blood vessels (angiogenesis) and signals to stop the formation (angiogenesis inhibitors). Hypoxia is the strongest stimulation for tissues to form new blood vessels, and angiogenesis is common in healthy wound healing, monthly female menses, and formation of the placenta in pregnancy.

Solid tumors can grow up to 2–3 mm and be supported by simple diffusion to bring in nutrients, such as oxygen and glucose, and remove waste products. However, at this point, the tumor must develop new blood vessels or starve (Bergers and Benjamin 2003). It has been shown that the most powerful stimulus to grow new blood vessels is given by VEGF, or bFGF (McMahon 2000). Figure 5.23 depicts the process of angiogenesis.

VEGF binds to receptors on the endothelial cells of nearby blood vessels and activates them through signal transduction, as shown in Figure 5.24. This causes the cells to divide to make new endothelial cells and to make enzymes, which will be used to dissolve tiny holes in the tissue surrounding the existing blood vessels. The newly produced endothelial cells migrate out through these holes in the basement membrane toward the malignant tumor, as shown in Figure 5.25. Integrins help pull the new blood vessel tube forward toward the tumor, and the enzymes (matrix metalloproteinases) dissolve the tissue in front of the blood vessel tube so it can move forward, just like a tank clearing the way for an army of men. After the vessel moves forward, the tissue moves back to surround the new vessel. The blood vessel tube then closes, special muscle cells stabilize the vessel, and blood begins to flow toward the tumor. Figure 5.26 shows potential targets to stop or prevent angiogenesis.

Angiogenesis has been found to correlate with certain growth characteristics in colon and rectal cancers if VEGF is overexpressed. This relates to vascular density in the tumor and predicts invasiveness, metastases, recurrence, and confers a poor prognosis (Doggrell 2004). It makes sense, then, that administration of a monoclonal antibody to block VEGF will help prevent tumor growth. The first angiogenesis inhibitor, bevacizumab, was FDA approved in 2004 for first-line treatment of metastatic colorectal cancer in combination with a 5-fluorouracil–containing regimen (Food and Drug Administration 2004). This occurred after a landmark clinical trial that showed that patients receiving the bevacizumab-containing regimen had a significantly higher response rate and longer survival compared with patients not receiving bevacizumab (Hurwitz *et al.* 2004). See Table 5.1 for details about bevacizumab (Avastin). Key nursing actions are to safely administer the drug and prevent, monitor for, and facilitate management of potential side effects such as hypertension, rare but potential arterial thrombus, bleeding, gastrointestinal perforation, and delayed wound healing.

Proteasome Function

Proteasomes are involved in a variety of critical cell functions, including degradation of protein waste and recycling it for further use, antigen presentation, regulation of cell metabolism and cell differentiation, and control of the cell cycle (Hilt and Wolf 2001). Probably the most notable function is regulation of protein homeostasis in the cell. The proteasome degrades "ubiquinated"

TABLE 5.1 Molecular Targeted Therapy

Drug Name	Mechanism of Action	Indications	Common Side Effects	Key Nursing Interventions
Alemtuzumab (Campath)	MoAb against CD52	B-cell chronic lymphocytic leukemia	Infusion reactions, BMD with risk of infection and bleeding, pain, peripheral edema, headache, dysesthesias, hypo- or hypertension	Premedicate prior to each treatment and monitor for reaction, cardiac changes; teach patient/family: anti-infective prophylaxis, self-care measures for bone marrow depression to prevent infection and bleeding, importance of birth control while receiving the drug
Azacitidine (Vidaza)	Causes hypomethylation of DNA, which may restore bone marrow gene function	Myeleodysplastic syndrome (MDS)	Severe nausea and vomiting, BMD with risk of infection and bleeding, constipation, diarrhea, stomatitis, fevers with rigors, fatigue, injection site irritation	Assess efficacy of antiemetics, and revise plan as needed; teach patient/family: self-care measures for BMD to prevent infection and bleeding, self-administration of antiemetics, importance of birth control while receiving the drug, to monitor temperature and self-administer antipyretics; self-injection technique, to monitor injection site and to rotate sites, to report diarrhea, constipation, or nausea and vomiting that do not respond to recommended management
Bevacizumab (Avastin)	MoAb neutralizes VEGF	First-line for advanced CRC, in combination with 5-FU–based regimen	Nose bleeds, hypertension, delayed wound healing, bleeding; rare arterial thrombus, rare GI perforation, nephritic syndrome; rare hypersensitivity reactions	Monitor BP prior to every treatment, and discuss antihypertensive treatment with MD for elevations; assess urine for protein baseline and as needed; teach patient/family to report: abdominal pain, and bleeding; avoid elective surgery or colonoscopy within 28 days of drug

Drug	Action	Indication	Side Effects	Nursing Considerations
Bortezomib (Velcade)	Inhibits proteasomes, which breakdown and recycle intracellular proteins	Treatment of patients with multiple myeloma who have progressed after 2 prior therapies	Peripheral neuropathy (PN), BMD with risk of infection and bleeding, nausea, vomiting, diarrhea, constipation, asthenia, hypotension	Assess efficacy of antiemetics, and revise plan as needed; assess for hypotension and PN; teach patient/family: self-care measures for BMD to prevent infection and bleeding; self-administration of antiemetics; importance of birth control while receiving the drug; to report symptoms that do not resolve, worsening of PN, dizziness
Cetuximab (Erbitux)	MoAb against EGFR-1	EFGR+ CRC, second-line in combination with irinotecan or single agent	Uncommon hypersensitivity including anaphylaxis, acne-like skin eruptions, rare nausea, diarrhea	Premedicate prior to each treatment and monitor for reaction; assess skin reaction prior to each treatment, and increase infusion time based on severity of reaction; teach patient/family skin care and self-administration of antibiotics as needed
Erlotinib (Tarceva)	Tyrosine kinase inhibitor (TKI) of EGFR, oral agent	Investigational, studied in colorectal, breast, and lung cancers	Acne-like skin eruptions, mild diarrhea, mild stomatitis, rare eye problems, headache	Assess skin reaction prior to each treatment; teach patient/family: self-administration of drug, skin care, and self-administration of antibiotics as needed, to report symptoms that do not resolve and any eye problems right away
Gefitinib (Iressa)	TKI of EGFR, oral agent	Lung cancer	Acne-like skin eruptions, mild diarrhea, nausea and vomiting	Assess skin reaction prior to each treatment; teach patient/family: self-administration of drug, skin care, and self-administration of antibiotics as needed, to interrupt treatment if severe diarrhea or skin reaction, and to report symptoms that do not resolve
Gemtuzumab ozogamicin (Mylotarg)	MoAb against CD33, linked to poison calciamycin	AML that is CD33+, for patients aged 60+	Acute infusion reactions, BMD with risk of infection and	Premedicate prior to each treatment and monitor for reaction;

(Continued)

TABLE 5.1 (Continued)

Drug Name	Mechanism of Action	Indications	Common Side Effects	Key Nursing Interventions
		years old in first relapse	bleeding, anemia; nausea, vomiting, hepatotoxicity, constipation or diarrhea, rash	teach patient/family: self-care measures for BMD to prevent infection and bleeding, importance of birth control while receiving the drug, to report symptoms that do not resolve
Imatinib (Gleevec)	TKI of c-ABL, oral	CML	BMD with risk of infection and bleeding, fluid retention, nausea, vomiting, diarrhea, muscle cramps, headache, fatigue, arthralgias, multiple drug interactions	Teach patient/family: self-administration of drug, self-care measures for BMD to prevent infection and bleeding, importance of birth control while receiving the drug, to report symptoms that do not resolve, potential drug interactions and implications
Rituximab (Rituxan)	MoAb against CD20	B-cell NHL, low grade or follicular, that has relapsed or progressed or initial therapy for patients with bulky disease	Infusion reactions, potential for infection, rare severe mucocutaneous reactions, uncommon nausea and vomiting, itching, asthenia, dizziness	Premedicate prior to each treatment and monitor for reaction, slowly increase infusion rate; teach patient/family: self-care measures to prevent infection, importance of birth control while receiving the drug, to report symptoms that do not resolve
Thalidomide	Inhibits TNF-α and angiogenesis	FDA approved for leprosy, but being studied in multiple myeloma	Peripheral neuropathy, birth defects, drowsiness, rash, constipation	Teach patient/family: self-administration of drug, self-care measures for drowsiness, constipation, and PN, importance of birth control while receiving the drug, to report symptoms that do not resolve

Tositumomab (Bexxar)	MoAb against CD20, radioisotope	Refractory NHL that is CD20+	Infusion reaction; BMD with risk of infection, bleeding, and fatigue	Premedicate patient, and monitor closely for reaction; teach patient/family: procedure and radiation precautions, self-care measures for BMD to prevent infection and bleeding, fatigue management, to report any symptoms that do not resolve
Trastuzumab (Herceptin)	MoAb against EGFR-2	HER-2 + BC	Infusion reactions; rare cardiomyopathy; rare pain, asthenia, dyspnea	Slowly increase infusion rate over first few weeks and monitor for reaction; teach patient/family: need for cardiac evaluation, importance of birth control, to report symptoms that do not resolve
Y ibritumomab tiuxetan (Zevalin), given with, rituxinab, (Rituxan)	MoAb against CD20, radioimmunoconjugate	Refractory low-grade follicular lymphoma or transformed NHL that is CD20+	Risk of infusion reaction; BMD with risk of infection, bleeding, and fatigue; asthenia, nausea, abdominal pain, second malignancies	Premedicate patient, and monitor closely for reaction; teach patient/family: procedure and radiation precautions, self-care measures for BMD to prevent infection and bleeding, fatigue management, to report any symptoms that do not resolve

MoAb, monoclonal antibody; TKI, tyrosine kinase inhibitor; BMD, bone marrow depression; GI, gastrointestinal; PN, peripheral neuropathy; AML, acute myelocytic leukemia; NHL, non-Hodgkin's lymphoma; BP, blood pressure; 5-FU, 5-fluorouracil; CRC, colorectal cancer; CML, chronic myeloid leukemia

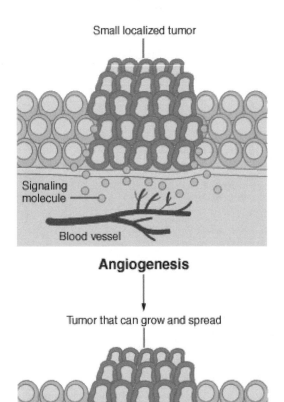

Angiogenesis

Small localized tumor

Signaling molecule

Blood vessel

Tumor that can grow and spread

FIGURE 5.23 Angiogenesis in tumor growth and metastases. Angiogenesis is the formation of new blood vessels. Malignant tumors cannot grow beyond 2–3 mm without establishing blood vessels. To get their nutrition (oxygen and glucose) and remove the cell's waste products, simple diffusion no longer works, and supplies must be brought in via new blood vessels. New blood vessels form when the tumor releases substances, such as vascular endothelial growth factor (VEGF), which stimulates the blood vessel cells (endothelial cells) to proliferate and migrate toward the tumor. Image reproduced from: http://press2.nci.nih.gov/sciencebehind/angiogenesis/angio04.htm. Reproduced with permission.

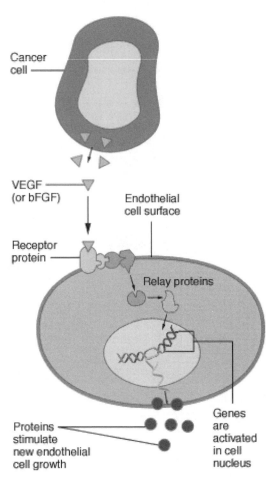

Cancer cell

VEGF (or bFGF)

Endothelial cell surface

Receptor protein

Relay proteins

Proteins stimulate new endothelial cell growth

Genes are activated in cell nucleus

FIGURE 5.24 The message asking for new blood vessels. The tumor releases vascular endothelial growth factor (VEGF) or beta-fibroblast growth factor (bFGF), which seeks endothelial cells in a nearby blood vessel. The growth factor binds to a cell surface receptor on the endothelial cell and starts a cascade of relay proteins that transmit the signal to the nucleus of the endothelial cell. The genes on the DNA in the cell nucleus are transcribed and make the proteins needed to produce more endothelial cells and to make them migrate toward the tumor. Image reproduced from: http://press2.nci.nih.gov/sciencebehind/angiogenesis/angio14.htm. Reproduced with permission.

proteins, which is a tag that is placed on the protein to tell the proteasome it can be broken down and the component parts can be recycled. The proteasome is found in all cells, and its function is tightly regulated. However, if the proteasome

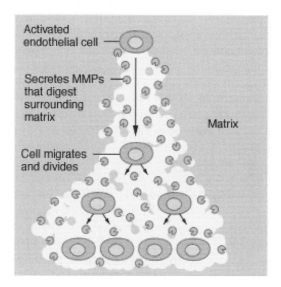

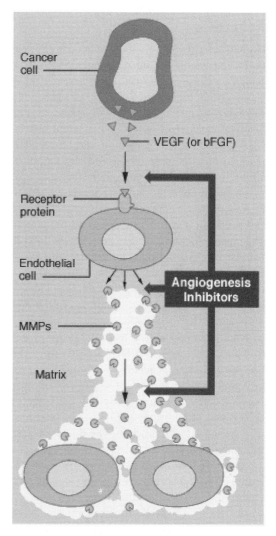

FIGURE 5.25 Making the new blood vessel. Once activated by VEGF or bFGF, the endothelial cell produces enzymes that will help clear the path in the surrounding tissue (extracellular matrix) for the new blood vessel to travel to the tumor, called metalloproteinases or MMPs. MMPs work like a military tank, breaking down the support material that lies between cells so that the army of new endothelial cells can migrate into the tissue between the tumor and the blood vessel. As the endothelial cells proliferate, they roll into hollow tubes that ultimately form the mature blood vessels. However, these new blood vessels are not as good as normal blood vessels; they are leaky, and some lead to nowhere. Image reproduced from: http://press2.nci.nih.gov/sciencebehind/angiogenesis/angio15.htm. Reproduced with permission.

FIGURE 5.26 Potential molecular flaws to target in angiogenesis. This image identifies many potential molecular targets for therapeutic intervention. Currently being studied are inhibitors of (1) endothelial cells, (2) proteins in angiogenesis signaling cascade, (3) MMPs, and (4) VEGF and bFBF. Image reproduced from: http://press2.nci.nih.gov/sciencebehind/angiogenesis/angio21.htm. Reproduced with permission.

process is inhibited, the cell receives conflicting regulatory signals and cannot function. It has been found that malignant cells cannot tolerate the overload of conflicting signals, and the cell goes into apoptosis or programmed cell death. In addition, inhibition of this process by the drug bortezomib (Velcade) stabilized cell cycle–regulatory proteins, inhibited NF-κB activation, limited angiogenesis, and induced apoptosis (Dalton 2004).

Normal cells are less sensitive and can recover from a temporary inhibition of proteasome inhibition. Bortezomib is an effective proteasome inhibitor and has been FDA approved for the treatment of multiple myeloma after progression on at least two previous regimens (Food and Drug Administration 2003). See Table 5.1 for more details on bortezomib. Key nursing functions are related to drug administration and the prevention and monitoring of potential side effects.

Apoptosis

Human cell growth and division is carefully regulated based on the body's needs. More than 100,000 cells are produced every second in the human body, and about 100,000 cells die every second by apoptosis, so that cell birth equals cell death (Vaux and Korsmeyer 1999). Mutations occur frequently, but the meticulous scrutiny of DNA prior to mitosis (restriction and checkpoints) allows the cell to weed out and destroy any cells in which the DNA mutations cannot be repaired by repair genes. These cells undergo programmed cell death, or apoptosis, which is an organized, systematic process leading to the death of the cell. An example is a young lady of fair complexion who goes out in the sun, develops a sun burn, and then finds her skin peeling the next day. The UV light from the sun caused mutations in the epidermal cell DNA; the mutations were unable to be repaired, so the skin cells undergo apoptosis, die, and are sloughed off. Well, how does the process of apoptosis occur?

Apoptosis is an important step in making sure that the cells no longer needed by the body, or cells which might injure the body, are destroyed in a systematic and efficient way that avoids an inflammatory response.

Apoptosis can occur by intrinsic or extrinsic stimulation, and both come together at caspase 3, an enzyme that is called the "henchman that executes the cell" (MedicineNet.com, accessed October 2, 2005). The extrinsic pathway is initiated when factors outside the cell determine that the cell must die—there is binding of the Fas ligand to the Fas receptor on the cell membrane (Fas belongs to the death receptor family as does the TNF receptor). This begins the death-induced signaling complex, which proceeds through a number of steps to produce active caspase 3, which brings about apoptosis.

In the intrinsic pathway, there is injury inside the cell and the cell's internal machinery goes to work to prevent inflammation by neatly packaging and removing the injured cell. If the mitochondria (powerhouse of the cell) is injured, it overcomes the pro-survival protein effect of Bcl-2. The membrane becomes permeable and cytochrome c escapes, along with other proapoptotic enzymes, and after a number of steps, results in the formation of active caspase 3. Bcl-2 is a proto-oncogene, and its gene product is a protein that sits on the outer membrane of mitochondria. The protein Bcl-2 regulates the release of cytochrome c, so that prior to its release, high levels of the protein Bcl-2 can halt the apoptotic process by preventing cytochrome c release. However, once cytochrome c is released, it is irreversible. Cytochrome c then promotes the activation cascade of capases. Bax is a protein that also lies in the mitochondrial membrane and opposes Bcl-2, pushing the cell toward apoptosis. When Bax prevails, the cell undergoes disintegration through the fragmentation of the nucleus, the cytoplasm, and the DNA is broken up, forming blebs or apoptotic bodies. These bodies are formed and enclose within their membranes the fragments of condensed chromatin from the nucleus, cell organelles, and cytoplasm, which are then phagocytized without inflammation. The small, neat packages are taken up by neighboring cells. Another participant in the apoptotic process is NF-κB, a transcription factor that is critical for apoptosis, cell cycle control, and malignant transformation.

Chemotherapy-induced cell death follows the intrinsic pathway, leading to apoptosis of the cancer cell. However, if the cell becomes resistant to chemotherapy, it does so by blocking the apoptotic process at some point. In some patients with lymphoma the mutated *BCL-2* gene on chromosome 18 is translocated to chromosome 14 and vice versa [an equivalent portion of chromosome 14 is translocated to chromosome 18; reciprocal translocation, t(14;18)]. The *BCL-2* proto-oncogene is now located near the antibody heavy-chain gene locus. With the mutation of the proto-oncogene *BCL-2* to form the *BCL-2* oncogene, its location next to the antibody gene causes the Bcl-2 protein to be synthesized in large quantities. This confers resistance to apoptosis and resistance to many chemotherapeutic agents. Research continues to underscore the importance of targeting the overexpression of the Bcl-2 family proteins that block apoptosis which leads to increased mutations (genomic instability) and tumor formation (Nelson *et al.* 2004).

To find effective strategies to reestablish apoptosis in the malignant cell, a number of drugs have been studied. One approach is to find an effective inhibitor of caspase, and one agent being studied is XIAP (X inhibitor of apoptosis), the most potent caspase inhibitor. Another approach is using an antisense mechanism, such as oblimersen sodium (Gentasense or Genta). In this approach, antisense RNA is substituted for normal RNA, so when the DNA of *Bcl-2* oncogene is transcribed, the messenger RNA attempts to be translated at the ribosome level to make the Bcl-2 protein and it cannot be translated. Thus the protein is not made. The result of decreased or absent Bcl-2 protein is increased effectiveness of chemotherapy. This drug is currently being studied in malignant melanoma, chronic lymphocytic leukemia, multiple myeloma, lymphoma, and lung cancer (Stahel and Zangemeister-Wittke 2003). Table 5.1 provides details on oblimersen sodium. Nursing implications focus on drug administration, managing flu-like symptoms, monitoring for hypersensitivity reactions, and patient self-care.

Targeted Therapy: Malignant Lymphocytes

A number of diseases involve B lymphocytes. Lymphocytes are a type of white blood cell that provides protection from invading organisms. Bursa-dependent or B cells are those lymphocytes that specialize and eventually mature and form plasma cells, which produce antibody. B cells originate in the bone marrow, arising from a pluripotent stem cell, which then differentiates or specializes and forms a B lymphocyte. As the B cell matures in the bone marrow, at the stage of a pre-B cell, it develops a protein or antigen on its

membrane, called CD20. CD stands for cluster of differentiation antigen (National Institute of Health 2004), and each protein is given a number for identification. Once the B lymphocyte matures from an immature cell to an activated B cell, it leaves the bone marrow and circulates in the blood. Fortunately, the stem cell and early precursors of the pre-B cell do not have a CD20 antigen (Rieger 2001). This is important because targeted therapy that kills all CD20-positive B lymphocytes will spare the stem cell and precursors, and new, nonmalignant CD20 positive B cells can be made to replace those killed by treatment. B-cell malignancies include B-cell leukemia (involving B-cell precursor cells), B-cell lymphomas, chronic lymphocytic leukemia (involving immature and early activated B-cell lymphocytes), and multiple myeloma (involving plasma cells). Another CD antigen that may be targeted for treatment of B-cell malignancies is the CD52 antigen in chronic lymphocytic leukemia. Because the CD52 antigen is also found on thymocytes, Thymus-dependent lymphocytes or T cells, monocytes, macrophages, natural killer (NK) lymphocytes or NK cells, granulocytes, and spermatozoa, treatment results in profound immunosuppression as all cells with a CD52 antigen are destroyed.

Acute myelocytic leukemic cells often have the CD33 antigen on their surfaces, especially the very immature blast cells, as do normal immature myeloid cells. Again, fortunately, the pluripotent stem cells that give rise to all the blood cells do not have this antigen.

Monoclonal antibodies have been developed that specifically target the CD antigen. Monclonal antibodies work like a lock and a key; they are very specific and will only bind to the antigen that fits the antibody. An antibody is a gycloprotein, called an immunoglobulin, that circulates in the blood to help protect the body from invading micro-organisms (antigens) or other threats to the body.

The antibody is composed of two parts as shown in Figure 5.27: one, a longer constant region (Fc) does not change but signals the immune

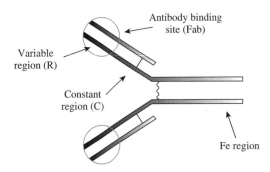

FIGURE 5.27 Antibody formation. An antibody is composed of two major regions: the constant region, which is most of the fork, and the variable region, which is the tips of the fork. The constant region attracts the immune system to the site of infection or invasion, while the variable region fits like a "lock and key" to the antigen or invading micro-organism.

system to destroy the cell of the invading micro-organism that the antibody has attached to, and second, the ends of the Y-shaped figure called the variable regions, or Fab portion, recognizes and then binds to the cell of the invading micro-organism. It is the variable region that changes form to perfectly fit the protein or antigen of the invading micro-organism and it is called the antibody-binding site. When the circulating antibody encounters this antigen again, it will automatically bind to it and mark it for destruction by the macrophages. The antibody can also work with complement, which is found in the blood plasma, and kill the micro-organism. To fight cancer, many of these specific antibodies are made to zero in on only one CD antigen (e.g., the CD20, CD33, or CD52 antigen). Because the many antibodies are made to target only one antigen, they are called monoclonal antibodies.

To make a monoclonal antibody, as shown in Figure 5.28, a mouse is used. Tumor cells (antigen) are injected into a mouse, which stimulates the production of B cells which make antibodies against the injected cancer antigen. The mouse B lymphocyte is fused together with an immortal multiple myeloma B-lymphocyte cell (which

becomes an antibody factory). The fused cell (hybridoma) will now produce the specific antibody (clone) in large quantities against the cancer antigen. As expected, murine or mouse monoclonal antibodies can cause an allergic reaction in the recipient or may cause the person to reject the mouse monoclonal antibody as foreign, with resulting high clearance of the drug. In addition, the person may develop antibodies against the monoclonal antibody, which it sees as foreign, and neutralize the effect, especially after the second treatment (Rieger 2001). This led to engineering of the monoclonal antibody so that most of the mouse antibody is removed, creating a chimeric (having up to 33% mouse protein) or humanized (having about 10% mouse protein) antibody. Newer methods have resulted in the production of 100% human monoclonal antibodies. The name of the monoclonal antibody will tell the amount of mouse or murine antibody in the agent:

- *U*mab: Fully humanized, no mouse or murine protein
- *Z*umab: Humanized antibody (2–5% mouse or murine protein)
- *X*imab: Chimeric, or up to 33% mouse protein
- *M*omab: fully murine

Now, how do monoclonal antibodies kill a cancer cell? Well, there are a variety of ways. First, monoclonal antibodies can be either *naked*, that is, not attached to anything, or *conjugated*, that is, attached to a poison or a radioisotope. Examples of a naked monoclonal antibody are rituximab (Rituxan), which targets CD20 antigens on B lymphocytes in non-Hodgkins' lymphoma, and alemtuzumab (CamPath), which targets CD52 antigens on B lymphocytes in patients with chronic lymphocytic leukemia.

Naked monoclonal antibodies attach to a cell of the invading micro-organism and then kill cells by one or more mechanism, as shown in Figure 5.29. After the monoclonal antibody specifically binds to the target antigen on the cancer cell, it inactivates or destroys the cancer

Monoclonal Antibody Production

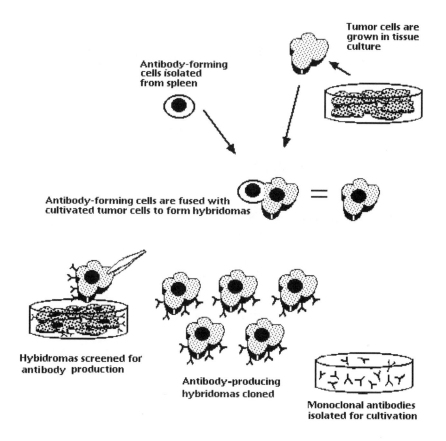

Tumor cells are grown in tissue culture

Antibody-forming cells isolated from spleen

Antibody-forming cells are fused with cultivated tumor cells to form hybridomas

Hybidromas screened for antibody production

Antibody-producing hybridomas cloned

Monoclonal antibodies isolated for cultivation

FIGURE 5.28 Manufacture of monoclonal antibodies. As shown in this figure, fused B lymphocytes will make antibody, and they are fused with cultivated tumor cells to form hybridomas. These are then cloned. Image adapted from: Access Excellence @ The National Health Museum, http://www.access excellence.org/RC/VL/GG/monoclonal.html.

cell through one or more of the following possible mechanisms:

- Blocks the cell's normal biologic function, like signal transduction. This causes the cell to stop growing (cytostatic) but doesn't kill the cell; it may also sensitize the B lymphocytes to chemotherapy, when given together or in sequence. An example is R-CHOP (rituximab plus cyclophosphamide, doxorubicin, vincristine, and prednisone), a treatment for non-Hodgkin's lymphoma

- Kills the cell by antibody-dependent cell-mediated cytotoxicity (ADCC), where the Fc portion of the antibody signals phagocytes,

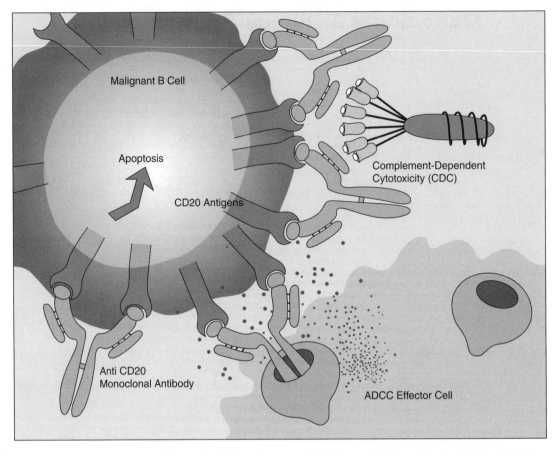

FIGURE 5.29 Monoclonal antibody–induced death of a malignant B-cell lymphocyte. Naked monoclonal anti-bodies directed against the CD20 antigen on a B-cell lymphocyte can cause cell death through four mechanisms: (1) antibody-dependent cytotoxicity (ADCC), (2) complement-dependent cytotoxicity (CDC), (3) direct activation of apoptosis or programmed cell death, and (4) block normal function of the antigen, such as growth signal transduction, which together with chemotherapy, results in cell kill.

T lymphocytes, NK cells, and other immune cells that secrete cytokines and kill the cell

- Kills the cell by joining with complement in the plasma (complement-dependent cytotoxicity or CDC) via the activated complement cascade

- Direct activation of apoptosis, or programmed cell death, of the antibody-bound cell

A conjugated monoclonal antibody is attached to something. A radioimmunoconjugate is attached to either a radioisotope, such as tositumomab and iodine I[131] (Bexxar), or a radiation source, such as yttrium-90, which emits gamma ray's (ibritumomab tiuxetan; Zevalin). Here, the monoclonal antibody attaches to the CD20 antigen on B-cell lymphocytes, releases the radiation, and kills the cells. Finally, gemtuzumab ozogamicin (Mylotarg) acts like a Trojan horse, and once bound to the CD33 receptor, the monoclonal antibody with its attached poison, calicheamicin, is brought into the cell, the poison is released and binds to the cell's DNA, causing double strand breaks and cell death.

Table 5.1 lists monoclonal antibodies used in cancer treatment. Nursing implications in caring for the patient receiving monoclonal antibody therapy focuses on the following:

- Preventing and managing infusion-related reactions
- Preventing and managing hypersensitivity reactions (higher risk in murine and chimeric monoclonal antibodies)
- Prevention of infection and its complications
- Side-effect management of conjugated substances, such as bone marrow suppression

Nursing Implications in Caring for Patients Receiving Molecular Targeted Therapy

The nursing role in caring for patients receiving targeted therapy and their families is crucial. Initially, helping the patient and family understand the differences between conventional therapy, such as chemotherapy, and molecular targeted therapy is the focus of teaching. Then, once the type and mechanism of treatment are understood, helping the patient and family to develop a plan for anticipating and managing potential side effects takes center stage. Many side effects occur after the patient has left the hospital, so an ongoing partnership in teaching and management between the patient and nurse is important. Patients should know when and whom they should call if questions or unmanageable side effects arise. The nurse plays a pivotal role in medication administration. If the patient will self-administer the molecular targeted agent, such as an oral tyrosine kinase inhibitor, the patient must know how and when to take the drug. If the drug is administered in the clinic or hospital, the nurse teaches the patient what to expect and what to report and continues to monitor the patient during the treatment. Infusion reactions and hypersensitivity reactions may occur during the infusion of monoclonal antibodies and require immediate nursing action to assure patient safety. The nurse needs to assess for and be able to manage acute reactions together with physician colleagues. Key points are shown in Table 5.2.

Patients and their family must understand the potential side effects, strategies to manage side effects to minimize complications, and when to call the nurse or physician for more effective interventions. If bone marrow suppression is a possible side effect, then the patient and family need to learn potential sources of infection, strategies to avoid infection, signs and symptoms of infection, and when to report them. For example, patients should be able to verbalize actions to prevent infection, such as strict handwashing and body hygiene, avoiding crowds and people with a cough or infection, and drinking 2–3 quarts of fluid a day. Patients should also be able to self-assess for signs and symptoms of infection, such as taking their temperature twice daily, and to report a temperature $\geq 100.5°F$ and/or signs or symptoms of dysuria or productive cough. If thrombocytopenia is a potential side effect, the nurse reviews and provides written information about avoiding aspirin or aspirin-containing over-the-counter drugs and physical injury and reporting any bleeding. Table 5.1 reviews each of the molecular targeted agents and their mechanisms of action, indications, common side effects, and key nursing interventions.

Future Horizons

Microarray technology has greatly expedited the search for key gene mutations and their protein products. A specific mutation can be compared to known mutations in a specific type of cancer so that a definite diagnosis of the type of cancer can be made and the treatment tailored to that individual patient with those specific mutations. New agents targeting different parts of the malignant process will need to be combined to shut down cancer at vulnerable points. In addition, by knowing what mutations cause which cancers, and in what order they happen, screening for changes in the cell or DNA can be done before the

TABLE 5.2 Nursing Actions in Managing Infusion and Hypersensitivity Reactions

Type of Reaction	Mechanism	Nursing Actions
Infusion-Related Reactions	Acute immune response: antigen-antibody binding complex activates immune effector cells: 1. cytokines in the plasma: TNFα, IL-6, IL-8, interferon-α 2. Complement in the plasma: C3, C4, CH50 Usually seen with the first infusion; most infusion-related reactions decrease in intensity with subsequent infusions Signs and symptoms are those of an inflammatory response: ■ Fever, chills, rigors, nausea, headache, flushing ■ pain at tumor site	1. Premedication as ordered with acetaminophen and diphenhydramine hydrochloride 2. Assess for signs and symptoms 3. Monitor vital signs at baseline and during infusion; notify physician or advanced practice nurse if symptoms occur 4. Slow down or stop infusion depending upon severity of signs/symptoms 5. If severe, stop and disconnent drug, and keep vein open with 0.9% NS; administer IV NS as ordered if hypotensive 6. Administer support medications as ordered, including meperidine for rigors 7. Blankets and other comfort measures 8. Resume ordered rate once infusion reaction resolves, usually at 50% of the previous rate
Hypersensitivity Reaction	Patient's immune system perceives drug as a foreign invader and mounts an immune response against it Murine monoclonal antibodies (MoAb) have highest risk, followed by chimeric and rarely humanized MoAb Signs and symptoms: urticaria, pruritis, rhinitis, vomiting, throat irritation or swelling, and more severe dyspnea, angioedema, wheezing, bronchospasm, and hypotension	1. Monitor vital signs at baseline and during infusion; have emergency equipment nearby 2. Assess for signs and symptoms; notify physician or advanced practice nurse if they occur 3. Slow down or stop infusion depending upon severity of signs/symptoms 4. If severe, stop drug and disconnent tubing; keep vein open with 0.9% NS; administer IV NS as ordered if hypotensive 5. Administer support medications as ordered, including meperidine for rigors, steroids and bronchodilators as needed, SQ or IM epineprine 1:1000 for hypotension 6. If anaphylaxis, do not rechallenge

cancer even starts growing (malignant transformation), with the hope of correcting or removing the mutation to prevent cancer. This is being studied in colorectal cancers using DNA screening for mutations in fecal specimens.

As complex as genetic inheritance is, new evidence supports the fact that additional mutations caused by environmental forces can be inherited (epigenetic changes). Epigenetics is the study of heritable changes in gene function that do not from a change in DNA sequencing. Hochedlinger *et al.* (2004) reported their success in transferring the nucleus of a melanoma cell into a mouse egg cell, from which mice were then cloned. The nucleus with malignant melanoma mutations (activation of oncogenes and silencing of tumor-suppressor genes) was able to be reprogrammed into a pluripotent embryonic stem cell that was normal. This demonstrates that mutations can be reprogrammed, and future research will identify ways to achieve this. Key in bringing about epigenetic changes are DNA methylation, histone acetylation, and RNA interference. The first chemotherapy drug approved for myelodysplastic syndrome that corrects an epigenetic change is azacitidine (Vidaza), which restores normal growth and differentiation in bone marrow cells (Food and Drug Administration 2004). Azacitadine is a DNA methylation inhibitor.

The 21st Century in Cancer Care

With the deciphering of the human genome, the possibilities of fingerprinting each malignancy by virtue of its mutations and proteins made by the mutated gene (proteonomics) are becoming a reality. Similarly, individually tailored antineoplastic treatment will become a reality, based on microarray technology and identified mutations. New technology has also helped health care professionals evaluate the patient's response to usual treatment. Some patients do not respond, and this may be the result of polymorphisms or genetic alterations in metabolism, so that traditional antineoplastic agents do not achieve the usual response or the patient experiences significant toxicity from the drug as with irinotecan. Patients will need to be identified and this information factored into the treatment equation. Great strides have been accomplished in understanding the molecular biology of malignancy and developing molecular targeted therapy in the new millennium. Other technological advances, such as nanomedicine, will assist in achieving the NCI 2015 target of elimination of death and suffering from cancer.

References

Bergers, G., and Benjamin, L.E. 2003. Tumorigenesis and the angiogenic switch. *Nature Reviews: Cancer* 3:401–410.

Cunningham, D., Humblet, Y., and Siena, S. 2004. Cetuximab monotherapy and cetuximab plus irinotecan in irinotecan-refractory metastatic colorectal cancer. *New England Journal of Medicine* 351:337–345.

Dalton, W.S. 2004. From targets to therapy: Proteasome. http://www.medscape.com/viewprogram/3034.

Daly, R.J. 1999. Take your partners, please: Signal diversification by the erbB family of receptor tyrosine kinases. *Growth Factors* 16:255–263.

DiBacco, A., Keeshan, K., McKenna, S.L., and Cotter, T.G. 2000. Molecular abnormalities in chronic myeloid leukemia: Deregulation of cell growth and apoptosis. *The Oncologist* 5(5):405–415.

Doggrell, S.A. 2004. Vascular biology support for the use of bevacizumab in colorectal cancer. *Expert Opinion on Investigational Drugs* 13(6):703–705.

Downward, J. 1998. Ras signaling and apoptosis. *Current Opinion in Genetics and Development* 8(1):49–54.

Ellis, L.M. 2003. A targeted approach for antiangiogenic therapy of metastatic human colon cancer. *The American Surgeon* 69:3–10.

Fadeel, B., Orrenius, S., and Zhivotovsky, B. 1999. Apoptosis in human disease: A new skin for the old ceremony? *Biochemical and Biophysical Research Communications* 266(3):699–717.

Fearon, E.R., and Vogelstein, B. 1990. A genetic model for colorectal tumorigenesis. *Cell* 61:759–767.

Food and Drug Administration (FDA). 2003. Velcade (bortezomib) information. http://www.fda.gov/cder/drug/infopagedrug/velcade/default.htm, accessed October 2, 2005.

Food and Drug Administration (FDA) News. 2004. http://www.fda.gov/bbs/topics/news/2004/NEW01069.html.

Genome Glossary. 2004. http://www.ornl.gov/sci/techresources/Human_Genome/glossary/glossary.shtml#geneexpression.

Goldie, S.J., Grima, D., Kohli, M., *et al.* 2003. A comprehensive natural history model of HPV infection and cervical cancer to estimate the clinical impact of a prophylactic HPV-16/18 vaccine. *International Journal of Cancer* 106(6):896–904.

Gribbon, J., and Loescher, L.J. 2000. The biology of cancer, chapter 2. In C.H. Yarbro, M.H. Frogge, M. Goodman, and S.L. Groenwald (Eds): *Cancer Nursing Principles and Practice* (ed 5). Sudbury, MA: Jones and Bartlett Publishers.

Hilt, W., and Wolf, D. 2001. *Proteasomes: The world of regulatory proteolysis.* Berlin: RG Landes Inc.

Hochedlinger, K., Blelloch, R., Brennan, C., *et al.* 2004. Reprogramming of a melanoma genome by nuclear transplantation. *Genes and Development* 18:1875–1885.

Hurwitz, H., Fehrenbacher, L., and Novotny, W. 2004. Bevacizumab plus irinotecan, fluorouracil, and leucovorin for metastatic colorectal cancer. *New England Journal of Medicine* 350:2335–2342.

Johnstone, R.W., Ruefli, A.A., and Lowe, S.W. 2002. Apoptosis: A link between cancer genetics and chemotherapy. *Cell* 108(2):153–164.

McMahon, G. 2000. VEGF receptor signaling in tumor angiogenesis. *The Oncologist* 5(Suppl 1):3–10.

Nelson, D.A., Tan, T.T., Rabson, A.B., *et al.* 2004. Hypoxia and defective apoptosis drive genomic instability and tumorigenesis. *Genes and Development* 18:1223–1226.

Okada, H., and Mak, T.W. 2004. Pathways of apoptotic and non-apoptotic death in tumor cells. *Nature* 4:592–604.

Pistoi, S., and Palmerini, C. 2002. Quiet celebrity: Interview with Judah Folkman. http://www.sciam.com/article.cfm?articleID=00077C61-DE6E-1DC2-AF71809EC588EEDF.

Rieger, P.T. 2001. *Biotherapy: A Comprehensive Overview* (ed 2). Sudbury, MA: Jones and Bartlett Publishers.

Rodrigues, N.R., Rowan, A., Smith, M.E., *et al.* 1990. p53 mutations in colorectal cancer. *Proceedings of the National Academy of Sciences of United States of America* 87(19):7555–7559.

Stahel, R., and Zangemeister-Wittke, U. 2003. Antisense oligonucleotides for cancer therapy: An overview. *Lung Cancer* 41:S81–S88.

Starling, N., and Cunningham, D. 2004. Monoclonal antibodies against vascular endothelial growth factor and epidermal growth factor receptor in advanced colorectal cancers: Present and future directions. *Current Opinion in Oncology* 16(4):385–390.

Sundaresan, S, Penuel, E, and Sliwkowski, M. 1999. The biology of human epidermal growth factor receptor 2. *Current Oncology Report* 1:16–20.

Thesaurus for cluster of differentiation antigen. http://crisp.cit.nih.gov/Thesaurus/00001384.htm.

Vaux, D., and Korsmeyer, S.J. 1999. Cell death in development. *Cell* 96:245–254.

von Eschenbach, A.C. 2003. 2015: A target date for eliminating suffering and death due to cancer. *Benchmarks* 3(2). http://www.cancer.gov/newscenter/benchmarks-vol3-issue2.

Welzel, N., Le, T., Marculescu, R., *et al.* 2003. Templated nucleotide addition and immunoglobulin JH-gene utilization in t(11;14) junctions: Implications for the mechanism of translocation and the origin of mantle cell lymphoma. *Cancer Research* 63(7):1722–1723.

Weinberg, R.A. 1996. How cancer arises. *Scientific American* 275:62–72.

Wilkes, G.M., and Barton-Burke, M. 2004. *Oncology nursing drug handbook*. Sudbury, MA: Jones and Bartlett Publishers, pp 443–504.

Hematopoietic Stem-Cell Transplantation

Janice P. Maienza, R.N., M.S.N., A.O.C.N.

Introduction

Hematopoietic stem-cell transplantation (HSCT) is a rapidly expanding, extremely challenging subspecialty of oncology nursing. Myeloablative HSCT allows lethal doses of chemotherapy to be administered to kill the tumor cells with rescue of normal bone marrow function through stem-cell repopulation of the bone marrow. It requires expert nursing care of patients undergoing the procedure, together with collaboration among multiple disciplines and settings. With the trend towards nonmyeloablative stem-cell transplantations (NST), nurses in the inpatient, outpatient, home, and community settings must understand this therapy. No longer do patients stay in the tertiary setting until their symptoms are resolved and their immunity is restored. They now travel home, receiving only their intensive therapy in the tertiary hospital setting. This chapter will review key points of HSCT and present strategies for nurses to effectively and efficiently assess, plan, intervene, and revise treatment depending upon the patient responses to HSCT. Because patients undergoing HSCT may have rapid changes in their physical status, nurses must be able to make quick but accurate assessments to effectively intervene when subtle changes occur. Refer to Table 6.1 for the various types of HSCT.

Bone marrow transplantation (BMT) is now called HSCT. In the early days of transplantation and for many years, the only source of the stem cells was the donor's bone marrow. In the operating room under general anesthesia, physicians collected the bone marrow from the donor's iliac crests. Now, however, physicians and advanced practice nurses collect stem cells from peripheral blood, bone marrow, or umbilical cord blood. Hence, the more general term hematopoietic stem-cell transplantation is more accurate.

The donor further defines the procedure. When the patient donates the cells, the transplantation is termed autologous; when the patient's sibling or someone other than the patient donates cells, it is termed allogeneic; when the donor cells come from umbilical cord blood, it is termed an umbilical cord blood transplantation (UCBT). For example, when a patient is admitted to receive an autologous peripheral stem-cell transplantation, it is clear that the patient is the donor and the cells were pheresed from the patient's peripheral blood using a pheresis machine in the blood bank. The collected cells are stored and later infused into the patient. An allogeneic peripheral stem-cell transplantation uses cells from a donor other than the patient. The donor's stem cells are collected from the donor's peripheral blood, readied, and stored for later use after the patient receives a preparatory regimen. Table 6.2 outlines the phases of HSCT.

TABLE 6.1 Types of Hematopoietic Stem-Cell Transplantations

Transplantation	Description
Autologous	Stem cells are retrieved from the patient and stored; stem cells are collected from the patient's peripheral blood or the bone marrow
Syngeneic	The donor is an identical twin; stem cells are collected from the peripheral blood or the bone marrow of the twin donor
Related allogeneic or matched related donor	The donor is a family member of the donor and not a genetically identical twin; stem cells are collected from the peripheral blood or the bone marrow of the family member donor
Matched unrelated donor (MUD)	An unrelated, allogeneic donor; donors are usually drawn from the National Marrow Donor Program (NMDP) registry; stem cells are collected from the peripheral blood or the bone marrow of the donor and transported immediately to the patient
Umbilical cord blood transplantation (UCBT)	Collected at the time of delivery and saved for the patient (autologous), family member (related allogeneic), or matched unrelated recipient (MUD); stem cells are collected from the placenta via the umbilical vein after delivery
Nonmyeloablative stem-cell transplantation (NST) ■ matched related ■ matched unrelated	Stem cells are collected from the peripheral blood or the bone marrow of the allogeneic donor; UCB may also be used

History

Active interest in stem-cell transplantation began after World War II, when the atomic bomb was developed and actually detonated in Japan. Research began on the effects of high-dose radiation and ways to survive these effects. In mice, protecting the spleen resulted in survival from high-dose radiation. Further study led to a more complete understanding of the hematopoietic system and engraftment. The first transplantation successes were in animals receiving autologous transplantations. Graft rejection and graft-versus-host disease (GVHD) did not complicate these procedures. Patients underwent these transplantations in the late 1960s for acute leukemia and aplastic anemia. During this time, further discovery, study, and understanding of the immune system in dogs led to successful allogeneic transplantations in animals. By understanding the dog leukocyte antigen (DLA) system and successfully transplanting dogs, scientists were able to then understand the human leukocyte antigen (HLA) system. This led to successful allogeneic transplantations in humans. In the 1970s and early 1980s, patients with immune deficiency and leukemia successfully underwent allogeneic transplantations. Now, since the early 1980s, HSCT has grown exponentially as major centers throughout the country become expert with the technique and patient support. HSCT is now the standard of care for certain cancers. Research continues to better elucidate the physiology so that efforts to prevent GVHD, opportunistic infections, and sequelae that impact the morbidity and quality of life of patients undergoing these therapies can be improved (Appelbaum 2003; Thomas 2000).

TABLE 6.2 Phases of Hematopoietic Stem-Cell Transplantation

Phase	Description
Pretransplantation	Patient work-up ■ HLA testing ■ Laboratory studies ■ ECG ■ Heart function studies—MUGA/ echocardiogram ■ Dental consult ■ Disease work-up Donor selection ■ HLA testing ■ Patient ■ Sibling ■ Unrelated donor ■ Umbilical cord donation Stem-cell collection ■ Bone marrow ■ Peripheral stem cells ■ Cord blood Patient/family teaching Informed consent
Transplantation	Preparatory regimen Stem-cell infusion ■ Autologous ■ Allogeneic ■ Umbilical cord blood
Posttransplantation	Engraftment Symptom management Blood product support

Rationale for Transplantation

An autologous transplantation rescues the patient from high-dose radiation or chemotherapy. This chemotherapy attacks and kills the cancer and ablates the patient's bone marrow. At the appropriate time, the patient receives back their stem cells, which migrate to the bone marrow, engraft, and restore the patient's hematopoietic system.

A syngeneic transplantation is a transplantation from an identical twin. Strictly defined, this is an allogeneic transplantation. Because identical twins are genetic doubles, this type of transplantation behaves like an autologous transplantation. The benefit of having an identical twin is assurance that the marrow is free of disease, and there is very little risk of GVHD.

An allogeneic transplantation gives the donor a new immune system by repopulating the bone marrow with new hematopoietic stem cells. These transplantations cure diseases incurable by chemotherapy alone, regardless of the dose. An example of this is chronic myelogenous leukemia (CML) in chronic phase. The patient receives high-dose chemotherapy, irradiation, and then stem cells from another person. The benefit of a new immune system is that it recognizes the leukemia as "foreign" and eliminates any residual disease that escapes the chemotherapy. Other diseases treated by allogeneic transplantations are listed in Table 6.3. Allogeneic transplantation donors are either matched related donors, termed allogeneic, or matched unrelated donors (MUD).

Patients undergoing an umbilical cord blood transplantation (UCBT) receive stem cells extracted from the placenta at a normal birth. These newborns no longer need their placenta to grow. Placental stem cells have a unique hematopoietic capacity different from their adult counterparts. Patients experience less morbidity from infection and GVHD with UCBT. Fewer cells are necessary for engraftment, but research is concentrating on ways to expand cells successfully *in vitro* and in vivo. In addition, when UCBT is used, patients are able to tolerate HLA mismatches. The donors are mothers consenting to give their placenta after birth, so the process is noninvasive and risk free. The cells are extracted from the umbilical cord in the laboratory. Collaboration between the obstetrical and hematology oncology practitioners is critical to the success of this process (Barker and Wagner 2003).

NSTs are allogeneic transplantations. Donor sources are from the patient's family or unrelated donors selected from the National Marrow Donor Program (NMDP) registry. Patients receive a low dose of radiation or a purine analog agent together with chemotherapy to suppress the patient's immune

TABLE 6.3 Diseases Treated with Hematopoietic Stem-Cell Transplantation

Transplantation Type	Disease Treated
Autologous	Inflammatory breast, melanoma, ovarian, testicular, sarcoma, multiple myeloma, amyloidosis (light chain), AML (first remission), NHL, Hodgkin's disease
	Autoimmune diseases: rheumatoid arthritis, systemic lupus erythematosis (SLE), multiple sclerosis, scleroderma
	Germ cell tumors (pediatric), neuroblastoma (pediatric)
Allogeneic	Aplastic anemia, AML, ALL, CML, NHL, multiple myeloma, myelodysplastic syndrome, aplastic anemia, sickle cell disease, severe combined immunodeficiency disease
Nonmyeloablative	Lymphoma (low grade)
	CML (older patients)
	Multiple myeloma
	CLL
	Patients with poor prognosis, patients ineligible for myeloablative transplantations, older patients

Source: Adapted from Burcat 2004; Williams and McCarthy 2004; Gertz 2004.

system, particularly T cells, and to make room for the new stem cells to engraft. In these transplantations, the patient hopes that this new immune system will "take charge" and eradicate the disease. This graft-versus-tumor (GVT) effect takes time to establish, and at present, an NST is most effective in indolent diseases or in those cancers in remission (Bearman 2003). These transplantations may be called mini, mini allo, mini MUD, reduced-intensity, and nonmyeloablative transplantations. Transplantation physicians are struggling to designate a term that accurately names the procedure. The term "mini" leads health care professionals to believe that these transplantations are less toxic and without risk. NSTs have their own sets of toxicities requiring careful assessment and action. Because these toxicities often occur later, patients are often in community settings when first experiencing side effects. Therefore, NST patients require focused education about the treatment, self-care strategies, and who to contact if there is a problem. In addition, a wider collaboration is required among health care providers.

To clearly understand a NST, the nurse must have a basic understanding of the immune system and chimerism. The word chimera has its roots in Greek mythology and pertains to an animal with a lion's head, goat's body, and serpent's tail. Full chimerism occurs in full allogeneic transplantations when the blood and marrow become that of the donor. Mixed chimerism occurs in NST regimens when both donor and host cells exist in the blood and marrow. In NST and depending on the goal of treatment, the end point is either mixed or full chimerism. In transplantations requiring full chimerism after transplantation, a donor lymphocyte infusion (DLI) is sometimes administered to augment the donor system and achieve full chimerism. Chimerism is responsible for GVT effect. Donor dendritic cells or antigen-presenting cells (APCs) present antigen or tumor fragments to donor T and natural killer (NK) cells. This process orchestrates the GVT effect on the host disease (Solomon and Komanduri 2001).

Nursing Care

The care of the HSCT patient depends on many factors. As described, there are many types of transplantations, and the first step in assessing the patient is understanding the patient and his comorbidities, the target disease, and the source of the stem cells. It is very important to know whether the transplantation is a full transplantation or a nonmyeloablative regimen. This basic information provides the foundation for individual assessment and care planning.

The transplantation process is divided into three phases: the pretransplantation, transplantation, and posttransplantation phases. Each particular phase guides the nursing assessment, nursing plan, interventions, and overall care of the patient.

Pretransplantation Phase

In this phase, the recipient prepares for their HSCT. The patient donates and stores their own stem cells (autologous transplantation), or prepares their body to receive the donor's cells (allogeneic). Table 6.3 identifies diseases that are currently treated with HSCT.

Autologous HSCT

The intent of HSCT is to rescue patients with their own stem cells after receiving very high doses of chemotherapy. To be successful, the patient's malignant cells must be sensitive to the chemotherapy or radiation. The chemotherapy regimen chosen has a high dose-response curve, meaning the more chemotherapy given, the more malignant cells are killed. Also, the type of chemotherapy chosen has the marrow as its major dose-limiting toxicity. Hence, this is the reason for the rescue using the patient's own stem cells. Targeted diseases include the solid tumor cancers such as breast, ovarian, and testicular cancer, melanoma, and sarcoma. Patients with multiple myeloma, acute myelocytic leukemia (AML, first remission), non-Hodgkin's lymphoma (NHL), and Hodgkin's disease (salvage therapy) are also candidates to receive this treatment to either cure or control their disease (Williams and McCarthy 2004).

Several autoimmune diseases have been successfully treated with autologous transplantation (Table 6.3). Autologous HSCT is a very active treatment in the pediatric population against germ cell cancers, sarcoma, and neuroblastoma (Schmit-Pokorny and Nuss 2004).

Allogeneic HSCT

Allogeneic HSCT treats disorders and malignancies in patients who require a rescue after a lethal dose of chemotherapy and a new immune system to combat the disease. This new immune system provides the GVT effect and is equally or more important than the high-dose chemotherapy/rescue component. GVT is the focus of NSTs. The chemotherapy/radiation given in the pretransplantation phase attacks the disease and prepares the marrow for the new transplanted immune system.

Aplastic anemia and immune disorders require a new immune system that contains the missing components of the recipient's own deficient system. AML and acute lymphocytic leukemia (ALL) require a new immune system that will replace their malfunctioning components. Multiple myeloma (MM) and myelodysplastic syndrome (MDS) are complicated by older age and comorbidities. In MM, tandem transplantations are under investigation. The patient may undergo two autologous transplantations, or one autologus to debulk the disease and, after recovery, a NST for the immunologic effect.

Currently, there are no defined diseases where NST is the first treatment choice. NST offers another treatment approach for patients who are otherwise excluded from a myeloablative, high-dose transplantation because of older age, refractory disease, and comorbidities. Because it takes time for the immunologic effect to occur, NST may be an option in treating low-grade indolent lymphomas (Hinds and Minor 2004).

Chronology of Transplantations

Once the type of transplantation and the disease treated are clear, the nurse can anticipate a predictable sequence of events. Understanding the sequence adds data to the assessment and drives nursing interventions (Figures 6.1 and 6.2).

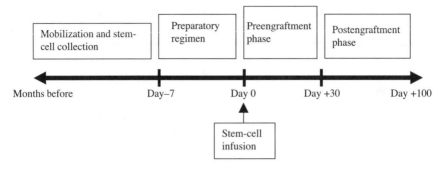

FIGURE 6.1 Chronology of autologous stem-cell transplantation.

Autologous Pretransplantation Mobilization Phase

Months before the transplantation, the patient's peripheral stem cells are collected and stored. This is the mobilization phase of autologous transplantation. In most centers, peripheral blood is the source of stem cells. Peripheral blood contains older stem cells. These cells engraft earlier, resulting in fewer days of absolute neutropenia and less risk for opportunistic infection. The patient receives chemotherapy (alkylating agents) to further treat the disease and to stimulate the marrow to produce stem cells. At an appropriate interval after chemotherapy (usually 24 hours), growth factor injections stimulate the marrow to produce stem cells and recover the blood counts. High doses of granulocyte colony-stimulating factor (G-CSF) or granulocyte-macrophage colony-stimulating factor (GM-CSF) cause the stem cells to spill into the peripheral blood. Through the process of stem-cell pheresis, these cells are collected and frozen. Sometimes, there may not be enough cells collected. The patient then travels to the operating room and has cells collected directly from the bone marrow. Cyclophosphamide, a chemotherapy agent, is commonly used for stem-cell mobilization.

During this pretransplantation phase, multiple tests are done to evaluate the patient's organ function and extent of disease. Ideally, the patient enters the transplantation procedure with good to excellent performance status and minimal disease. A psychiatric evaluation is often done to ensure that the patient will be able to psychologically tolerate the HSCT.

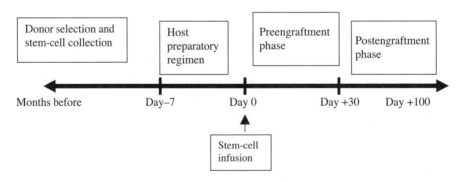

FIGURE 6.2 Chronology of allogeneic stem-cell transplantation.

Allogeneic Pretransplantation Phase

Multiple caregivers are involved in the transplantation process. The patient is prepared by receiving chemotherapy that will reduce tumor burden and, ideally, place the patient in remission, as in AML transplantations in first remission. During this time, the blood of the patient and family is typed for HLA. HLA is the major histocompatibility complex (MHC) in man. Matching the donor and recipient HLA type by serology is the focus of family donor selection. A person's HLA type is determined genetically. Antigens encode on these genes, and these HLA antigens identify cells as self or foreign to the body. Class I antigens are HLA-A, HLA-B, and HLA-C. These are found on all nucleated cells and platelets. HLA-DR, HLA-DQ, and HLA-DP constitute the class II antigens found on B-cell macrophages and activated T cells. In determining a suitable donor, the HLA-A, HLA-B, and HLA-D antigens are the primary focus. Each person has six antigens, three from each parent. Patient siblings have a one in four chance to match. A 6/6 matched is a perfect match. A 5/6 match means there is a mismatch with one of the antigens. This is sometimes acceptable, depending on the antigen, when the donor is related. Most centers have guidelines regarding the acceptability of the mismatch. The major morbidity with mismatched transplantations is GVHD (Solomon and Komanduri 2001).

If there is not a satisfactory match with family members, the search extends to unrelated donors. The National Marrow Donor Program (NMDP) keeps a registry of potential donors. The patient's HLA type is entered into the system, and the database searches for potential donors throughout the world. Because the donor is unrelated, high resolution typing examines the HLA molecule at the allele or gene level. Different alleles can encode the same antigens. Typing at high resolution uncovers these allele differences and identifies the ideal donor (Petersdorf et al. 2001).

Donors are chosen based on their HLA type, age, sex, medical history, number of pregnancies, cytomegalovirus (CMV) status, and blood types ABO compatibility. The preferred donor is an HLA and ABO compatible, CMV-negative young healthy male. ABO compatibility is not a contraindication. If necessary, the recipient's ABO antigen and red cells are removed from the collection by plasma pheresis to avoid a transfusion reaction (Kernan and Confer 2000; Bleakley and Riddell 2004).

If the donor is a family member, this donor becomes a patient of the transplantation center. The donor-patient receives a complete history and physical and is seen and evaluated by a transplantation physician. A donor-patient who donates bone marrow also donates autologous blood. The donor-patient fills out a thorough health questionnaire and is evaluated by the transplantation social worker, who also interviews the donor. Donors are carefully protected and supported throughout the transplantation process.

As in an autologous transplantation, the donor will donate stem cells from their peripheral blood or directly from the bone marrow. Most centers now prefer peripheral-blood stem cells. This is because peripheral stem cells engraft earlier, shorten the period of neutropenia, and lower the risk of opportunistic infection (Devine et al. 2003). However, these stem cells are older than those found in the bone marrow. This increases the risk (to the recipient) of GVHD. To collect peripheral stem cells from an allogeneic donor, the stem cells are also mobilized. The donor receives either G-CSF or GM-CSF to mobilize the cells into the periphery for collection via stem-cell pheresis (Devine et al. 2003).

Nursing Care during the Pretransplantation Phase

Nurses in outpatient clinics coordinate the care and educate the patient and family. The transplantation coordinator helps with coordinating appointments, works with the NMDP by sending the necessary studies to facilitate donor identification, and

TABLE 6.4 Pretransplantation Nursing Care Plan

Nursing Diagnosis	Defining Characteristics	Nursing Interventions	Expected Outcomes
Knowledge deficit related to transplantation experience	Patient asks many questions about transplantation experience	Written and verbal eduation regarding transplantation; interview with transplantation survivor if available Review of Informed Consent	Patient will verbalize understanding of transplantation and course of therapy
Anxiety regarding transplantation experience	Patient verbalizes anxiety about upcoming transplantation experience and fear of the unknown	Address patient's concerns Designation of Health Care Proxy Discussion regarding fears and self-care strategies to address these fears Social service consult Pastoral care consult Psychiatry consult	Patient will verbalize anxiety and self-care strategies to cope with these anxieties
Anxiety related to tobacco and alcohol cessation	Patient with history of tobacco and alcohol intake	Assessment of tobacco and alcohol use Tobacco cessation program including patches and aids to stop smoking Develop plan to address alcohol withdrawal while inpatient	

educates the patient regarding the whole transplantation process. The transplantation nurse coordinator begins the education that is reinforced throughout the patient's experience. The patient receives, reads, and signs the informed consent at this time. The patient and family require support from the extended family and community to prepare for the procedure ahead. The patients become overwhelmed and often feel as though they are hearing information for the first time when it has actually been told to them multiple times by multiple caregivers (see Table 6.4).

In addition to the extensive teaching required, outpatient clinic nurses administer the chemotherapy necessary for mobilization of peripheral stem cells in the autologous patient. These high-dose regimens have their own morbidity, with patients experiencing fever and neutropenia, nausea and vomiting, anemia, mucositis, and fatigue. It is important for patients to progress through mobilization with sufficient functional status to endure the actual transplantation. Therefore, the nurse advocates for the patient by providing effective antiemetic regimens, mucositis management, and fever guidelines. In addition, patients learn a safe, self-injection technique and administer their own growth factor at home. For patient convenience as well as insurance purposes, these pretransplantation chemotherapy regimens often occur in the patient's own community. Communication between centers is imperative to provide the best continuous care.

The transplantation team must also teach unrelated donors extensively. Growth factor will cause the physically well donor to feel ill with flu-like symptoms. To collect their cells, the donors will have a central pheresis line placed. In some centers, the request is for bone marrow. In this case, the donor consents to general anesthesia and the operating room procedure. Whether giving peripheral stem cells or bone marrow, risk is involved for this often very healthy donor. It is important for nurses to ensure that the donor understands the risks and benefits involved. There is a point of no return when the donor must give cells to rescue the patient. The nurse helps ensure that the patient's consent is an informed consent.

A transplantation social worker interviews donors. The NMDP has very strict guidelines regarding donor identification. Social workers counsel the donor regarding their commitment and responsibility to the recipient. They also educate the donor about the whole process and the feelings they may have should the recipient become sick or even die. Many family donors have feelings that their marrow was not good enough or that their marrow was the cause of the recipient's demise. This is addressed early by professional counselors. Many recipients of unrelated transplantations want to contact their donor to thank them for their life-saving gift. The NMDP protects donors for at least the first year. This is because not all transplantation patients have favorable outcomes. It is important for the donor to not feel guilt should the transplantation prove unsuccessful. Therefore, the patient is encouraged to send a simple thank you note that does not contain any identifying information.

Transplantation Phase

For purposes of the discussion about the transplantation phase, this section includes the preparatory regimen and the infusion of stem cells.

Preparatory Regimens

Preparatory regimens (Table 6.5) kill the malignant cells in preparation for the transplantation, and immunosuppress the patient so that the donor stem cells will engraft in their bone marrow. Time is designated in negative days until the stem cells are administered on day 0. For example, the patient may receive preparative chemotherapy on day −6. This means that, in 6 days, the patient will receive their stem cells. Preparatory regimens are synonymous with conditioning regimens. All transplantation types have some kind of preparatory regimen, although they may differ in their purpose. It is important from this point on for the nurse to know what treatment day the patient is receiving. Because most toxicity is time dependent, this helps the nurse understand symptoms and will direct the patient's assessment, interventions, and plan.

Autologous Preparatory Transplantation Regimens

Because the purpose of an autologous transplantation is to rescue the patient from high-dose chemotherapy with their own stem cells, the preparatory regimen chosen will focus on attacking

TABLE 6.5 Transplantation Preparatory Regimens: Common Agents and Treatments

Transplantation Type	Common Agents	Treatment
Autologous and allogeneic	Cyclophosphamide, busulfan, melphalan, carmustine, etoposide, thiotepa, cisplatin, cytarabine	Total-body irradiation (TBI)
Nonmyeloablative	Fludarabine, cladribine, cytarabine, pentostatin, alemtuzumab, gemtuzumab ozogamicin, ATG, busulfan, melphalan, idarubicin, cyclophosphamide	TBI (low dose) Photopheresis with UVA Thymic radiation

the disease. Alkylating chemotherapy agents are the major class of drugs used in the preparatory regimens (see Table 6.5). Total-body irradiation (TBI) destroys malignant cells as well as the bone marrow. Together, these agents treat the whole body, including the central nervous system (CNS), leaving no sanctuary for malignant cells.

Allogeneic Transplantation Preparatory Regimens

In full allogeneic and MUD transplantations, the patient must prepare to receive the donor's stem cells (graft) and establish a new immune system. Preparatory regimens have two purposes: (1) immunosuppression in the host so that the graft will transplant into the bone marrow, and (2) making room in the recipient's bone marrow for the new graft. The patient receives drugs to which the malignant cells are sensitive, which further reduces tumor burden. Chemotherapy and radiotherapy penetrate every organ, so there will be no sanctuary for disease. If TBI is contraindicated, the patient receives alkylating agents that penetrate the CNS as well as ablate the marrow. Examples are busulfan, carmustine, and melphalan (see Table 6.5).

The purpose of the preparatory regimen in NST is to establish the GVT effect. Drugs that target T-cell immunity are in the preparatory regimen to suppress the host so that the graft is accepted. T cells mediate GVHD as well as the GVT effect. In these transplantations, it is helpful to have some degree of GVHD. It provides clinical evidence that the donor graft and the new donor T cells are attacking the host tumor. Agents and therapies that suppress host T cells are the purine analogs, some monoclonal antibodies, and extracorporeal photopheresis with ultraviolet A light. Extracorporeal photopheresis is a photoimmune therapy where T cells are deactivated in the presence of UVA methoxypsoralen (injected into the pheresed bag of leukocytes). These therapies, in combination with low-dose TBI or an alkylating chemotherapy agent, make up the preparatory regimens for NST therapy. The major morbidity of these regimens is chronic GVHD, and efforts aim to define a regimen that will limit this long-term morbidity.

Nursing Considerations during the Transplantation Phase

During the transplantation phase, the patient is quite anxious and requires constant support from professional caregivers and family members. Expected outcomes of patient teaching are that the patient will understand the chemotherapy and radiation side effects and will learn self-care measures. Assessment of prior experience with chemotherapy provides the basis for the antiemetic regimen. These regimens, in combination with TBI, are highly emetogenic and require HT_3 antagonists (palonosetron, ondansetron, granisetron, and dolasetron) with or without aprepitant (substance P antagonist) and benzodiazepines, particularly lorazepam. Table 6.6 displays the nursing considerations during the transplantation phase.

Input and output (I/O) is strictly measured. Many alkylating agents (e.g., cyclophosphamide) require extensive hydration to prevent renal failure and hemorrhagic cystitis as a complication. Safety becomes a concern when patients are aggressively hydrated while on drugs that sedate and confuse the patient.

During the transplantation phase, the nurse introduces an aggressive mouth care regimen. Alkylating agents and TBI cause debilitating mucositis. Many centers have their own unique regimens for this toxicity. All regimens concentrate on careful cleansing of the mouth with saline, sodium bicarbonate, or plain water at least every 4 to 6 hours. The patient and clinician carefully examine the mouth and treat appropriately for fungal and viral infections. The University of Pennsylvania Health System Nursing (2003) published evidenced-based guidelines for oral care. The investigational growth factor palifermin has shown a significant protective effect, with

TABLE 6.6 Transplantation Phase Nursing Care Plan

Nursing Diagnosis	Defining Characteristics	Nursing Interventions	Expected Outcomes
Nausea and vomiting related to preparatory regimen	Patient has previous experience with uncontrolled nausea and vomiting or ineffective antiemetic regimen Patient experiences anticipatory nausea	Establish plan for highly emetogenic chemotherapy, including benzodiazepine, $5HT_3$ antagonists, and steroids Assess and instruct patient and family regarding side effects specific to high-dose chemotherapy Assess ways for patient to be distracted, and offer movies, relaxation techniques, and visualizations	Patient tolerates chemotherapy with minimal or no nausea and vomiting
Fluid volume excess related to high-volume IV fluid and chemotherapy	Laboratory values outside normal limits Weight gain Edema Signs of congestive heart failure (CHF) Arrhythmias	Monitor vital signs Monitor fluid balance, measure I/O urine, Cardiac monitor for abnormal electrolyte values and signs of CHF Monitor edema	Vital signs WNL Weight returns to baseline Hemodynamically-stable Stable fluid balance with electrolytes within normal limits
Fluid volume excess related to SIADH	Hyponatremia, confusion, irritability hyporeflexia, diarrhea, weight gain, decreased urine output, decreased serum osmolality	Monitor serum sodium and electrolytes Urine osmolality Serum osmolality Fluid free water restriction Daily weights Strict I/O Hypertonic saline if indicated Diuretics as indicated Seizure precautions Renal consult	Stable fluid balance with electrolytes within normal limits
Pain related to central line insertion and infection	Newly inserted central line upon admission Difficult insertion	Assess pain prn and maintain comfort at # using visual analog scale (0–10) Monitor for signs and symptoms of infection and obtain blood cultures as soon as possible with chest x-ray and urine culture Change dressing as per hospital policy and prn	Patient will have minimal pain with no signs or symptoms of infection

enhanced healing of mucositis (Peterson and Cariello 2004).

Depending on the transplantation center and the type of transplantation, patients receive the preparatory regimens in inpatient or outpatient settings. In the outpatient setting, careful and simple instruction is given at the patient's and family's appropriate learning level. Patients are taught to come to the emergency department if they experience fever, which is a medical emergency in a neutropenic patient.

During the transplantation phase, all patients receive some type of central line. Unfortunately, these lines are a primary source of infection, and the patient learns to carefully assess their line every day. Pain is often the first sign of infection, and patients are taught to report this right away. If the patient is in the hospital during this preparative phase, nurses are responsible for dressing changes. For the outpatient setting, nurses teach the patient and family to change dressings.

With the completion of the preparatory or conditioning regimen, the patient next experiences 1 or 2 days of rest. Rest means there is no planned clinical intervention at this time. This period allows for the elimination of the chemotherapy from the patient's body. During this time, the patient generally experiences fatigue and may still experience nausea and vomiting, depending on the effectiveness of the antiemetic regimen (see Table 6.6).

Transplantation Phase: Day 0

Day 0 is the day the patient receives their stem cells, which may be their own (autologous) or a donor's (allogeneic) cells. The day is much more eventful psychologically than clinically. Many patients view day 0 as a new beginning and forever mark the day as one of celebration.

Autologous Day 0

For the autologous stem cells to be frozen prior to chemotherapy, a preservative, dimethylsulfoxide (DMSO), is used. DMSO is the major cause of side effects during the stem-cell infusion. DMSO is a cardiotoxin with a direct negative inotropic effect. This can cause bradyarrhythmias and heart block. The patient is placed on a cardiac monitor. Emergency drugs are in the room in the event of anaphylaxis to the DMSO. Rapidly infusing the thawed marrow contributes to nausea, abdominal cramping, and chest tightness. The patient is vigorously hydrated to help the kidneys eliminate the preservative as well as any nonfunctional damaged cells. The patient receives antiemetics to prevent nausea and vomiting. Hard candy provides comfort for the dry throat and cough. Facial flushing and a strong garlicky smell emanates from the patient's breath and secretions. Because of newer, sophisticated methods for freezing cells, patients rarely experience the more dangerous side effects of cardiac arrhythmias and anaphylaxis. However, patients with cardiac disease require very close monitoring. A clinician (either a physician or nurse) thaws the collection in a warm water bath. The infusion is very similar to a blood transfusion, except the product is unfiltered. The infusion depends on the number of bags collected and lasts 1 to 2 hours (Horak and Forman 2001).

Allogeneic Day 0

Infusion of allogeneic, including nonmyeloablative, stem cells is very much like a blood product transfusion, except the product is unfiltered. The patient receives the cells freshly prepared and without the preservative DMSO. Preparation involves vigorous hydration prior to the infusion. The stem cells infuse over 1 to 2 hours.

Nursing Care Day 0

Day 0 is a landmark for the patient. It is the nurse's challenge to support the patient physically and emotionally. Family members often celebrate the day as a new beginning full of hope. Clergy and social work professionals attend to the psychological and spiritual needs of the whole family system.

Posttransplantation Phase

Posttransplantation care is the last phase of the process and is composed of three stages. The period of the first 30 days is termed the engraftment phase. The other two phases are the postengraftment phase (30–100 days) and the last posttransplantation phase (100+ days after transplantation), which continues until the patient discontinues immunosuppressive therapy.

Using homing mechanisms, the donor stem cells travel to the recipient's bone marrow and engraft. Engraftment is confirmed when the patient has at least 500 neutrophils/μl in the white blood cell differential. During this time, the patient is at risk for a variety of complications. Acute complications occur within the first 100 days. Chronic complications, particularly from GVHD, occur after 100 days. Chronic effects from transplantation are identified years after a patient's stem cells are infused (Figure 6.2).

Engraftment Phase: Day 0 to Day 30

For autologous and allogeneic transplantations, the engraftment phase is the time of careful monitoring while the patient awaits bone marrow engraftment. Patients experience side effects from the preparatory regimen including profound pancytopenia. Infection, mucositis, fluid and electrolyte imbalances, pulmonary complications, acute GVHD (aGVHD with allogeneic recipients), organ compromise, and nutritional deficits are common. The patient requires multiple antibiotics, blood products, fluids, electrolytes, analgesics, and, sometimes, nutritional support with total parenteral nutrition (TPN). At some centers, patients go home or to a nearby site with close, daily follow-up. Patients enter the hospital when complications require close intervention and monitoring. In the outpatient setting, the patient requires a center with 24-hour direct admission to transplantation or separate oncology units and clinics with liberal hours or a pathway for emergency department triage nurses to notify appropriate physicians and expedite admission to the specialty unit.

Because NST preparatory regimens do not rely on high-dose chemotherapy, patients experience less severe side effects during these first 30 days after transplantation. In many instances, the patient goes home to the care of their local community physicians. During this time, the patient should be taught the signs and symptoms of infection, self-care measures, line care, skin hygiene including meticulous mouth care, and how to recognize early signs of aGVHD.

Mucositis

Mucositis is a progressive inflammatory response of the mucosal body surfaces. It encompasses the patient's total alimentary tract from the mouth to the anus. Autologous and allogeneic transplantation patients experience severe mucositis. TBI and the ablative chemotherapy regimens have both a direct and indirect effect on the mucosa. Stem cells within the mouth are directly affected by irradiation and chemotherapy. Destruction of stem cells in the tongue and salivary gland results in changes in taste and ability to chew, speak, and digest. The protective function of saliva is altered. Indirectly, by ablating the marrow with chemotherapy and radiotherapy, neutrophils are absent or limited, with a consequent decrease in ability to fight bacteria or repair cell damage. Damage to the oral mucosa causes growth of opportunistic organisms, particularly candida (yeast). Damage to the esophageal and stomach mucosa causes loss of appetite as well as debilitating nausea. Damage to the small and large intestinal mucosa causes alterations in absorption, digestion, and elimination. Patients may experience painful, watery diarrhea without any infection or immune-mediated etiology.

Many factors contribute to mucositis. Radiation therapy has a direct effect on the mucosa. The depth of penetration, total dose delivered (gray), and the number of treatments influence the severity. Radiation of the parotid gland causes xerostomia and problems with swallowing and digestion.

TBI is a major contributor to damaged mucosa. Chemotherapy directly affects the mucosa by damaging cells undergoing mitosis (Beck 2004). Indirectly, chemotherapy and radiotherapy contribute to mucositis by affecting the bone marrow and causing myelosuppression. Patients with hematologic malignancies are at higher risk. In the allogeneic patient, aGVHD causes severe mucositis, or conversely, severe mucositis may increase the risk of AGVHD. Young patients tend to develop mucositis more often than older patients. This may be a result of the higher turnover rate of basal cells in children (Woo and Treister 2001). In the high-dose setting, poor dentition and decreased renal function place patients at increased risk of mucositis (Berger and Eilers 1998). To summarize, the severity of mucositis depends on direct, local damage and, indirectly, on the degree of myelosuppression and extent of patient comorbidities. The biologic model for mucositis involves four phases (Table 6.7) which are discussed in the following paragraph.

The first phase, inflammatory phase, causes the release of cytokines. These cytokines mediate the inflammation and dilatation of blood vessels. Tumor necrosis factor alpha (TNF-α) causes tissue damage. In the second phase, chemotherapy and radiation retard cell division, causing decreased cell turnover and renewal. These first two stages cause erythema from increased vascularity and a thinning epithelial layer. The trauma from eating, speaking, swallowing, and chewing causes further ulceration (third phase). Bacteria congregate in the ulcers, causing release of endotoxins and local cytokines. In the fourth phase, as counts recover, reepithelialization occurs with control of local bacteria and healing (Woo and Treister 2001; Shih et al. 2002).

Both the patient and clinician carefully examine and grade the degree of mucositis daily. There are many scales and guides. The National Cancer Institute (NCI) Common Toxicity Criteria addresses BMT stomatitis/pharyngitis specifically. The grade range is from 0 to 4 and ranges from normal to severe ulceration requiring parenteral and enteral support (Table 6.8). There are other NCI criteria for mucositis graded in the gastrointestinal category under the specific sites (colitis, gastritis, vaginitis, and radiation-induced mucositis). Eilers Oral Assessment Guide (OAG) is a more extensive assessment guide that assesses the gingival, tongue, teeth, and buccal mucosa (Berger and Eilers 1998; Worthington et al. 2001).

Interventions for grade 4 mucositis are limited. Being such a sensitive part of the body, the mouth has many pain receptors. The inability to eat without pain and the nausea accompanying treatment regimens cause significant changes in the patient's quality of life (Borbasi et al. 2002). Bellm et al. (2000) interviewed 38 subjects undergoing transplantation. Nearly all (90%) reported a change in taste during their experience. Patients reported that solids and liquids simply tasted horrible. Nearly all patients (100% allogeneic, 71% autologous) experienced changes in their oral pharyngeal mucosa. Oral pain, soreness, tender/sensitive mouth, and thick ropy mucous were the symptoms most frequently mentioned.

TABLE 6.7 Biologic Phases of Mucositis

Phase	Description
Inflammatory	Cytokine release, TNF-α, interleukin–1, interleukin-6
	Inflammation and tissue damage
Epithelial	Reduced epithelial renewal from radiation; increased vascularity, epithelial, thining, atrophy, and ulceration
Ulcerative	Further damage and ulceration from release of cytokines and mechanical trauma; bacterial infection
Healing	Tissue repair and epithelial proliferation and differentiation as white blood cell count recovers

Source: Shih et al. 2002.

TABLE 6.8	National Cancer Institute (2004) Common Toxicity Criteria for Stomatitis/ Pharyngitis in BMT Population
Toxicity Grade	Description
0	None
1	Painless ulcers, erythema, or mild soreness in the absence of lesions
2	Painful erythema, edema, or ulcers and can swallow
3	Painful erythema, edema, or ulcers preventing swallowing or requiring hydration of parenteral nutrition
4	Severe ulceration requiring prophylactic intubation or resulting in documented aspiration pneumonia

Source: http://ctep.cancer.gov/forms/ CTCv20_4-30-992.pdf.

Patients stated that mouth sores were the single most debilitating side effect of their transplantation experience. Borbasi *et al.* (2002) quote patient descriptions of mucositis as ". . . feels like I have razor blades there" or "living with foul breath" or "feeling tired and having to talk with effort" or "a complete loss of appetite" and "definite changes in taste" (p. 1054).

Treatment involves the management of infection, pain control, nutritional support, and meticulous mouth care. The most effective preventive treatment involves keeping the mouth as clean as possible. Normal saline and water are as effective as the more expensive nonalcoholic mouth rinses. Antifungals and antiviral medications treat opportunistic growth. Hydrogen peroxide is not beneficial because it causes the breakdown of new granulation tissue (Worthington *et al.* 2001). Oral agents and systemic opioids control the pain. "Miracle Mouthwash" (viscous lidocaine, diphenhydramine, and aluminum hydroxide suspension) is a preparation familiar to most nurses, but its effectiveness is controversial. Although the

lidocaine may be helpful for local lesions, the diphenhydramine may actually cause further dryness and delay healing. Gelclair is a new product recently approved for mucositis. It acts as a "liquid band aid" in the mouth and when swallowed. It has no systemic effects. Gelclair is comprised of three ingredients: (1) polyvinylpyrrolidone, a muco-adherent and film-forming agent; (2) hyaluronic acid, which hydrates the damaged tissue and accelerates healing; and (3) glycyrrhetinic acid, an anti-inflammatory agent (Gelclair Product Information 2002).

Finally, systemic opioids are helpful when local analgesic treatment does not effectively control the pain. The pain related to grade 4 mucositis often requires an opioid administered by patient-controlled analgesia (PCA). Unlike many patients with cancer, the stem-cell transplantation patient may be new to opioids, and the side effects of this treatment add to the distress of the mucositis. Untoward side effects of opioids include hallucinations, decreased mental acuity, and feelings of total loss of control. Some patients discontinue the opioid because of these distressing side effects. Some transplantation patients may require PCA for more than 7 days. This causes physical dependence and escalating doses. Parran and Pederson (2000) developed an opioid taper algorithm useful in discontinuing the opioid once the mucositis resolves. This algorithm tapers the opioid by 10% of the pretaper dose every 8 to 12 hours based on the length of time on PCA, the amount of pain during the taper, and withdrawal symptoms.

Mucositis is a major cause of debilitation during the transplantation process and causes compromised nutritional status. Patients receive TPN or enteral feeding to maintain positive nitrogen balance and promote healing. Glutamine, a conditionally essential nutrient, is helpful when added to parenteral or enteral nutrition. It selectively targets the gastrointestinal tract and provides fuel for intestinal epithelial cells as well as macrophages and lymphocytes. It is given orally as a rinse, in enteral therapy, and intravenously in TPN (Murray and Pindoria 2000;

Peterson *et al.* 2004). Although more randomized trials are necessary, it may be of benefit in this population to reduce infection and length of stay and to decrease the incidence and severity of mucositis (Murray and Pindoria 2000).

Mucositis causes gastrointestinal problems, such as nausea, vomiting, and diarrhea, during the engraftment period. Treatment with 5-HT$_3$ antagonists as well as low-dose steroids may help, but the patient often eats very little during this time. As blood counts recover, so does the ability to taste and eat. With the intestines, the patient experiences diarrhea. After cultures, the patient may receive loperamide or diphenoxylate with atropine to combat the diarrhea. In some instances, octreotide is prescribed. Recombinant human keratinocyte growth factor (palifermin) is also showing promise. It selectively stimulates growth of basal epithelial cells and may be a valuable tool to prevent and heal mucositis (Meropol *et al.* 2003).

Nursing Care

Nursing care involves careful assessment, education, and diligence with the treatment plan. Patients learn to inspect their mouth at least daily and report any new lesions or areas of breakdown. The nurse also inspects the mouth every shift if the patient is hospitalized and recommends the best mouth care regimen to the health care team. If the patient is on PCA, pain assessment is a significant part of the assessment, and the dose is adjusted to maintain adequate pain control and allow for local care. Brushing is discouraged once platelets drop below 50,000, and spongy toothettes can be substituted. Frequent rinsing with normal saline, bicarbonate, or plain water helps thin the ropy saliva and keep the oral mucosal clean. Ice chips can sometimes reduce the pain.

The nurse encourages the patient to persevere and helps the patient understand that the physical pain will subside once the bone marrow engrafts and neutrophils are available to help heal the oral mucosa. Unfortunately, the sequelae of mucositis may persist for months, with difficulty eating because of changes in taste, xerostomia, and persistent nausea and vomiting.

Patient education for mucositis during this period closely resembles the teaching for any neutropenic patient receiving chemotherapy. A clean mouth (teeth and oral mucosal) is the goal of daily care. Patients rinse with saline, a dilute solution of sodium bicarbonate, or plain water at least every 4 hours and particularly after any eating and at bedtime. In addition, antifungal rinses or troches are self-administered 5 times a day to prevent fungal opportunistic infections.

Noninfectious Pulmonary Complications

In the first 30 days after transplantation, infection, the preparatory regimen, mucositis, and aGVHD cause damage to the lungs. In the pancytopenic patient, these pulmonary complications can result in mortality. Pulmonary edema is common, with the patient experiencing weight gain and hypoxemia. The nurse assesses for bilateral rales on auscultation and observes diffuse bilateral infiltrates on chest x-ray. Engraftment syndrome occurs around days 7 to 14, just when the patient begins to show signs of neutrophil return. The patient experiences fever, hypoxemia, pulmonary infiltrates, and rash. Diffuse alveolar hemorrhage (DAH) occurs around day 12 and manifests as sudden onset of dyspnea, fever, hypoxemia, and nonproductive cough. There is usually no evidence of bleeding, and DAH is confirmed only with bronchoalveolar lavage (BAL) (Huaringa *et al.* 2000). These noninfectious complications occur after autologous and allogeneic transplantations, including NST, and can be fatal if not recognized and treated immediately. High-dose preparatory regimens containing cyclophosphamide, carmustine, busulfan, thiotepa, TBI, and nonmyeloablative regimens with antithymocyte globulin, thymic radiation, and cyclosporine increase risk (Yen *et al.* 2004; Spitzer 2001; Wong *et al.* 2003).

The etiology of engraftment syndrome is multifactoral and globally includes DAH. Increased cytokine production and release, T-cell interactions, and damage to local and systemic tissue result in damage to the lung parenchyma. The cytokines necessary for neutrophil recovery are the same cytokines implicated in capillary leak syndrome, acute respiratory distress syndrome (ARDS), aGVHD, and multiorgan failure (Spitzer 2001; Shankar and Cohen 2001; Schots *et al.* 2003). In the allogeneic patient, engraftment syndrome may be an indication of a host-versus-graft effect or graft rejection (Spitzer 2001).

Nursing Care

Table 6.9 highlights the nursing necessary during the immediate posttransplantation period. The nurse is alert to signs and symptoms of engraftment syndrome when the patient's white blood cell count begins to recover. It may start as simply as a dry cough. The patient becomes flushed because of dyspnea and increasing oxygen requirements. Chest x-ray shows diffuse pulmonary infiltrates. Whatever the cause of this noninfectious syndrome, platelets, high-dose steroids, and oxygen reverse the syndrome when given promptly. If unrecognized and untreated, the patient will require intubation and will be transferred to an intensive care environment. This major lung complication after transplantation is a major cause of transplantation related mortality within 1 year, with death rates as high as 61% (Schots *et al.* 2003; Spitzer 2001; Wong *et al.* 2003).

Infection

Protecting and preventing opportunistic infection is the focus during the first 30 days after the transplantation and continues for the first year. Initially, the patient is at risk from the preparatory regimen and the presence of central lines. The preparatory regimen and the resulting neutropenia deplete neutrophils, monocytes, and macrophages in the body and severely compromise the mucosal barrier. The gastrointestinal tract, which normally houses bacteria and fungus, is a reservoir of pathogens. B- and T-cell immunity is lost, and the patient's immune system no longer fights using the arsenal of antibodies accumulated over a lifetime. Mucositis, the presence of aGVHD, and further immunosuppression (allogeneic recipients) with cyclosporine or tacrolimus, steroids, and methotrexate exacerbate the problem. Shortening the time to engraftment is helpful and effective with the autologous population and in some allogeneic regimens using growth factors and peripheral stem cells (Dykewicz *et al.* 2000; Yen *et al.* 2004).

Gram-negative and gram-positive bacteria, herpes simplex virus (HSV), CMV, and fungal infections are common pathogens during this period of engraftment. Mucositis causes the gastrointestinal tract to be an ideal portal of entry for opportunistic microorganisms of the skin and mucosa. Gram-positive and -negative bacteria are usually the first infections suspected and treated during this time. With continued temperature elevation, early fungal infection with *Candida* (*tropicalis* and *albicans*) is suspect. The seropositive HSV patient is at risk for reemergence of HSV1 painful oral, esophageal, and tracheal ulcers that can lead to HSV pneumonitis. These ulcers also cause breaks in the mucosal surface and allow entry for other opportunistic microorganisms.

CMV pneumonia usually occurs 6 weeks after transplantation but may occur early in the seropositive patient, in the seronegative patient receiving seropositive stem cells, or in patients receiving contaminated blood products (Dykewicz *et al.* 2000; Yen *et al.* 2004).

Early recognition and empirical treatment of infection, often without identification of the actual source, are the standard approach. Initially, the patient receives antibiotic prophylaxis with an oral quinolone until the first fever spike. The seropositive HSV patient receives oral acyclovir. For *Candida tropicalis* and *albicans*, the patient receives fluconazole or an oral antifungal troche or mouth rinse. The seropositive CMV patient receives ganciclovir or close observation with weekly antigenemia testing.

With the first temperature spike, the antibiotics, a fourth generation cephalosporin or a carbepenem with vancomycin, are given to provide gram-positive and gram-negative coverage, including pseudomonas. This regimen broadly covers bacteria originating on the skin and in the

TABLE 6.9 Posttransplantation (days 0–30+) Nursing Care Plan

Nursing Diagnosis	Defining Characteristics	Nursing Interventions	Expected Outcomes
Infection related to central line infection and neutropenia	Very low WBC Pain and slight erythema around central line site Fever	Neutropenia precautions No live plants Freshly cooked foods only Strict hand washing No young children (minimum age deteremined by transplantation center) Meticulous attention to ADLs with daily showers Mouth care as per unit policy Administer antibiotics/antifungals/antivirals	Patient recovers from neutropenia without sepsis
Potential for bleeding related to thrombocytopenia	Platelets < 20,000 Petechiae Bruising	Thrombocytopenic precautions No IM injections or enemas Pressure to phlebotomy sites for at least 5 minutes (teach patient to apply pressure after phlebotomist leaves) Assess fall risk Administer platelets as ordered	Remains free of injury related to thrombocytopenia throughout hospitalization
Fatigue related to chemotherapy, anemia, pain, sleep deprivation, bed rest, poor appetite, fluid and electrolyte imbalance, steroids,	High-dose chemotherapy altering fluid and electrolyte balance Mucositis pain and opioid medication	Offer and administer pain medication as needed to achieve a level of ≤ 3 with visual analog scale (0–10) Mouth care	Pain ≤ 3 with visual analog scale (0–10) Patient is satisfied with amount of sleep/rest in 24 hours

Nursing diagnosis	Findings	Interventions	Outcomes
disease, and transplantation experience	Weight gain Muscle wasting Sleep deprivation Decreased calorie intake Anxiety	Tailor antiemetics for nausea and vomiting Monitor daily electrolyte values and replete per protocols Daily weights Assess sleep pattern and develop plan to allow for uninterrupted sleep Schedule steroids to avoid late evening/night administration Nutrition consult to address caloric intake Physical therapy to address deconditioning and muscle wasting Social service consult and plan to address anxiety	Independently executes self-care strategies that address anxiety Fluid and electrolytes are maintained in balance Nausea and vomiting is at tolerable level Weight stabilizes
Potential for injury/safety related to medications	Medications for nausea and vomiting and pain Cyclosporine and steroids for immunosuppression	Assess safety every shift Monitor neuro status Safety precautions when necessary Cyclosporine levels as per hospital policy	Cyclosporine level remains therapeutic Patient mental status remains at baseline throughout transplantation experience
Alteration in comfort related to aGVHD	Rash with pruritus and pain Diarrhea Elevated bilirubin with jaundice	Assess rash every shift Topical treatments as prescribed for rash and dry skin Strict I/O Daily weight Monitor electrolytes and replete as necessary NPO if experiencing diarrhea	Rash, diarrhea will disappear, and bilirubin will return to normal

(Continued)

TABLE 6.9 Posttransplantation (days 0–30+) Nursing Care Plan (Continued)

Nursing Diagnosis	Defining Characteristics	Nursing Interventions	Expected Outcomes
		Culture diarrhea	
		Antidiarrheals as prescribed	
		Sitz baths prn	
		Nutrition consult to assess for TPN	
		Grade aGVHD weekly	
		Immunosuppressants as prescribed	
Fluid volume deficit related to anemia and dehydration	Low blood pressure	Do orthostatic blood pressure every morning	Patient remains euvolemic with vital signs at baseline
	Increased heart rate	Daily weight	Hgb is maintained at ≥ 11
	Orthostatic hypotension	Strict I/O	
	Fatigue	Fluid and blood component administration as prescribed	
	Low Hgb (< 11)	Monitor for safety	
	Negative fluid balance	Nutrition consult	
	Dry skin		
Decreased cardiac output related to arrhythmia, and decreased ejection fraction	Conditioning regimens containing potentially cardiotoxic therapies including carmustine, cyclophosphamide, cytarabine, etoposide, ifosfamide, cisplatin, busulfan, and radiation	Left ventricular ejection fraction study prior to preparatory regimen	Patient's cardiac function will be maintained at preadmission status
		Baseline EKG and daily during preparatory regimen	
		Cardiac isoenzymes daily during preparatory regimen	
		Assess respiratory status and heart sounds every shift and prn	
		Monitor oxygen saturation	
		Maintain fluid balance	

Nursing Diagnosis	Assessment	Interventions	Expected Outcome
Ineffective breathing related to engraftment syndrome	Patient experiences rash, dry cough, and increased oxygen requirements around time of engraftment (days 7–15)	Assess lung sounds every shift and prn Assess temperature, vital signs, and oxygen saturation every 4 hours and prn as patient shows signs of engraftment syndrome Monitor skin for rash, particularly on face, torso, hands, and feet Watch for laboratory increases in liver enzymes Monitor patient feelings of anxiety and sense of doom Alert medical team at first sign of decreased respiratory status, fever, and rash	Patient will have minimal clinical symptoms as engraftment occurs and is treated emergently at the first signs of the syndrome
Mucositis related to preparatory regimen	Preparatory regimens, includes alkylating agents and radiation, painful mouth, sore throat, nausea and vomiting, and diarrhea	Assess Herpes Simplex Virus (HSV) status before transplantation Oral assessment every shift with documentation of mucositis grade Local treatment to lesions with topical anesthetics or Gelclair Meticulous oral hygiene at least every 4 hours while awake with normal saline or sodium bicarbonate rinses (1 tsp/8 oz. water) Antifungal rinses/troches for mouth candidiasis;	Patient will have tolerable mucositis during the preengraftment phase of transplantation

(Continued)

TABLE 6.9 Posttransplantation (days 0–30+) Nursing Care Plan (Continued)

Nursing Diagnosis	Defining Characteristics	Nursing Interventions	Expected Outcomes
		systemic antifungals if local therapy not effective or noncompliance	
		Culture for HSV if suspected and administer appropriate medication	
		Treat pain aggressively with patient-controlled analgesia (PCA)	
		H_2 blocker or proton pump inhibitor for GI upset	
		Administer antiemetics	
		Strict I/O, nutrition consult	
		Culture diarrhea for Clostridium difficile and medicate with diphenoxylate or loperamide if cultures negative	
		NPO if aGVHD suspected	
Hyperglycemia related to medications	High-dose steroids	Monitor serum glucose daily with morning laboratory values; determine need for insulin sliding scale and fingerstick schedule with transplantation team if hyperglycemic	Blood sugar will remain within normal limits
		If on TPN, add insulin to bag	
Alteration in urinary elimination related	Preparatory regimen contains renal toxic	Assess BUN and serum creatinine and electrolytes	Patient's renal status will remain at

			pretransplantation levels
to impaired renal function, diuretics, hemorrhagic cystitis, and dehydration	drugs; for example, cyclophosphamide, cisplatin, and radiation Cyclosporine and methotrexate for continued immunosuppression Renal toxic antibiotics Renal toxic diuretics	daily with morning laboratory values Daily weight Monitor I/O Monitor cyclosporine levels; consult with team and adjust antibiotics per renal status Renal consult to evaluate for dialysis	
Activity intolerance related to fatigue and bed rest	Ineffective sleep Patient is deconditioned Fluid and electrolyte imbalance Anemia High-dose steroids	Teach patient regarding the dangers of bed rest and strategies for energy conservation Monitor fluid balance and replete fluids Transfuse as directed Daily weight Diuretics and electrolytes as prescribed PT consult for exercise regimen Encourage patient to get out of bed during the day particularly when visiting with family	Patient will have adequate conditioning during hospital stay
Alteration in coping related to hospitalization and isolation from family support system	Depression and sadness Verbalizing social isolation	Social service consult Pastoral care consult Encourage family visits, cards, letters, and telephone conversations with children	Patient will develop and use strategies to keep in touch with family and friends during hospitalization

gastrointestinal tract. Further medications, most empirically prescribed based on assessment, are added as the patient continues to have temperature spikes. Patients with *Clostridium difficile*, identified by stool culture or with a suspected intestinal source, receive oral or intravenous metronidazole. Antifungals are added if the patient has persistent fevers. Despite multiple blood cultures, organisms may never be identified, and the patient is treated until the neutrophil count returns to at least 500 neutrophils/μl (Dykewicz *et al.* 2000).

Patients are tested for HSV, Epstein-Barr virus (EBV), and CMV before transplantation. Respiratory syncytial virus (RSV), which is a seasonal virus in children and adults, can lead to RSV pneumonia and death in a transplantation patient. The patient is cultured (nasal washings) at the earliest sign and begins antiviral therapy with ribavirin.

Nursing Care

As part of the pretransplantation workup, the patient undergoes a dental evaluation. The goal is for the patient to have the healthiest mouth (teeth and oral mucosa) possible. Meticulous hand washing is taught and reinforced to all families and caregivers. Because bacteria are on the hands, this simple routine prevents multiple complications if carried out habitually.

The nurse's careful assessment is the best tool for early and aggressive treatment. Fever is often the only sign of infection. Steroids mask this obvious sign in the allogeneic population. Careful recognition of trends in vital signs and liver, respiratory, and kidney function provide early subtle clues of infection. The nurse assesses the mouth and rectal area and reinforces mouth care regimens and daily performance of activities of daily living (ADL) with showers and sitz baths. Central lines are examined, and early treatment begins with the first signs of infection. With no white blood cells, the early sign may be pain, with minimal palpation at the central line entry site. Table 6.10 highlights the organisms causing infection after transplantation in this patient population. Once recognized, treatment begins

promptly with antibiotics. Assessments continue, and antibiotics, antivirals, and antifungals are added when fevers do not respond to treatment (Dykewicz *et al.* 2000; Buchsel 1998).

Hepatic Venoocclusive Disease

Hepatocytes are the cells of the liver. At the cellular level, hepatocytes interact directly with the liver's end point blood vessels (sinusoids) as well as tiny venules. Endothelial cells line the sinusoid. Damage to these cells by cytokines, chemotherapy metabolites, and alloreactive mechanisms begin the cascade of events in hepatic venoocclusive disease (VOD). VOD is also termed sinusoidal obstruction syndrome (Kumar *et al.* 2003; Schots *et al.* 2003). VOD occurs in the first week or two after HSCT. It is more severe in allogeneic patients. One of the major risk factors is the preparatory regimen. High-dose conditioning regimens, particularly with busulfan, or TBI and cyclophosphamide, with methotrexate as part of GVHD prophylaxis, place the patient at risk for VOD. Preexisting hepatic dysfunction with elevated transaminases, advanced age, CMV status, and mismatched and unrelated donors are also risks (Kumar *et al.* 2003).

The clinical features of VOD are sometimes confused with aGVHD. The standard procedure for diagnosis is histologic examination by biopsy, which is often impossible in pancytopenic patients. The patient presents with unexplained, symptomatic weight gain, followed in a few days by hyperbilirubinemia (elevated direct bilirubin). Pain is in the right upper quadrant, and in later stages, jaundice and ascites develop. As hepatic function declines, the patient experiences coagulation factor deficiencies and prolonged prothrombin time. The patient may experience DAH or engraftment syndrome simultaneously. This may all progress to multisystem organ failure and death (Schots *et al.* 2003).

No treatments are uniformly effective, but some agents that are promising include defibrotide and ursodeoxycholic acid. Low molecular weight heparin and heparin may help, but these are difficult to administer to thrombocytopenic patients (Pallera and Schwartzberg 2004).

TABLE 6.10 Organisms Causing Infection After Transplantation (days 0–100+)

Phase (day)	Organism	Prevention	Treatment
0–30	Gram-positive bacteria	Hand washing Vaccinate at 12, 14, and 24 months for *Haemophilus influenzae* Dental consult before transplantation	Fourth-generation cephalosporins or carbepenems
0–30	Herpers simplex virus 1 (HSV1)	Acyclovir in seropositive patients	Acyclovir
0–100+	Cytomegalovirus (CMV)	CMV-negative blood products, antigenemia testing or ganciclovir in seropositive patients	Ganciclovir, foscarnet
0–100+	Fungal infections *Aspergillus,* candida	Hand washing, protective environment, avoid construction and renovation	Azoles, amphotericin, echinocandins
30–100+	*Pneumocystis carinii* pneumonia (PCP)	Trimethoprim/sulfamethoxazole prophylaxis or pentamidine by inhalation	Oral, intravenous trimethoprim/ sulfamethoxazole
30–100+	Respiratory syncytial virus (RSV)	Hand washing, protective environment	Ribavirin
100+	Varicella zoster virus (VZV)	Vaccination of seronegative family members, varicella zoster immunoglobulin within 96 hours in exposed seronegative patients	Acyclovir Valacyclovir Famciclovir

Source: Adapted from Pallera and Schwartzberg 2004.

Nursing Care

Supportive care is currently the standard treatment for VOD. This includes managing fluid and electrolytes, managing ascites, managing drugs affected by diminished liver and kidney function, and treating any coagulopathies. The overall goal of supportive care is to restore blood flow to the liver. Ongoing research is underway to identify effective interventions (Kumar *et al.* 2003).

aGVHD

aGVHD occurs within the first 100 days after HSCT. In aGVHD, donor T lymphocytes recognize MHC and minor histocompatibility antigen (mHA) mismatches on host cells. These T lymphocytes attack and kill the host cells and are defending the donor against foreign invasion. Unfortunately, the foreign invader is the host.

Two pathways cause destruction of host cells. The preparatory regimen consisting of high-dose chemotherapy and radiation causes direct damage to the liver, gastrointestinal tract, and skin. Cytokines are released with this damage. These cytokines up-regulate MHC and mHA, promoting interaction between host APCs and mature donor T lymphocytes. Further release of cytokines causes helper T cells to recruit and stimulate natural killer cells and cytotoxic T lymphocytes. This causes programmed cell death.

Intestinal cell damage provides a second pathway for aGVHD. Lipopolysaccharide from the damaged intestinal mucosa initiates monocyte activation and the release of cytokines. Targeted cell death (apoptosis) furthers the release of cytokines, perpetuating the cycle of uncontrolled damage and tissue necrosis (Davies 2003; Ferrara 2003; Reddy 2003; Mitchell 2004).

Preparatory regimens and damage to mucosa are predictors of aGVHD severity. It may be a part of or be confused with the engraftment syndrome as cell counts begin to rise. Full chimerism is necessary for aGVHD. Mixed chimerism evident in NST causes a tolerance between the donor and host immune system and delays the presentation of aGHVD. Consequently, aGVHD may present as late as day +100. NST is challenging the definition of aGVHD temporally.

Factors influencing the severity of aGVHD include donor-recipient histocompatibility and whether the stem-cell source is peripheral blood or bone marrow. Peripheral blood contains more donor T lymphocytes than donor bone marrow or cord blood and contributes to more aGVHD. Depleting T cells in the graft either in the lab or by the administration of agents like Campath-1H reduces the risk of aGVHD but may increase the likelihood of disease relapse. Female to male transplantation results in more aGVHD, as does CMV seropositivity in either donor or recipient. Older recipients also experience more aGVHD (Mitchell 2004).

aGVHD attacks the skin, liver, and gut. The stage defines the severity in each system and, considered together, determines the grade (Tables 6.11 and 6.12). The grade of aGVHD is a strong predictor of mortality. Grade 4 aGVHD is a very poor prognostic indicator for survival to 1 year (Cutler *et al.* 2001).

Preventive treatment for aGVHD begins on or before day 0 with combination immunosuppressant regimens including cyclosporine or tacrolimus and methotrexate. Steroids are added to suppress the immune system further at the first sign of rash, noninfectious diarrhea, or otherwise unexplained elevated bilirubin.

Nursing Care

The patient may initially exhibit a slight rash appearing on the palms, soles of feet, or tip of ears. If the rash appears on the trunk, it may be mistaken for a drug rash. Understanding the whole picture of where the patient is in their engraftment aids with the identification and prompt treatment. Local treatment with topical and systemic steroids adds to the immunotherapy regimen at this first sign. Careful monitoring is part of the daily routine

TABLE 6.11 Staging of Acute Graft Versus Host Disease

	Stage 1	Stage 2	Stage 3	Stage 4
Skin	Erythema (sunburn-like) on hands, feet, earlobes, trunk with pain or pruritus on less than 25% of body surface	Erythema on hands, feet, earlobes, trunk with pain or pruritus on more than 25% but less than 50% of body surface	Erythema on more than 50% of body surface	Erythroderma–generalized erythema over all of body surface area with skin blistering and desquamation
Liver	Total bilirubin up to 3 mg/dL	Total bilirubin up to 6 mg/dL	Total bilirubin up to 15 mg/dL	Total bilirubin more than 15 mg/dL
Gut	Watery, mucoid, green diarrhea more than 500 mL/day	Watery, mucoid, green diarrhea less than 1.5 L/day	Watery, mucoid, green diarrhea more than 1.5 L/day	Intense abdominal pain with or without ileus with watery, mucoid, green diarrhea more than 2 L/day

Source: Przepiorka *et al.* 1995; Mitchell 2004.

TABLE 6.12 Grading of Acute Graft Verses Host Disease Based on Stage

Grade 1	Grade 2	Grade 3	Grade 4
Erythema (sunburn-like) with pain or pruritus on up to 50% of body surface area (Stage 1–2) with no liver or gut involvement	Erythema on more than 50% of body surface area (Stage 3) **OR** Total bilirubin no greater than 3 mg/dL (Stage 1) **AND/OR** Green, watery, mucoid diarrhea more than 500 mL/day but less than 1 L/day (Stage 1)	Erythema on more than 50% of body surface area (Stage 3) **AND** Total bilirubin up to 15 mg/dL (Stage 3) **AND/OR** Green, watery, mucoid diarrhea but more than 1.5 L/day (Stage 3)	Generalized erythroderma (Stage 4) **OR** Total bilirubin greater than 15 mg/dL (Stage 4) **AND/OR** Intense abdominal pain with or without ileus and diarrhea greater than 2 L/day (Stage 4)

Source: Przepiorka *et al.* 1995; Mitchell 2004.

for the nurse and patient. If the patient experiences aGVHD of the gastrointestinal tract, careful measurement of I/O with aggressive fluid repletion and TPN is required. The patient receives nothing by mouth (NPO) to totally rest the gut. During this time period, the patient is allowed only ice chips and, even then, in only modest amounts. Liver GVHD does not usually appear first. The bilirubin begins to rise, and the symptoms progress and resemble VOD. Jaundice with high bilirubin and further skin changes cause alterations in appearance and overall discomfort.

aGVHD is a major cause of treatment-related mortality in the allogeneic population. Patients with grade 1-2 aGVHD survive, whereas those with higher grades (3 or 4) develop multisystem organ failure and die within the first year after transplantation.

In the NST population, many patients are home shortly after their preparatory regimen and stem-cell infusion. They are then cared for collaboratively by their community and major center physicians. Because aGVHD may appear later, these patients may present to their local emergency room with a rash that is misdiagnosed as an allergy to medicine, food, or the environment. This rash can quickly escalate to a high stage and influence mortality if not treated quickly and appropriately with steroids. Patients and community health care providers must be educated regarding the early signs and treatment for aGVHD.

Cardiac Disease

The preparatory regimen, the specific disease treated, alterations in hemodynamic balance (fluid and electrolyte shifts and blood product transfusions), and anemia cause cardiac stress. The patient's comorbidities (hypertension, diabetes, preexisting heart disease, poor functional status, and poor nutritional status) exacerbate the possibility for cardiac complications during HSCT. Cyclophosphamide, in doses of 120–200 mg/kg, damages the heart's endothelial lining, leading to myocardial hemorrhage and necrosis. Cardiomegaly with thickening of the left ventricular wall, pericarditis, pericardial effusion, and cardiac tamponade are all possibilities of chemotherapy-induced cardiac changes. TBI is synergistic with chemotherapy and adds to the cardiac toxicity. TBI in fractions greater than 300 cGy/day and targeting more than 33% of the heart results in cardiac complications. Shields provide reduced exposure to the heart, but complications involve pericardial effusions, cardiac tamponade, and constrictive pericarditis. Assessment includes careful monitoring of heart sounds, jugular venous distention (JVD), and blood pressure.

Anemia stresses the heart. Most transplantation centers establish transfusion parameters based on the daily hemoglobin. Careful assessment of heart function prior to HSCT establishes a baseline, and most regimens require a left ventricular ejection fraction (LVEF) of at least 50% as a baseline requirement for therapy initiation. History of hypertension, diabetes, and preexisting heart disease as comorbidities all impact and influence the patient's course.

Nursing Care

Prior to each dose of cyclophosphamide, the patient's team obtains and reads the electrocardiogram (ECG). During the chemotherapy phase, daily CPK with MB isoenzymes are monitored. Electrolytes are carefully monitored throughout the transplantation. Fevers, diarrhea, anorexia, nausea, vomiting, and chemotherapy all contribute to fluid and electrolyte shifts. Laboratory values are evaluated daily, and electrolytes and fluids are repleted and adjusted. Careful I/O recording, changes in weight, and renal status are noted. Fluid shifts and electrolyte imbalances lead to cardiac dysrhythmias and congestive heart failure (CHF). In the allogeneic patient, aGVHD and immunotherapy with cyclosporine contribute to electrolyte imbalance and acute renal failure.

The signs and symptoms of CHF are shortness of breath, weight gain, pedal edema, and cough. CHF is managed with oxygen, diuretics, daily weight, strict I/O, and fluid restriction with the concentration of medications as well as the concentration of blood products, particularly platelets, in minimal fluid.

Arrhythmia management involves a cardiology consult, careful adjustment or addition of medications, and close monitoring. Atrial fibrillation is a very common dysrhythmia associated with heart disease and chronic heart failure. It increases with age and is seen in patients receiving NST. ST complex and changes in T waves are also common.

Acute Renal Failure

Acute renal failure is the sudden deterioration of renal function. The etiology of acute renal failure may be prerenal, intrarenal, or postrenal, and Table 6.13 highlights the causes and the management. The kidney is very sensitive to blood flow, and any condition that diminishes blood flow prerenally will contribute to renal failure. Intrarenal failure results when drugs, syndromes, or conditions directly insult the kidney. Postrenal failure results when there is damage or obstruction in the bladder or ureters.

TABLE 6.13 Acute Renal Failure

Type	Causes	Management
Prerenal	Decreased blood flow, sepsis, decreased cardiac output, hypotension	Vital signs, I/O, weight, monitor for signs of infection
Intrarenal	Nephrotoxic drugs, prolonged ischemia, hypertension, SIADH, tumor lysis syndrome (TLS)	Monitor therapy with nephrotoxic drugs, including cyclosporine, diuretics, antibiotics, antifungals, antivirals, and chemotherapy
		SIADH: free water restriction, hypertonic saline, diuretics
		TLS: allopurinol, hydration with sodium bicarbonate, diuretics
Postrenal	Hemorrhagic cystitis, bladder obstruction, ureteral obstruction	Hydration, bladder irrigation, mesna

Nursing Care

Prerenal causes of acute renal failure require careful monitoring of laboratory values, vital signs, I/O, and weight to identify problems that will affect the kidney early. Tumor lysis syndrome (TLS) with hyperuricemia causing crystallization obstructs and damages the kidney. Aggressive hydration with sodium bicarbonate, diuretics, and allopurinol prevent this syndrome. Syndrome of inappropriate antidiuretic hormone (SIADH) is the result of therapy with cyclophosphamide and causes fluid shifts and electrolyte imbalances. Free water restriction is necessary when this occurs, along with treatment with diuretics and electrolyte repletion. Postrenal complications require aggressive hydration and bladder irrigation to relieve obstructions or rid the bladder of toxic chemotherapy and metabolites (e.g., acrolein).

Discharge Planning

Discharge planning is a complicated process and begins very early in the patient's transplantation experience. It involves many disciplines including medicine, social work, physical therapy, nutrition, home infusion therapy companies, the local Visiting Nurses Association (VNA), the local community hospital, and nursing and family caregivers. While patients are in the hospital, family caregivers prepare the home.

Carpets, drapes, and bathrooms are thoroughly cleaned. If there is more than one bathroom in the home, the patient has his or her own. This bathroom is cleaned daily. Pets are permitted but are not allowed to sleep on the patient's bed. The patient may stroke the cat or dog but may not allow the animal to lick his or her face. Litter boxes are confined, and the patient does not clean this area. Plants are allowed but placed in rooms that are not predominantly occupied by the patient. The patient may not dig or transplant plants.

Teaching

The Nutrition Service closely follows the patient while in the hospital and teaches the patient and family regarding the preparation of food at home.

Although the patient has engrafted, the graft is young, and this new immune system needs time to develop. In the home, food is freshly prepared, and the patient is discouraged from eating leftovers. Food is well cooked, and someone other than the patient prepares salads. Hand washing is central when handling food, and caregivers wash hands before and after handling food. Waterless, alcohol-based soaps are acceptable when hands are not obviously soiled. Otherwise, soap and water, with attention to all surfaces and between fingers, is recommended. Thick-skinned fruit like oranges and bananas are permitted. The patient or caregiver must once again wash hands before and after peeling, and the fruit is washed before peeling. The allogeneic HSCT patient avoids grapefruit, whole or as juice. Grapefruit juice interferes with the cytochrome P450 enzyme system in the liver and is involved in many drug interactions, particularly cyclosporine.

Throughout the inpatient experience, the patient learns about oral and central line care. The hospital's mouth care routine begins during the transplantation phase while the patient is receiving the preparatory regimen. The patient assesses his or her mouth and self medicates with troches or antifungal rinses after careful brushing (when platelet counts are adequate), swabbing (spongy applicators), and rinsing with normal saline or sodium bicarbonate. This continues at home, and the patient reports any new lesions or evidence of candida.

During nonclinic days, the patient or designated family member carefully inspects the patient's central line. This includes visual inspection of the site with palpation. The patient reports any new tenderness, discharge, or redness to the transplantation center; this may result in a trip to the clinic. Dressings are changed after showering if the site becomes wet. Port flushing becomes a task of the patient or caregiver once the patient is at home. Nurses teach this procedure while the patient is in the hospital, and reinforce the teaching with videos or printed materials that are taken home. Patients sometimes require TPN, antibiotics, and immunosuppressants after discharge, which requires caregivers to learn their safe administration. Initial teaching is done in the hospital or clinic, with follow-up by VNA nurses in the home. TPN is cycled to allow freedom during the day with hook-up and administration through the night. This requires learning the pump system and line care.

Some protocols require the administration of growth factor (G-CSF or GM-CSF) to stimulate production of white blood cells and shorten the engraftment period. This is taught in the hospital or clinic and reinforced by the VNA or home infusion company.

Signs and symptoms of aGVHD and sepsis are taught early in the transplantation process and reinforced during clinic visits. Often, patients return to their home communities. The patient and family caregivers must be knowledgeable regarding their transplantation experience and be able to articulate clearly to the local emergency room physicians the disease, type of transplantation, and emergent need for attention when the patient comes unannounced to the emergency room with a fever, rash, new pain, or any symptom suggesting aGVHD or sepsis. At the first sign, the patient calls the transplantation center for direction. There is a clear communication plan that is carefully explained regarding how to contact the transplantation team members during weekdays, evenings, nights, and weekends. There is never a gap in contact. In emergency situations, the transplantation physician may direct the patient to a local emergency room and will call ahead to the local physician to help initiate a plan of care.

Patients often require blood products, including platelets, after discharge. The patient and family learn about the signs and symptoms of bleeding and to avoid any trauma. Stumbling, tripping, stubbing, and hitting or bumping the head require calling the transplantation center. Cutting fingernails, avoiding hangnails, and noticing headaches are important to reinforce before returning home. Patients also purchase or are given ID bracelets that state the need for irradiated blood products.

Sexuality is an important part of any partner relationship and is addressed early in the transplantation experience. Isolation while in the hospital is very debilitating. The patient avoids kissing on the mouth during the engraftment phase. Hugging and snuggling is safe, but penetration anally or vaginally is not allowed during this time. Once platelets exceed 50,000 and the neutrophil count is safe (individual centers determine the number, but it is at least 500), the couple may have intercourse with protection. Vaginal mucosa is often tender, and the female transplantation patient may require lubrication.

Clinic Visits

Upon discharge, and depending on the transplantation center protocol, the patient visits the clinic frequently at first and gradually becomes more independent as their hematologic system, physical strength, and endurance improve. Many centers manage the whole transplantation, particularly autologous regimens, in outpatient clinics. Patients visit daily, have their laboratory values checked, and receive the necessary blood products, IV fluid, and electrolyte repletion before returning home. If they have a fever, they may be admitted or they may get antibiotics in the clinic and continue them at home with caregiver support. This requires a great deal of coordination with professional and family support.

Some centers institute administration of intravenous gamma globulin to help provide the necessary humoral immunity against certain viral infections, particularly CMV. The first dose is administered in the clinic setting, with subsequent doses administered in the home and coordinated by a home infusion company and their nurses.

Postengraftment Period: Day 30 to Day 100

During this time, the patient is closely followed by the transplantation center. Patients are monitored for signs of infection, aGVHD, and late complications from the preparatory regimen.

Idiopathic pneumonia syndrome (IPS) is alveolar injury in the absence of active lower respiratory tract infection or any identified pathogen. It occurs in 10–12% of autologous and allogeneic transplantation patients whose preparatory regimens include TBI and high-dose chemotherapy with alkylating agents, particularly cyclophosphamide and carmustine. Symptoms include fever, tachypnea, nonproductive cough, and hypoxemia. BAL demonstrates no infectious etiology. Chest x-ray and chest computed tomography (CT) show multilobar infiltrates. The syndrome often occurs at the same time the patient experiences GVHD. The cytokine-mediated inflammation followed by fibrosis is very similar (Shankar and Cohen 2001). Treatment consists of steroids and antibiotics, as well as antiviral and antifungal coverage for opportunistic pathogens (Wong *et al.* 2003).

Radiation pneumonitis occurs during this time period after transplantation. It presents as a dry nonproductive cough, and infiltrates develop on x-ray and CT scans as symptoms progress. Radiation pneumonitis is treated with steroids and antibiotics, antivirals, and antifungals (Keller 2004).

Opportunistic Infections

Bacterial infections with gram-positive bacteria originating in sinopulmonary sites are suspect throughout the posttransplantation period. Patients are treated with third- and fourth-generation cephalosporins and quinolones.

CMV Pneumonia

CMV is part of the herpes family, and over 50% of the population is seropositive. Both patient and donor are tested before transplantation, and CMV-negative blood products are administered to seronegative patients with seronegative donors. Because of the absolute neutropenia and its prolonged duration, patients may reactivate their own virus. The patient has a dry nonproductive cough, increasing oxygen requirements, fatigue, and dyspnea with progressive, diffuse interstitial infiltrates on chest x-ray. The pneumonia is treated with ganciclovir or foscarnet. Mortality from this pneumonia is high if not treated promptly. Older patients, seropositve patients, HLA-mismatched patients, and patients with aGVHD are at greatest risk for developing this pneumonia (Johnson and Quiett 2004; Keller 2004).

Respiratory Syncytial Virus (RSV)

RSV is a common virus in children and adults, particularly in the winter and early spring. Runny nose, congestion, cough, and fever are the symptoms. In the HSCT patient, however, RSV can rapidly progress to pneumonia, with mortality as high as 80% (Keller 2004). Nasal washings are diagnostic and obtained early. Treatment includes aerosolized ribavirin and RSV immunoglobulin (Dykewicz *et al.* 2000).

Aspergillus

Aspergillus spores are found everywhere in the environment and are the most common cause of fungal pneumonia in HSCT patients. The more common species are *Aspergillus fumagatis, flavus, niger, clavatus,* and *nidulans.* Mortality from *Aspergillus* pneumonia approaches 90%. Inhalation of these spores causes infection in immunocompromised hosts. Prolonged neutropenia, steroid therapy, and aGVHD place patients at risk. To diminish exposure, patients avoid areas of construction, dust, fresh and dried plants, and any foods containing mold (Keller 2004; Horak and Forman 2001).

Clinically, *Aspergillus* pneumonia causes pleuritic chest pain with hemoptysis. Infections are also found in the sinuses, skin, and central nervous system. X-rays show rounded cavitary lesions, sometimes with a characteristic halo (Horak and Forman 2001). Treatment is complex, with many side effects. Drugs include amphotericin B, azoles, and echinocandins.

Pneumoncystis carinii Pneumonia (PCP)

PCP is a protozoal infection occurring primarily in the allogeneic population. Patients with prolonged immunosuppression from GVHD and cyclosporine and steroid therapy are at increased

TABLE 6.14 Posttransplantation (days 30–100+) Nursing Care Plan

Nursing Diagnosis	Defining Characteristics	Nursing Interventions	Expected Outcomes
Potential for infection related to opportunistic organisms: CMV, RSV, Aspergillus, PCP, and gram-positive and -negative bacteria	Allogeneic preparatory regimens that include TBI, alkylating agents, CMV-seropositive patient or donor Allogeneic patients on steroids and immuno-suppressant therapy Fever Dry cough Dyspnea on exertion Pain, redness, inflammation, discharge at central line site	During each clinic visit: Physical assessment of the respiratory system, GI system, and skin (particularly around central line sites) Evaluate laboratory tests Assess central line sites for signs and symptoms of infection Reinforce patient/family teaching concerning line care and infection, hand washing practices, and avoiding patient exposure to family when ill with colds or flu	Patient will be free from opportunistic infection
Potential for injury/bleeding related to thrombocytopenia	Platelets , 20,000, petechiae, bruising, and headaches	Transfuse platelets as necessary Teach patient about thrombocytopenia and risky behavior Reinforce that platelets will return to normal and this is temporary	Patient will have no bleeding from thrombocytopenia
Potential/actual injury related to IPS, radiation pneumonitis, and aGHVD	Allogeneic preparatory regimens with high-dose alkylating agents and TBI, fever Dry cough Dyspnea on exertion CT with multilobar infiltrates	Careful respiratory assessment, skin and GI assessment for diarrhea and increased LFTs, particularly bilirubin Blood cultures to rule out infection Respiratory therapy consult regarding pulmonary toileting and respiratory medications (inhalers)	Patient will manage symptoms related to IPS, radiation pneumonitis, and aGVHD with minimal impact on quality of life

Nursing Diagnosis	Signs/Symptoms	Interventions	Outcomes
Fluid volume deficit related to anemia, nausea and vomiting, and taste changes	Elevated BUN/creatinine; assess eating patterns at home, monitor Hgb	Administer fluids and transfuse as necessary Home referrals for fluids and TPN, arrange dietary consult during clinic visits	Patient will be euvolemic with normal electrolytes Patient will maintain/gain healthy weight
Ineffective patient/family coping related to fatigue, sexuality issues, and unclear family roles	Patient and family verbalize conflicts at home Patient fatigued and unable to assume prior roles at home and in the workplace Patient acknowledges impact of transplantation experience on family/work goals Patient and/or partner having difficulty with intimacy	Careful assessment of home environment and family coping, social service consult, and continued follow-up Explore issues of intimacy with patient and partner or refer to appropriate expert	Family system will stabilize, with patient adjusting to new role in family system and community
Knowledge deficit related to discharge	Missed clinic visits Questions about discharge and when to call transplantation center providers	Review discharge guidelines and answer questions; reinforce written material	Patient and family will communicate educational needs and demonstrate knowledge about discharge guidelines and when to call transplantation center to seek help

risk. Prophylactic treatment with trimethoprim-sulfamethoxazole (TMP-SMZ) or with aerosolized pentamidine has virtually eliminated this complication. This complication must be considered in those patients unable to undergo these preventive therapies (Dykewicz et al. 2000).

Nursing Care

The nursing for the patient after transplantation in the late acute phase of recovery is summarized in Table 6.14. With patients out of the hospital and frequently visiting the clinic, nurses must carefully assess for early signs of infection and complications from the preparatory regimen. Allogeneic patients are more at risk than autolgous patients. These patients are still on immunosuppressive medications, with some experiencing aGVHD. This predisposes them to opportunistic infections. Physical assessment of the respiratory system, gastrointestinal system, and skin and laboratory test evaluation are necessary at each visit. Central line sites are visually examined and palpated for early signs of infection. Pain at the site is often the first sign of infection. Careful listening helps the nurse understand the home environment and family coping. If patients are unable to eat, the nurse provides home referrals for fluids and coordinates dietary consults during clinic visits.

Medication teaching is complicated. Nurses direct their teaching to the patient and primary caregiver. Written material is a patient resource and reinforces the teaching. Many centers provide videos on infection, central line care, and nutrition for home viewing.

NST patients are at risk for aGVHD later than expected with full allogeneic transplantations. These patients are often at home when they experience the early rash or diarrhea. In the clinic, teaching focuses on early recognition and prompt intervention. If patients travel to their local emergency room, they must accurately describe their transplantation treatment and urge local providers to contact the transplantation center immediately to ensure proper treatment.

Postengraftment: Days 100+
Chronic GVHD

Chronic GVHD (cGVHD) is a major morbidity that affects up to 80% of allogeneic HSCT recipients (Przepiorka et al. 2001). Patients experiencing aGVHD are at greatest risk for cGVHD. Older patients and donors, HLA mismatches, aggressive myeloablative regimens, and peripheral versus marrow stem cells are also risk factors for this chronic disease.

All organ systems may be involved, with the skin involved most often. The eyes, mouth, gastrointestinal tract, and lung are most commonly involved. As more organ systems become involved, mortality increases. Models describe cGVHD based on pattern of onset, extent of disease, or histologic pattern. Patterns range from no prior aGVHD to explosive, with aGVHD and cGVHD occurring concurrently. Extent of disease may be limited to extensive involvement of multiple organ systems. Histologic pattern can be lichenoid or evolve into sclerodermatous. The highest morbidity and mortality occurs in patients with extensive, explosive disease with sclerodermatous characteristics (Mitchell 2004). Table 6.15 offers an assessment for and management of chronic GVHD.

Infection

Varicella zoster virus (VZV) may occur during this time period. VZV is commonly known as shingles and most often occurs in patients who have had chicken pox some time in their life. Lesions appear on the face and torso and follow the corresponding dermatome. This is quite painful and distressing to the patient. Patients are treated with acyclovir, valacyclovir, and famciclovir as soon as lesions appear (Johnson and Quiett 2004). Pain management is extremely important with this diagnosis and often overlooked. The pain is difficult to control with nonsteroidal analgesics and opioids. Pain regimens must also include drugs that address neuropathic pain such as garbapentin and tricyclic antidepressants. Early recognition of VZV may prevent long-term complications with postherpetic neuralgia.

TABLE 6.15 Chronic Graft-Versus-Host Disease: Assessment and Management

Organ System	Signs and Symptoms	Diagnosis and Management
Skin	■ Erythema ■ Dryness ■ Urticaria ■ Maculopapular rash ■ Pigment changes ■ Exfoliation ■ Lesions and ulcerations ■ Loss of sweat gland function ■ Joint contractures	■ Skin biopsy ■ Cultures and sensitivities for infection ■ Immunosuppressants ■ Avoid sun exposure; sun block; large hats and protective clothing ■ Pain management ■ Extracorporeal photopheresis with UVA
Oral	■ Dryness (xerostomia) ■ Mucositis ■ Hyperkeratotic changes toL mucosa and tongue ■ Pain ■ Sensitivity to hot and cold ■ Taste changes ■ Tooth decay	■ Immunosuppressant therapy ■ Pilocarpine for xerostomia ■ Topical steroids ■ Oral and systemic antifungals ■ Mouth care with Gelclair ■ Fluoride gels and rinses
Liver	■ Jaundice ■ Pain	■ Monitor liver function tests ■ Liver biopsy ■ Rule out infections ■ Ursodeoxycholic acid
Ocular	■ Photophobia ■ Corneal ulceration ■ Cataracts	■ Ophthalmology referral ■ Eye lubricants ■ Steroid eye drops
Lungs	■ Cough ■ Wheezing ■ Dyspnea on exertion ■ Fatigue ■ Hypoxia ■ Pleural effusions ■ Recurrent sinus infections ■ Hyperinflation of lungs with flattening of diaphragm	■ Pulmonary function tests ■ ABG ■ BAL ■ Chest CT ■ Lung biopsy ■ Steroids ■ Inhalation therapy with bronchodilators and steroids ■ Oxygen therapy
Gastrointestinal	■ Esophageal webbing or strictures ■ Odynophagia ■ Dysphagia ■ Early satiety ■ Anorexia ■ Nausea ■ Vomiting ■ Diarrhea ■ Weight loss	■ GI series ■ Swallowing studies ■ Total parenteral nutrition with electrolyte replacement ■ Antiemetics ■ Volume repletion ■ Pain management ■ Anti-infectives ■ Stool cultures ■ Antidiarrheals (loperamide, diphenoxylate with atropine)

(Continued)

TABLE 6.15 (Continued)

Myofascial	■ Joint and muscle pain ■ Stiffness ■ Muscle contractures ■ Pain and cramping ■ Erythema	■ Nerve and muscle biopsy ■ Immunosuppressants ■ Steroids ■ Clonazepam, klonopin, baclofen for muscle cramping ■ Physical therapy

Source: Adapted from Mitchell 2004; Neumann 2004.

TABLE 6.16   Posttransplantation (days 100+) Nursing Care Plan

Nursing Diagnosis	Defining Characteristics	Nursing Interventions	Expected Outcomes
Potential/actual injury related to cGVHD	See Table 6.15	See Table 6.15	Patient will be free of major symptoms related to cGVHD
Potential/actual infection related to varicella zoster virus (VZV)	History of chicken pox Immunosuppressant therapy	Pain management Antivirals as prescribed	Patient will be free of or have minimal distress from VZV
Anxiety related to transitioning care to local medical oncologist	Frequent phone calls to transplantation center with vague complaints Frequent social visits to transplantation center	Reassure patient about issues of abandonment Facilitate communication between local oncology nurses and transplantation center; supply local oncology practice with accurate telephone numbers for 24-hour coverage for questions; assure patient that this communication is complete and resources are continually available	Patient will feel comfortable with transition to local community

CMV, aspergillosis, and RSV continue to be risks particularly in allogeneic patients with GVHD on immunosuppressant therapy and steroids.

Follow-Up

During this time period and depending on complications, the patient transitions to home and their primary physician. Transition to their local medical oncologist is a huge step for the patient who has come to depend on the transplantation center. Ideally, the transplantation center has been in contact with the local physician, updating the physician with information regarding symptom management and response to therapy. Upon transition, the local physician receives detailed information regarding type of transplantation, complications, response to treatment, aGVHD and cGVHD grade, performance status, maintenance therapy including plans for immunizations, medications with current doses, and quality of life measurement.

Survivor and Quality of Life Issues

HSCT, whether autologous or allogeneic, affects patients in a profound way. Quality of life dimensions include physical, psychological, social, and spiritual well-being. Problems with physical well-being are related to the morbidities of transplantation, particularly cGVHD, and include fatigue and sexual difficulties. Psychological well-being relates to the ability to work and engage in physical and sexual activity. Patients experience uncertainty about the future and their health. Ability to return to work and perform family functions at the pretransplantation level affect this dimension. Social well-being and sexuality issues are often examined together. Concerns continue in this dimension regarding sexual function and infertility, with women experiencing more distress than men. The spiritual or existential dimension is described as reassessing values, hope, and being grateful for every day (Holmes 2004).

Nursing Care

Care focuses on survivor issues and issues related to long-term sequelae of the transplantation procedure. After a long relationship with the transplantation center, patients now transition to their community. Nurses focus on making the transition thorough and smooth Table 6.16.

Future Direction of HSCT

Research continues aggressively in this exciting field. The ideal NST regimen has yet to be determined. Graft manipulation and gene therapy using viral or nonviral vectors will target the GVT effect, minimize GVHD, and repopulate diseased marrow after preparative chemotherapy. Expanding treatment to include nonmalignant diseases will provide hope to patients suffering with these diseases as well. Identifying minor HLA antigens on diseased cells will lead to engineering donor T cells ex vivo and augment the GVT effect. This science will further define NST therapy. This graft manipulation will also effectively address GVHD and reduce the long-term morbidity and mortality associated with HSCT, impacting quality of life in a very profound way (Burcat 2004; Bleakley and Riddell 2004).

Glossary of Abbreviations

ADL	Activities of daily living
aGVHD	Acute graft-versus-host disease
AML	Acute myelocytic leukemia
APC	Antigen-presenting cell
ARDS	Acute respiratory distress syndrome
BMT	Bone marrow transplantation
C.DIFF	*Clostridium difficile*
cGVHD	Chronic graft-versus-host disease
CHF	Congestive heart failure
CML	Chronic myelocytic leukemia
CMV	Cytomegalovirus
CNS	Central nervous system
DAH	Diffuse alveolar hemorrhage
DMSO	Dimethylsulfoxide
EBV	Epstein-Barr virus
G-CSF	Granulocyte colony-stimulating factor

GM-CSF	Granulocyte-macrophage colony-stimulating factor
GVHD	Graft-versus-host disease
GVT	Graft-versus-tumor
HLA	Human leukocyte antigen
HSCT	Hematopoietic stem-cell transplantation
HSV	Herpes simplex virus
I/O	Intake and output
JVD	Jugular venous distention
MDS	Myelodysplastic syndrome
MHA	Major histocompatibility antigen
mHA	Minor histocompatibility antigen
MM	Multiple myeloma
NCI	National Cancer Institute
NHL	Non-Hodgkin's lymphoma
NMDP	National Marrow Donor Program
NST	Nonmyeloablative stem-cell transplantation
PCA	Patient-controlled analgesia
RSV	Respiratory syncytial virus
SIADH	Syndrome of inappropriate antidiuretic hormone
TBI	Total-body irradiation
TLS	Tumor lysis syndrome
TNF-α	Tumor necrosis factor alpha
TPN	Total parenteral nutrition
UCBT	Umbilical cord blood transplantation
UVA	Ultraviolet light A
VNA	Visiting Nurses Association
VOD	Veno-occlusive disease
VZV	Varicella zoster virus

References

Appelbaum, F. 2003. Hematopoietic stem cell transplantation. In M. McLaughlin, and H. Lazarus (Eds): *Allogeneic Stem Cell Transplantation*. Totowa, NJ: Humana Press, pp 1–9.

Barker, J., and Wagner, J. 2003. Umbilical cord blood transplantation. In M. McLaughlin, and H. Lazarus (Eds): *Allogeneic Stem Cell Transplantation*. Totowa, NJ: Humana Press, pp 129–147.

Bearman, S. 2003. Reduced intensity allogeneic stem cell transplantation. *Current Hematology Reports* 2(4):277–286.

Beck, S. 2004. Mucositis. In C. Yarbro, M. Frogge, and M. Goodman (Eds): *Cancer Symptom Management* (ed 3). Boston: Jones and Bartlett, pp 276–292.

Bellm, L., Epstein, J., Rose-Ped, A., Martin, P., and Fuchs, H. 2000. Patient reports of complications of bone marrow transplantation. *Supportive Care Cancer* 8:33–39.

Berger, A., and Eilers, J. 1998. Factors influencing oral cavity status during high-dose antineoplastic therapy: A secondary data analysis. *Oncology Nursing Forum* 25(9):1623–1626.

Bleakley, M., and Riddell, S. 2004. Molecules and mechanisms of the graft-versus-leukemia effect. *Nature Reviews: Cancer* 4(5):371–380.

Borbasi, S., Cameron, K., Quested, B., Olver, I., and Evans, D. 2002. More than a sore mouth: Patients' experience of oral mucositis. *Oncology Nursing Forum* 29(7): 1051–1057.

Buchsel, P. 1998. Allogeneic bone marrow transplantation. In S. Groenwald, M. Frogge, M. Goodman, and C. Yarbro (Eds): *Cancer Nursing Principles and Practice* (ed 4). Boston: Jones and Bartlett, pp 459–525.

Burcat, S. 2004. Current research and future directions in hematopoietic stem cell transplantation. In S. Ezzone (Ed): *Hematopoietic Stem Cell Transplantation: A Manual for Nursing Practice*. Pittsburgh: Oncology Nursing Society, pp 249–268.

Cutler, C., Giri, S., Jeyapalan, S., Paniagua, D., Viswanathan, A., and Antin, J. 2001. Acute and chronic graft-versus-host disease after allogeneic peripheral-blood cell and bone marrow transplantation: A meta-analysis. *Journal of Clinical Oncology* 19:3685–3691.

Davies, J.K. 2003. New advances in acute graft-versus-host disease prophylaxis. *Transfusion Medicine* 13(6):387–397.

Devine, S., Adkins, D., Khourty, H., Brown, R., Vij, R., Blum, W., and Dipersio, J. 2003. Recent advances in allogeneic hematopoietic stem cell transplantation. *Journal of Laboratory and Clinical Medicine* 141:7–32.

Dykewicz, C., Jaffe, H., and Kaplan, J. 2000. Guidelines for preventing opportunistic infections among hematopoietic stem cell transplant recipients: Recommendations of CDC, the Infectious Disease Society of America, and the American Society of Blood and Marrow Transplantation. *Morbidity and Mortality Weekly Report* 49: RR-10.

Ferrara, J.L. 2003. The pathophysiology of graft-versus-host disease. *International Journal of Hematology* 78(3):181–187.

Gelclair product information. 2002. Melville, NY: Cell Pathways.

Gertz, M. 2004. Therapy for immunoglobulin light chain amyloidosis: The new and the old. *Blood Review* 18(1):17–37.

Hinds, M., and Minor, S. 2004. Nonmyeloablative transplantation: Reducing toxicity utilizing an immunologic approach. In P. Buchsel, and P. Kapustay (Eds): *Stem Cell Transplantation: A Clinical Textbook*. Pittsburgh: Oncology Nursing Society, pp 19.3–19.28.

Holmes, W. 2004. Quality of life issues in hematopoietic stem cell transplantation. In S. Ezzone (Ed): *Hematopoietic Stem Cell Transplantation: A Manual for Nursing Practice*. Pittsburgh: Oncology Nursing Society, pp 237–247.

Horak, D., and Forman, S. 2001. Critical care of the hematopoietic stem cell patient. *Critical Care Clinics* 17(3):671–695.

Huaringa, A.J., Leyva, F.J., Signes-Costa, J., Morice, R.C., Raad, I., Darwish, A.A., and Champlin, R.E. 2000. Bronchoalveolar lavage in the diagnosis of pulmonary complications of bone marrow transplant patients. *Bone Marrow Transplantation* 25:975–979.

Johnson, G., and Quiett, K. 2004. Hematologic effects. In S. Ezzone (Ed): *Hematopoietic Stem Cell Transplantation: A Manual for Nursing Practice*. Pittsburgh: Oncology Nursing Society, pp 133–143.

Keller, C. 2004. Cardiopulmonary effects. In S. Ezzone (Ed): *Hematopoietic Stem Cell Transplantation: A Manual for Nursing Practice*. Pittsburgh: Oncology Nursing Society, pp 177–188.

Kernan, N., and Confer, D. 2000. Unrelated donor stem cell transplantation therapy. In R. Hoffman, E. Benz, J. Sanford, B. Furie, H. Cohen, L. Silberstein, *et al.* (Eds): *Hematology: Basic Principles and Practice* (ed 3). New York: Churchill Livingstone, pp 1609–1615.

Kumar, S., DeLeve, L., Kamath, P., and Ayalew, T. 2003. Hepatic veno-occlusive disease (sinusoidal obstruction syndrome) after hematopoietic stem cell transplantation. *Mayo Clinic Proceedings* 78:589–598.

Meropol, N.J., Somer, R.A., Gutheil, J., Pelley, R.J., Modiano, M.R., Rowinsky, E.K., Rothenberg, M.L., Redding, S.W., Serdar, C.M., Yao, B., Heard, R., and Rosen, L.S. 2003. Randomized phase I trial of recombinant human keratinocyte growth factor plus chemotherapy: Potential role as mucosal protectant. *Journal of Clinical Oncology* 21:1452–1458.

Mitchell, S. 2004. Graft versus host disease. In S. Ezzone (Ed): *Hematopoietic Stem Cell Transplantation: A Manual for Nursing Practice*. Pittsburgh: Oncology Nursing Society, pp 85–122.

Murray, S.M., and Pindoria, S. 2000. Nutrition support for bone marrow transplant patients. *Cochrane Review*. http://www.update-software.com/abstracts.

National Cancer Institute. 2004. NCI Common Toxicity Criteria for Stomatitis/Pharyngitis in BMT Population. http://ctep.cancer.gov/forms/CTCv20_4-30-992.pdf.

Neumann, J. 2004. Graft-versus-host disease. In P. Buchsel, and P. Kapustay (Eds): *Stem Cell Transplantation: A Clinical Textbook*. Pittsburgh: Oncology Nursing Society, pp 22.1–22.13.

Pallera, A., and Schwartzberg, L. 2004. Managing the toxicity of hematopoietic stem cell transplant. *The Journal of Supportive Oncology* 2(3):223–237.

Parran, L., and Pederson, C. 2000. Development of an opioid-taper algorithm for hematopoietic cell transplant recipients. *Oncology Nursing Forum* 27(6):967–973.

Petersdorf E., Hansen, J., Martin, P., Woolfrey, A., Malkki, M., Gooley, T., *et al.* 2001. Major histocompatibility-complex class I alleles and antigens in hematopoietic-cell transplantation. *New England Journal of Medicine* 345(25):1794–1800.

Peterson, D., Beck, S., and Keefe, D. 2004. Novel therapies. *Seminars in Oncology Nursing* 20(1):53–58.

Peterson, D., and Cariello, A. 2004. Mucosal damage: A major risk factor for severe complications after cytotoxic therapy. *Seminars in Oncology* 31(3 Suppl 8):35–44.

Przepiorka, D., Weisdorf, D., Martin, P., Klingmann, H., Beatty, P., Hows, J., and Thomas, E. 1995. 1994 consensus conference on acute GVHD grading. *Bone Marrow Transplantation* 15:825–828.

Przepiorka, D., Anderlini, P., Saliba, R., Cleary, K., Mehra, R., Khouri, I., *et al.* 2001. Chronic graft-versus-host disease after allogeneic blood stem cell transplantation. *Blood* 98(6):1695–1700.

Reddy, P. 2003. Immunobiology of acute graft-versus-host disease. *Blood Review* 12(4):187–194.

Schmit-Pokorny, K., and Nuss, S. 2004. Pediatric stem cell transplantation. In P. Buchsel, and P. Kapustay (Eds): *Stem Cell Transplantation: A Clinical Textbook*. Pittsburgh: Oncology Nursing Society, pp 16.3–16.24.

Schots, R., Kaufman, L., Van Riet, I., Ben Othman, T., De Waele, M., Van Camp, B., and Demanet, C. 2003. Proinflammatory cytokines and their role in the development of major transplant-related complications in the early phase after allogeneic bone marrow transplantation. *Leukemia* 17:1150–1156.

Shankar, G., and Cohen, D. 2001. Idiopathic pneumonia syndrome after bone marrow transplantation: The role of pre-transplant radiation conditioning and local cytokine dysregulation in promoting lung inflammation and fibrosis. *International Journal of Experimental Pathology* 82:101–113.

Shih, A., Miaskowski, C., Dodd, M., Stotts, N., and MacPhail, L. 2002. A research review of the current treatments for radiation-induced oral mucositis in patients with head and neck cancer. *Oncology Nursing Forum* 29(7):1063–1078.

Solomon, S., and Komanduri, K. 2001. The immune system. In P. Rieger (Ed): *Biotherapy: A Comprehensive Overview*. Boston: Jones & Bartlett, pp 39–61.

Spitzer, T.R. 2001. Engraftment syndrome following hematopoietic stem cell transplantation. *Bone Marrow Transplantation* 27:893–898.

Thomas, E. 2000. Landmarks in the development of hematopoietic cell transplantation. *World Journal of Surgery* 24:815–818.

University of Pennsylvania Health System Nursing. 2003. *Guidelines for oral care for oncology patients.* Philadelphia: University of Pennsylvania.

Williams, L., and McCarthy, P. 2004. Diseases treated with peripheral stem cell transplantation. In P. Buchsel, and P. Kapustay (Eds): *Stem Cell Transplantation: A Clinical Textbook.* Pittsburgh: Oncology Nursing Society, pp 3.3–3.21.

Wong, R., Rondon, G., Salba, R., Shannon, V., Giralt, S., Champlin, R., and Ueno, N. 2003. Idiopathic pneumonia syndrome after high-dose chemotherapy and autologous hematopoietic stem cell transplantation for high-risk breast cancer. *Bone Marrow Transplantation* 31:1157–1163.

Woo S.B., and Treister, N. 2001. Chemotherapy induced oral mucositis. http://www.emedicine.com/derm/topic682.htm.

Worthington, H.V., Clarkson, J.E., and Eden, O.B. 2001. Interventions for treating oral mucositis for patients with cancer receiving treatment. Cochrane Review. http://www.update-software.com/abstracts.

Yen, K., Lee, A., Krowka, M., and Burger, C. 2004. Pulmonary complications in bone marrow transplantation: A practical approach to diagnosis and treatment. *Clinics in Chest Medicine* 25:189–201.

Cancer Therapy in Malignant and Nonmalignant Conditions: Safety and Administration Issues

Ann Marie B. Peterson, R.N., M.S., C.N.S., and Margaret Barton-Burke, Ph.D., R.N.

Introduction

The cancer therapies being used in the 21st century range from traditional chemotherapy to biotherapy, monoclonal antibodies, targeted therapies, and investigational vaccines. Additionally, more than ever before, we are witnessing the use of old drugs being used in new ways and newer drugs being used differently as well. The focus of this chapter is the safe administration of cancer therapies. The drugs that were formally thought of as cancer chemotherapeutic agents are being used as cancer treatment, but they are also commonly being used for treatment of autoimmune disorders such as rheumatoid arthritis and systemic lupus erythematosus, making administration and safety issues of these drugs paramount in the minds of all members of the multidisciplinary team.

Current trends in patient safety (Institute of Medicine 1999) and the tragic events in the field of oncology from the mid-1990s underscore the importance of the roles of all members of the multidisciplinary team in the safe administration of cytotoxic agents. In the mid-1990s, national attention was given to cancer chemotherapy overdoses at one of the leading comprehensive cancer centers in the United States. This episode emphasized the reality of the risk of drug errors and heightened

the awareness of the public, media, patients, and health care professionals (Fischer *et al.* 1996).

The multidisciplinary team still works together to administer chemotherapeutic drugs, but the roles have changed such that each role is integral to every other role; the roles have become a series of checks and balances to ensure the safe administration of these agents. The roles of nurses and pharmacists as well as other members of the multidisciplinary team have expanded over the years. In major health care centers today, generally only nurses with specialized education and competencies within an institutional program safely administer these powerful drugs. Whether the site is a major inpatient hospital or institution, a busy outpatient chemotherapy facility, or a physician's office, decisions are made each day concerning standards for staff education and competency to increase safety for patients.

Drugs once known by the broad category of chemotherapy were often agents that exerted cytotoxic effects to cells, organs, and body systems. Today, the category of chemotherapy has grown to include not only the cytotoxic agents but also other classes of medications such as biologic response modifiers and monoclonal antibodies. The people receiving these therapies include patients with malignancies and also individuals with conditions such as rheumatic disorders.

The powerful drugs that are given to patients with or without malignancies continue to provide the possibility of disease remission or cure. Along with hope for success is the real potential for harm from either the adverse effects of the agents themselves or the challenges to the management of the effects of the therapy. Clinicians caring for these patients must have a comprehensive knowledge base about the medications, intended actions, potential side effects, dosage, route, administration time, dose modification variables, drug contraindications, recommended predrug therapies, safe handling and disposal measures, compatible intravenous flushes, and specialized tubing and filters. The clinician requires expertise in the recognition and management of complications such as infection and hypersensitivity to drugs. The well-being of our patients depends on the accountability of both the institution and the clinician for following the standards and guidelines for staff education. The staff must also provide evaluation and maintenance of competency for the administration of these therapies. It is imperative that the institution is committed to safe staffing practices to support a high standard of care. Nothing less is acceptable.

The Need for an Infrastructure for Safe Administration of Cytotoxic Agents

Standards are written value statements of the expectations of practice and outcomes for patients that staff members put forward by the legal and regulatory bodies, professional organizations, and the employing institution. A standard of care defines the desired results to be achieved with the patient (an outcome), whereas the standard of practice defines what the caregiver does to help achieve the outcome. When giving cancer therapies, clinical practice guidelines, policies, and procedures are recommended to ensure that standards of care and standards of practice are met. Safe practice is established when there is effective use of

cytotoxic agents for patients being treated for malignant and nonmalignant conditions. These guidelines should be reviewed and updated as needed, but at least yearly, by members of the multidisciplinary team.

In most cases, cytotoxic agents are administered through a systemic route. This trend is increasing, with more and newer agents being ordered and given by either oral or intravenous routes. In addition to the considerable knowledge about the drugs to be administered, all members of the oncology team, especially the nurses, require substantial technical skills and knowledge of drug administration. The management of chemotherapy administration includes technical information such as prescription, assessment (including patient information, specific steps to take prior to administration, and venous access), the actual administration of the drug, and postchemotherapy evaluation (including observation and management of side effects). Competency is the key to safe practice when working with these agents. It is the knowledge, skills, abilities, and behaviors needed to care effectively for patients receiving cytotoxic agents.

Three primary disciplines are involved in the chemotherapy administration process and make up the multidisciplinary cancer team. They are the physician or health care provider who orders the drug, the pharmacist who prepares the drug, and the nurse who administers the drug. Each member of this team must have baseline knowledge of cancer chemotherapy before practicing in their specific areas.

The multidisciplinary team consists of a doctor of medicine or osteopathy, physician assistant or nurse practitioner, registered nurse, pharmacist, and pharmacy technician. These individuals must be specifically trained in chemotherapeutic procedures related to prescribing, preparing, administering, and spill management. The physicians should be board-certified and/or board-eligible hematologists or oncologists. The physician assistant or nurse practitioners should be board certified, experienced, and competent with the use, prescription, and side effect management of chemotherapeutic agents. Pharmacists and pharmacy technicians should be competent in the preparation of cytotoxic agents, and nurses should know how to administer the chemotherapeutic agents and monitor for side effects.

Physicians authorized to write chemotherapy orders for neoplastic disease should be board-certified and/or board-eligible hematologists or medical, pediatric, radiation (for specified drugs on protocol), or gynecologic oncologists and oncology fellows who are being taught the fine points of prescribing these cytotoxic agents. An attending physician must routinely check and counter-sign chemotherapy orders written by an oncology fellow or other licensed provider such as a nurse practitioner. Some systems vary in the latitude that the nurse practitioner is given regarding this privilege; as a general rule, all new chemotherapy and all biotherapy and monoclonal antibody therapy require a cosignature. Oncologists or oncology fellows should be responsible for writing chemotherapy orders and/or entering them into a computer on a specially authorized chemotherapy order form. To maintain a system of checks and balances, it is imperative that the physicians complete the first step of order writing, which includes dose calculations and modifications. The practice of chemotherapy order writing discourages and limits the use of verbal chemotherapy orders (American Society of Clinical Oncology [ASCO] 2004a; ASCO 2004b).

Pharmacists involved in chemotherapy practice must complete a pharmacy department staff development program on preparation of these agents. According to the American Society of Health-Systems Pharmacists (ASHP 2002) competency includes the successful completion of a written examination, demonstrated competency in safe and accurate chemotherapy compounding and handling, and attendance at a yearly update session.

Registered nurses handling and administering chemotherapeutic or biologic agents must be cancer chemotherapy competent. According to the Oncology Nursing Society (Brown *et al.* 2001), competency includes attending a chemotherapy course, successful completion of a written examination, demonstrated competency in administering chemotherapy, and a yearly assessment of both knowledge and skills to remain competent to administer these medications. Standard chemotherapy reference texts and handbooks and standard drug references should be readily available to physicians, nurses, and pharmacists on all patient-care areas and the pharmacy (Barton-Burke *et al.* 2001).

Ordering Cancer Therapies Safely

The chemotherapy, biotherapy, and monoclonal antibody order should be written in a standard format. Ideally, computer order sheets should be created and/or order sheets preprinted with standard and commonly used regimens. Drugs should always be ordered by the generic name, consistent with usage in the hospital formulary and the federally recognized compendia. Trade names or abbreviations are not an acceptable substitute for the generic name of a given cytotoxic agent, even though a cooperative group protocol may use it. Trade names and abbreviations may be used by placing them in parentheses only if this information will add to the clarity of the drug order. A reference to the source(s) that provides the basis for the order must be cited; this is especially important when free-form chemotherapy orders are written for unusual or nonstandard drug regimens. Whenever possible, a copy of the relevant source should be placed in the chart, and an explanation should be written in the chart, as to why this particular therapy was chosen. The initial creation of preprinted orders or order sets should be the responsibility of one discipline and verified independently by the other two.

This verification can be done in a number of ways. Journal articles, abstracts, outside institutional protocols, and any other potential treatment references that represent the source of the orders or clarify them should be made known to all involved professionals by placing a copy in the patient's chart before treatment begins. Copies of outside institutional protocols should also be made available to the pharmacist. The copy should contain at least the following information: generic drug name, dose, dosage schedule, side effects or toxicity, rationale for the regimen, necessary dose reductions, and administration guidelines.

An increasing number of patients are being treated on protocols. Any protocol that accrues patients must be approved by the institutional review board. When a new protocol is instituted, multidisciplinary education must take place before patient enrollment. This is especially important when protocols involve investigational agents, high-dose therapy, and unusual or new combination therapies. This education must ensure adequate communication between the principal investigator, outpatient nurses, research nurses, inpatient nurses, and all oncology pharmacists. Copies of all new protocols and amendments must be placed in designated patient-care areas, clinics, and central and decentralized pharmacies. Preprinted or computer order sets should be configured and in place before patient enrollment begins to avoid order variability and ambiguity. From a safe practice perspective, new protocols or unusual therapies should not begin off-hours or on weekends unless it is an acute emergency situation. New protocols should be initiated on weekdays when appropriate specialists and clinicians are available in case of untoward side effects.

Attending physicians who write the chemotherapy order should be required to include the cumulative dose of anthracycline, bleomycin, and mitomycin previously received by the patient. To avoid confusion and potential error, an ordering system must be part of the infrastructure to ensure safe practices with these cytotoxic agents. In the case of cumulative doses of chemotherapeutic agents, the current dose must be notated in a different place than the cumulative dose such that the two doses are not on the same order sheet or the same computer screen and cannot be confused with each other by the pharmacist, pharmacy technician, or nurse.

Orders should be written using the following format: generic drug name, dose to be given (in milligrams), dose used (milligrams per meter squared or per kilogram), frequency, days of administration, and infusion guidelines. Ordinarily, the total dose for the entire course should not be listed on the order sheet or the computer order screen, lest it be misinterpreted as a single dose to be administered at one time. For continuous infusion pump delivery, the total dose to be infused over the set period must be included, but there should be a notation of how much is to be delivered each day. All pertinent information must be supplied to ensure a safe and accurate order capable of verification (Opfer *et al.* 1999; Rogers 1999; Schulmeister 1999).

Order verification and/or double-checking improves safe chemotherapy practice, and there should not be any exceptions to this practice. The nurse and pharmacist are each independently responsible for the following:

- Check entire order set against an acceptable reference (protocol, journal article, chemotherapy text or handbook, abstract, computer hard copy of order set, etc.)
- Verify that current body surface area (BSA), height, and weight are correct
- Verify the final dose of each drug
- Check the rate of administration, amount, and type of solution
- Check the antiemetic regimen, before hydration and after hydration, for omissions or additions of ancillary medication therapy
- Compare current orders with previous therapy; consider any radical changes
- Check that an x-ray has been read to confirm central venous access for new line placements for continuous vesicant infusions
- If dose modification has been made, confirm parameters with a published reference or research protocol and then consult with prescriber to verify rationale if nonstandard modification was made
- Determine if appropriate laboratory values are within normal parameters, based on known

organ-specific toxicity of each drug, in addition to hematologic parameters; abnormal values should be called to the attention of the prescriber, and treatment modifications should be made after adequate discussion

For each patient, physicians and health care providers are expected to prescribe the appropriate drug and the appropriate solution. In addition to these expectations, pharmacists must ensure that the prescribed solution and administration parameters will enable adequate drug delivery and ensure compatibility of chemotherapy with intravenous solutions and/or additives. One safety recommendation that is suggested is that a pharmacy develops standard admixtures, that is, predetermined types and amounts of compatible solutions are developed for the most frequently prescribed chemotherapy. This list must be updated on a regular basis, but it can become a tool for learning to write chemotherapy orders safely by limiting the type, kind, and amount of drug that is diluted in different diluents (Womer *et al.* 2002).

Once orders are double-checked, they should be prepared and labeled following pharmacy compounding policies and safe handling procedures. For example, computer-generated labels are verified against the original order and the patient's pharmacy medication profile. All chemotherapy doses, lot numbers, premedications, and appropriate laboratory values are recorded in the patient's pharmacy medication profile, which is a valuable tool for tracking ongoing therapy and patient status ensuring uniformity from dose to dose, visit to visit, and pharmacist to pharmacist. Although the pharmacist chooses the drugs and intravenous fluids, the pharmacy technician compounds the preparation and verifies all calculations, drugs, and fluids. Another safety step is that all vials used by the pharmacy technician are placed in a zip-lock bag to be given back to the pharmacist, again verifying correct dose. An unused or "dummy" syringe is pulled back to the volume used in the final product to further verify the volume (ASHP 2002).

Nursing verification should be completed by two nurses, both of whom have attended a chemotherapy course. Each nurse should sign the chemotherapy order sheet. Nurses are also responsible for checking laboratory parameters that may be dictated by the research protocol or the chemotherapeutic agent. Upon delivery of the initial chemotherapy (cycle 1) to the clinic or nursing unit, the pharmacist and nurse recheck all calculations such as BSA, dose, and references used in the original physician's order.

Administering Cancer Therapies Safely

Administration practices vary according to institutional policies and procedures, state professional practice acts (i.e., pharmacy and nurse practice acts), and practice standards and guidelines proposed by national organizations. For example, the Oncology Nursing Society (ONS) regularly publishes and revises guidelines and recommendations for the administration of chemotherapy and biotherapy (Birner 2003; Barton-Burke *et al.* 2001; Brown *et al.* 2001; Langhorne and Barton-Burke 2001).

Chemotherapy administration begins once the final product, which has been checked with the pharmacist, arrives in the designated patient-care area. Two nurses, both of whom have attended a chemotherapy course, must check the final product against the original order before administration. In the clinic setting, one nurse and the chemotherapy pharmacist should check the final product before administration. The check should take place at the patient's bedside so that the two professionals can ensure that the correct drug is being given to the appropriate patient by using 2 patient identifiers, in the same fashion that a blood transfusion is checked. The attending oncologist and/or oncology fellow may also administer chemotherapy, when necessary, after following comparable procedures.

Chemotherapy administration should occur on dedicated oncology inpatient units and ambulatory oncology clinics that are staffed by competent chemotherapy nurses. On occasion, patients are on other units or must be transferred, such as a patient on continuous infusion to an intensive care unit.

That nursing staff should then be educated by a chemotherapy nurse. All oncology settings should have a standard oncology text, a chemotherapy handbook, copies of approved protocols, and a standard drug reference book (Wilkes and Barton-Burke 2005).

To prepare nurses to administer chemotherapy, the educational programs should include both didactic and supervised clinical experience. The didactic component should include a review of cancer pathophysiology, focusing on the pharmacology of cytotoxic agents, principles of safe handling and drug administration, and management of potential treatment side effects and complications related to drug administration. Tables 7.1 and 7.2 highlight the steps necessary prior to beginning the actual infusions of cancer chemotherapeutic agents. The clinical aspects of administration must provide skills in intravenous therapy, such as venipuncture and site selection; administration techniques and guidelines; management of various venous access devices, such as silastic catheters, implantable ports, and, as appropriate, the more complex drug delivery techniques of intraperitoneal, intracavitary, and intrathecal therapies; arterial lines; and internal and external infusion pumps. Although the nurse should be able to recall the side effects listed for a particular drug, it is more important that she or he anticipate and prevent side effects that the patient is actually at risk of developing.

Table 7.3 is one example of a standard of practice for care of the patient receiving intravenous cytotoxic or biologic agents. Each institution develops standards of practice based on individual institutional programs. This standard of practice was developed by the National Institutes of Health, a research institution, and elements of the standard may not apply in other centers.

Using Cytotoxic Agents in Nonmalignant Conditions

As mentioned earlier in this chapter, chemotherapeutic agents exert cytotoxic effects on cells, organs, and body systems. These cytotoxic agents include other classes of medications such as biologic response modifiers and monoclonal antibodies. Today, patients with malignancies as well as individuals with autoimmune disorders are receiving cytotoxic therapies.

These therapies, also called hazardous drugs by the National Institute for Occupational Safety

---

TABLE 7.1   Nursing Guidelines for Administering Cytotoxic Therapy

I. Prechemotherapy assessment
   A. Physical evaluation
      1. Pertinent past history
         a. Diagnosis and disease presentation
         b. Concomitant health conditions and allergies
      2. System review
         a. Pertinent laboratory data (hematopoietic function)
         b. Neurologic function
         c. Oral cavity and integumentary status
         d. Cardiovascular function
         e. Respiratory function
         f. Urologic function
         g. Gastrointestinal function
         h. Sexual function
         i. Dermatologic status
      3. Presence of prior cancer therapy toxicities
         a. Surgery
         b. Radiation therapy
         c. Chemotherapy
   B. Psychosocial evaluation
      1. Knowledge of cancer and chemotherapy
         a. Dispel myths
         b. Address feelings of anxiety and fear
      2. Prior (personal) experience with chemotherapy
      3. Support system and significant others
      4. Informed consent
   C. Patient and family education
II. Postchemotherapy assessment
   A. Review assessment as above for changes
      1. Tumor response
      2. Status improvements
      3. Abnormal findings
   B. Management of side effects; Appendix I (pp 312–350) for Major Care Plans
   C. Patient/family education

TABLE 7.2　A Chemotherapy Check List for Safe Administration of Cancer Therapies

1. Verify written informed consent. It is required before chemotherapy administration. Informed consent is a process of effective communication during which the physician or a health care provider assisting the physician must provide information and appropriate time to enable the patient (or other person authorized to consent on behalf of the patient) to make an informed decision about the proposed treatment.
2. Know the drug pharmacology: mechanism of action, usual dosage, route of administration, acute and long-term side effects, and route of excretion.
3. Review laboratory data keeping in mind acceptable parameters. Report abnormalities to the physician.
4. Complete prechemotherapy assessment of patient, medical history, and prior chemotherapy.
5. Check physician order for name of drug(s), dosage, route, rate, and timing of drug(s) administration. (Question anything that seems out of the ordinary.)
6. Recalculate dosage: check height and weight; calculate body surface area (BSA).
7. Verify physician orders and dosage calculations with another nurse.
8. Premedication: administer most premedications at least 20–30 minutes before chemotherapy starts. In some cases, you may want to start the patient on antiemetic therapy the night before or the morning of therapy.
9. Patient education: teach and review with the patient and family the details of the chemotherapy schedule, expected side effects, and self-care preventive management suggestions to minimize untoward side effects. Provide written explanations the patient can refer to later because this information may be overwhelming. Refer questions to physician as necessary.
10. Provide patient with telephone numbers for physician and clinic, as appropriate.
11. Reconstitute drug(s) according to manufacturer suggestions, NIOSH and OSHA guidelines, and institution procedures. May be the responsibility of the nursing or the pharmacy department depending on the institution's policy.
12. Gather appropriate equipment: D5W or normal saline (NS) are commonly used to infuse chemotherapy but not exclusively. Use the correct solution and volume. Protect from direct sunlight if applicable.
13. Administer agents according to written policies and procedures using proficient intravenous therapy skills and techniques.
    a. Administer all medications using the five rights:
       (1) Right Patient
       (2) Right Drug
       (3) Right Dose
       (4) Right Route
       (5) Right Time
    b. If no information is available, assume the drug you are giving is a vesicant and administer it with caution, according to institutional policy and procedure.
    c. Avoid drug infiltration; if unsure whether the IV is infiltrated, discontinue it, and restart another IV rather than risk extravasation. WHEN IN DOUBT, PULL IT OUT.
    d. Do not mix drugs together when administering combination therapy. Use syringe or intravenous NS to flush before first drug, in between drugs, and upon completion of all drugs.
    e. It is not optimal to administer vesicant drugs through an indwelling peripheral IV (one that has been in place 4–6 hours or more). It is important to preserve veins, but it is more important to prevent potential extravasation.
    f. Nonvesicant chemotherapy drugs may be administered through an existing IV once the site has been fully assessed for patency and lack of infiltration.
    g. If unable to start an IV after two attempts, consult a colleague for assistance.
14. Do not allow anyone to interrupt you during the preparation or administration of chemotherapy.
15. Do not foster a patient's dependency on one nurse.
16. Always have emergency drugs and an extravasation kit readily available should an adverse reaction occur.
17. Always listen to the patient; the patient's knowledge and preference should be used as frequently as possible. As the patient becomes more knowledgeable regarding IV techniques, his or her personal

(Continued)

TABLE 7.2   (Continued)

experience with successful IV sites, methods, and sensations can be a great aid to the nurse. There are times when the patient's preference may not be the best choice, but his or her participation should always be encouraged.

18. Dispose of intravenous supplies according to OSHA and NIOSH guidelines and institution policy and procedure.

19. Document drug administration according to institution policy and procedures. Use time savers in documentation (e.g., instead of writing step-by-step how a vesicant was given, write "[name of drug]" administered according to institution policy and procedure for vesicants").

20. Observe for adverse reactions.

21. Use the opportunity to teach and counsel the patient and the family while administering the chemotherapy.

and Health (NIOSH), pose a health risk for health care workers. Anyone preparing or administering hazardous drugs or working in areas where these drugs are used can be exposed to these agents by aerosolization and by contamination of work surfaces, work clothing, medical equipment, and by patient excreta. Workplace exposure can manifest as skin rash, infertility, spontaneous abortions, congenital malformations, and possibly leukemia and other cancers (NIOSH 2004). Thus it becomes imperative that health care workers be informed of their risk. In the past, health care workers were aware of these concerns as they related to chemotherapy administration. Changes in science and clinical practice now have cytotoxic agents being administered for non-malignant conditions, increasing the potential for hazardous exposure to many health care workers who are unaware of the risk presented by these drugs. Earlier in this chapter the need for competencies related to prescribing, preparing, and administering were discussed in detail. Those competencies must be applied to health care workers involved in the care of patients receiving hazardous drugs for nonmalignant conditions.

The ONS (Brown *et al.* 2001) recommends that specialized preparation of professional registered nurses can ensure a safe level of care for the individual receiving chemotherapy that is not administered solely in cancer centers. Many

nononcology specialties use antineoplastic drugs for treatment of nonmalignant conditions in dermatology (e.g., methotrexate for psoriasis) or rheumatology (cyclophosphamide for patients with lupus nephritis). The recommendations for the nononcology specialties that use cytotoxic chemotherapy include having the department or section register with the pharmacy department the usual agents, dose ranges, and indicated diseases, with provision of published reference sources and/or institutional review board–approved protocols for these treatments.

Examples of Rheumatic Disorders Using Drug Therapies: Cytotoxic Agents, Biologic Response Modifiers, and Monoclonal Antibodies

Although this book mainly covers cancer therapies, this specific chapter describes the uses, rationale, and consideration of some of the same therapies used for nonmalignant conditions. Similarities and differences between patient groups are presented. Staff education, competency validation, and institutional systems for safety are discussed.

Review of examples of rheumatic disorders, disease characteristics, and specific drug therapies is helpful in understanding the context for the use of these specific drug therapies to treat

National Institutes of Health Warren Grant Magnuson Clinical Center Nursing Department

Standards of Practice: Care of the Patient Receiving Intravenous Cytotoxic or Biologic Agents

I. Assessment

A. General
   1. Assess patient and/or parent or caregiver understanding of the treatment plan, expected treatment outcomes, and potential risks.

B. Medical Record Review
   1. Assess presence of a completed consent (assent for children when appropriate) form.
   2. Review prescriber progress note for documentation of dose level if appropriate, protocol exemptions, and/or rationale for dose modifications.
   3. Review prescriber orders against clinical trial protocol, clinical map if applicable, and research data sheets if applicable for all ancillary medications and therapies.
   4. Review pre-treatment lab. Confirm the treatment plan with the prescriber if any results are abnormal or exceed protocol specifications.
   5. Review prescriber orders for treatment of extravasation and/or adverse drug reaction if applicable.
   6. Review baseline assessment including height, weight, body surface area (BSA), vital signs, history, physical examination, and known allergies.
   7. Review history of chemotherapy-induced side effects and successful management strategies.

C. Calculations/Drug Label Verification With A Second RN:
   1. Calculate the drug dosage including any dose modification, and complete chemotherapy worksheet (refer to Figure 7.1).
   2. Compare calculated dose to prescribed dose. If there is a discrepancy of 10% or more for adults or 5% or more for pediatric patients, notify the prescriber and pharmacist. Hold drug administration until the dosage is verified and documented.
   3. Check the diluent type and the drug container's label against the prescriber order for:
      a. Patient name and medical record number
      b. Cytotoxic/biologic agent, diluent, route (e.g., IV push, IV piggyback, or continuous infusion), dose, volume, date, infusion start time, length of infusion, and drug expiration
      c. Verify the infusion or ambulatory pump program against the prescribed order.

D. Venous Access Devices
   1. Assess preexisting peripheral lines for patency, brisk blood return; flush solutions should flow freely to gravity. Inserting a peripheral IV just prior to administration of vesicant agents is strongly recommended.
   2. Assess central venous access device (CVAD) for patency, brisk blood return, and ease of flushing.

(Continued)

TABLE 7.3   Standard of Practice for Care of the Patient Receiving Intravenous Cytotoxic or Biologic Agents (Continued)

3. Assess site for swelling, erythema, pain, or drainage.
4. Assess for signs or symptoms of venous obstruction.
   a. Assess for previous therapy-related acute or delayed complications, specific toxicities or adverse reactions.
   b. Verify that emergency medications are readily available in the area where patient will receive treatment.

II. Interventions
   A. General (nonvesicants, nonirritants, vesicants, and irritants)
      1. Ensure that emergency equipment is available in patient's room:
         a. Normal saline flush solution
         b. Oxygen
         c. Suction machine
         d. Vital sign monitor
      2. Assemble personal protective equipment (gloves, goggles, gown).
      3. Verify spill kit readily available on unit.
      4. Dispose of hazardous drug supplies according to the Procedure: Safe Handling and Disposal of Hazardous Drugs (Table 7.5).
      5. Provide patient and family teaching, including information about self-care and potential symptoms requiring health care provider attention.
   B. Venous Access
      1. Obtain peripheral IV access in a vessel of the upper extremity. Peripheral venous access in a lower extremity is not recommended.
      2. Avoid:
         a. Areas of hematoma, edema, impaired lymphatic drainage, phlebitis, inflammation, induration, or obvious infection and sites of previous irradiation.
         b. Fragile, small, or low flow vessels such as the dorsal aspect of the wrist.
         c. Using veins that have been accessed within the previous 24 hours.
         d. Sites distal to previous IV sites or previous sites of extravasation.
         e. Vessels of the hand, wrist, and antecubital fossa for administration of vesicants/irritants.
      3. If local anesthetics, e.g. EMLA, are used to facilitate venous cannulation, ensure that the effects of anesthesia have subsided prior to administration of cytotoxic agents.
      4. IV site dressing must allow for continuous visual inspection before, during, and after drug administration.
      5. Verify patency and blood return of venous access before and after administration.
      6. At the completion of cytotoxic/biologic agent administration, flush the line with a compatible flush solution to ensure maximum drug delivery as per Nursing Department drug administration procedures. For specific research studies, check protocol and consult pharmacy for any special guidelines on drug administration.

C. Administration
   1. IV push administration of vesicants/irritants via peripheral IV and CVAD
      a. Infuse a free-flowing compatible flush solution during administration of the cytotoxic agent.
      b. Administer agent through the IV administration set at the most proximal port to the patient.
      c. Check for blood return before administration, after every 2 ml of drug administration, and after administration.
      d. Observe the IV site continuously.
   2. Peripheral piggyback administration of vesicants/irritants
      a. General
         i. Administer the cytotoxic agent as the secondary infusion piggybacked to the primary line at the most proximal port to the pump.
         ii. Secure the IV tubing using tape or a secure locking device.
      b. Vesicants
         i. Use of an infusion pump is prohibited.
         ii. Check for brisk blood return before administration, every 5 minutes during administration, and after administration.
         iii. Observe the IV site continuously.
      c. Irritants
         i. Check for brisk blood return pre- and post-administration.
         ii. Observe the IV site every 15 minutes until infusion completed.
   3. CVAD piggyback administration of vesicants/irritants
      a. Secure the IV tubing using tape or a secure locking device.
      b. Administer the cytotoxic agent as the secondary infusion piggybacked to the primary line.
      c. Observe the IV site and connections every hour for inpatients; for outpatients monitor the site frequently and instruct the patient to call for any complications.
   4. Peripheral continuous (large-volume) infusion of vesicants is strictly prohibited.
   5. Peripheral continuous (large-volume) infusion of irritants: an IV infusion pump is required.
   6. CVAD continuous (large-volume) infusion of vesicants/irritants
      a. An infusion device is required.
      b. Observe the IV site and connections every 4 hours for inpatients. Instruct outpatients to monitor site frequently.
D. Adverse Event
   1. General
      a. If adverse event occurs, stop infusion, and notify prescriber and/or other clinical resources (e.g., clinical pharmacy specialist or clinical nurse specialist); follow treatment guidelines.
      b. After resolution of adverse event, consult with prescriber before continuing with administration.
   2. Extravasation guidelines for vesicants/irritants
      a. Stop administration of the cytotoxic agent.
      b. Disconnect the IV line at the point closest to the vascular access device.
      c. Aspirate residual drug from the vascular access device.

(Continued)

TABLE 7.3 Standard of Practice for Care of the Patient Receiving Intravenous Cytotoxic or Biologic Agents (Continued)

    d. Estimate the amount of drug extravasated.

    e. Notify the prescriber and clinical pharmacy specialist.

    f. Administer an antidote if appropriate.

    g. Remove peripheral access device (this does **not** include PICCs or midlines). Remove needle from implanted port.

    h. Assessment of extravasation site

        i. Inpatients: RN uses an indelible marker to indicate any area of induration and swelling. Assess every 8 hours for 48 hours for pain, erythema, induration, mobility, skin changes, and necrosis. Complications are assessed until resolved.

        ii. Outpatients: Assess as described for patients. Nurse instructs patient/significant other to report any complications.

    i. Size the area of extravasation by measuring a perpendicular length and width at the widest points. Refer to Figure 7.2 for additional information on the procedure for determining measurements.

    j. Protect the site from undue pressure.

    k. Apply warm or cold compresses as indicated.

    l. Verify consent for photograph and then obtain photograph of site as indicated.

    m. Apply dressing as indicated.

    n. Elevate and rest the extremity.

    o. File an occurrence report.

3. Flare Reaction

    a. Stop the administration of the cytotoxic agent.

    b. Flush the IV line with a compatible flush solution.

    c. Administer hydrocortisone and/or diphenhydramine IV followed by IV flush solution according to prescriber orders.

    d. Once flare has subsided, resume administration at a slower infusion rate.

    e. Monitor for recurrence of flare reaction and repeat sequence listed above according to prescriber orders.

    f. For patients scheduled to receive the same cytotoxic agent in the future, discuss with prescriber strategies to minimize risk of another flare reaction, that is, premedications, slower infusion rate, and dilution of cytotoxic agent.

4. Hypersensitivity or anaphylatic reaction

    a. Discontinue drug administration immediately and maintain line with compatible flush solution.

    b. Notify prescriber STAT of reaction.

    c. Implement prescriber orders.

III. Documentation
A. Document in MIS
1. Protocol, cycle, day, week, and dose level if appropriate.
2. Laboratory test results reviewed.
3. Cytotoxic agent, dose, route, container number if applicable, lot number if applicable, time of administration, and length of infusion.
4. Rationale for dose modification.
5. Patient/family teaching.
6. Presence of a complete consent or assent (minors only) form.
7. Presence of Durable Power of Attorney document as required by treatment protocol.
8. Name of staff who double checked the cytotoxic agent dose calculations, drug label, and infusion device settings.
9. Venous access device, location, patency and site assessment before, during, and after administration.
10. Patient's tolerance of procedure and interventions.
11. Complications or adverse drug reactions as well as interventions provided.
B. In the Event of Extravasation Document,
1. Date and time of extravasation.
2. Patient complaints before, during, and after extravasation.
3. Estimated amount of extravasation.
4. Agent extravasated; antidote administered.
5. Document date, time and those notified (prescriber, clinical pharmacy specialist).
6. The dimensions of the injured site and the site assessment.
7. The date and time of any photographs.
8. Dates of any follow-up evaluations and/or consultations such as surgery, dermatology, or rehabilitation.

Source: Modified from National Institutes of Health 2002. Magnuson Clinical Center, Nursing Department. Each institution develops procedures based on individual institutional programs. This standard of practice was developed for a research institution and elements of the standard may not apply in other centers.

CYTOTOXIC/BIOTHERAPY WORKSHEET

ADDRESSOGRAPH

Protocol #: _____   Dose Level: _____   Ht: _____

CYCLE DAY/WEEK AND DATE	WEIGHT	BSA OR IBW	DRUG	PROTOCOL DOSE	DOSE ORDERED	RN'S CALC.	WITHIN 10% 5% (PEDS)	DOSE MOD'D?	INFUSION RATE/RTE	COMMENT	1ST AND 2ND RN INITIALS

FIGURE 7.1 Cytotoxic/Biotherapy Worksheet. *Source:* National Institutes of Health 2005. Warren Grant Magnuson Clinical Center, Nursing Department.

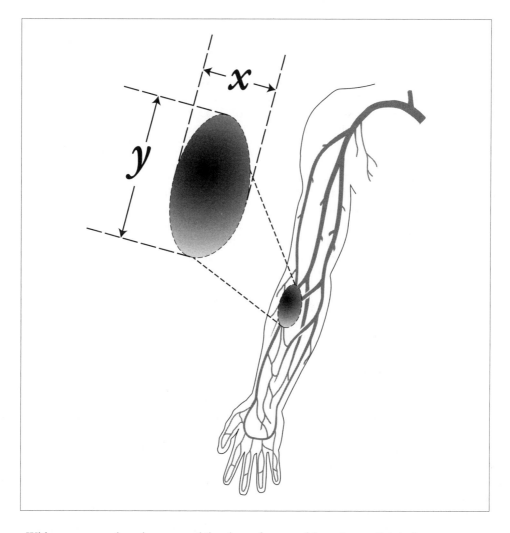

- With a pen or marker, draw around the circumference of the extravasation lesion.
- Measure the lesion at its greatest width and length (the 'x' and 'y' measurements, respectively, in the figure above). NOTE: Length and width measurements should be perpendicular to each other.
- Document initial and subsequent measurements explicitly. Identify what was measured (e.g., swelling, erythema, induration, ulceration, etc.) and when it was measured in relation to when extravasation occurred.

FIGURE 7.2 Guidelines for Measuring and Documenting Extravasation Injuries. *Source*: National Institutes of Health 2002. Warren Grant Magnuson Clinical Center, Nursing Department.

nonmalignant conditions. There are over 100 types of rheumatic diseases including rheumatoid arthritis (RA), systemic lupus erythematosus (SLE), and Wegeners granulomatosis (WG).

Rheumatoid Arthritis (RA) is a disease marked by inflammation in the synovial membrane of diarthrodial joints. It is a disease that affects organs throughout the body but concentrates on the peripheral synovial joints. Following the course of disease in RA allows discernment of several phases of the condition. The first phase involves accumulation of lymphocytes and mononuclear cells in the synovial tissue. Cytokines, such as TNF-α and interleukin-1, are released by macrophages into the joint. The joint inflammation causes pain and stiffness and may lead to joint destruction over time. Although treatments for RA often focus on relief of pain, some of the most exciting innovations in the treatment of RA therapies are directed at altering the progression of the disease. These types of medications are referred to as disease-modifying antirheumatic drugs (DMARDs). Examples of DMARDs for RA include methotrexate and biologic response modifiers.

Systemic Lupus Erythematosis (SLE) is an autoimmune disorder associated usually with antibodies to self. This condition is characterized by disease processes in potentially almost every organ or part of the body, including the skin, mouth, joints, lungs, kidneys, nerves, blood, and immune system. In SLE, clinical symptoms can range from mild skin rash to severe central nervous system involvement and end-stage kidney disease. Hematologic complications include hemolytic anemia and thrombocytopenia. Systemic Lupus Erythematosis is a disease with a pattern of waxing and waning of symptoms and complications. For example, the frequently occurring joint symptoms of pain and inflammation can change over time. The term "flare" is used to denote a worsening of condition in a rheumatic disorder. Flares can result in increasing pain in joints, increasing fatigue, or progression of inflammatory rashes and sudden worsening of hematuria

and kidney functions. Dr. Jill P. Buyon addressed examples of triggers that worsened disease in SLE when she wrote, "factors to consider that might precipitate the onset or exacerbation of systemic disease or isolated organ involvement include recent sun exposure, emotional stress, infection, and certain drugs such as sulfonamides" (Buyon 2001, 335).

The pathology of SLE is complicated and is characterized by an overreactive abnormal immune system. Genetics may play a role in the etiology of SLE. For example, specific genes are linked with SLE, including those associated with TNF and deficiencies in complement (Tse and Shaw 2004). Patients with SLE have higher titers of IgG antibodies to nuclear antigens, such as DNA and ribosomes. Tissue damage may result from cellular mechanisms associated with antinuclear antibodies. Autoantibodies can form immune complexes with their antigens that can be detected in the circulation and the target organs. Immune complexes can deposit in blood vessels and other target organs, such as the basement membranes of the glomeruli in the kidney, leading to inflammation. The subsequent damage explains a common complication of SLE, glomerulonephritis. Overactivation of T and B cells is also believed to be part of the disease pathology.

Treatments for SLE include cyclophosphamide (an inhibitor of activated T cells), methotrexate, mycophenylate mofetil, and azathioprine. Biologic immune modifiers, such as antibody to the CD40 ligand (CD40LmAb), anti-CD20, and MRA (anti–IL-6), are being evaluated in clinical trials. Monoclonal antibody therapies are used to prevent induction of antibodies and halt the progression of autoimmune disease (Tse and Shaw 2004).

The vasculitides are rheumatic disorders. One example of a vasculitic disorder is WG, a condition characterized by medium- and small-vessel destruction, leading to systemic inflammation. Individuals with WG may respond to treatments with anti-inflammatory agents in combination with cytotoxic agents. Currently, individuals with vasculitis and immune-mediated inflammatory and connective tissue disorders have a wider range of therapy options than in the past. Depending on the condition of the patient and the specific disease process involved in the disorder, a variety of agents may be used by the presciber for immunosuppressive and anti-inflammatory effects.

Some of these patients receive low-dose cytotoxic agents. Low dose means that the dosage of the cytotoxic agent is usually much less than the dosages used for malignancies.

Biologic response modifier therapies may also be a therapeutic option for individuals with vasculitic disorders. Treatment agents may be selected because of anti-TNF or cytokine effects. Examples of some of the drugs used in vasculitides include: cyclophosphamide, methotrexate, azathioprine, anakinra, etanercept, infliximab, cyclosporine, daclizumab (anti-CD25), and rituximab (anti-CD20). Table 7.4 summarizes some of the types of agents that are used for nonmalignant conditions in a variety of rheumatic diseases.

Infrastructure for Administering Cytotoxic Agents or Biologic Response Modifiers in Nonmalignant Conditions

Because oncology units are no longer the main or exclusive areas where chemotherapy is administered, nurses, physicians, and pharmacists caring for patients with rheumatic disorders require an infrastructure within the institution to help provide safe delivery of high-risk medications. The issues that institutions face include: comprehensive management of adverse effects; staff education; competency assessment; drug administration policies, standards, and procedures; guidelines for drug preparation; drug management (dispensing, administration, and dose checking); review of safety labs; and safe handling and disposal of hazardous agents (Connor *et al.* 1999; Department of Health and Human Services 2004; Fortenbaugh and Rummel 2004; Martin and Larson 2003; NIOSH 2004; Polovich 2003).

TABLE 7.4   Examples of Drugs and Drug Classifications Used in Nonmalignant Rheumatic Disorders

Drug Class/Mechanism	Cytotoxic Agents	Immuno-suppressant Agent	Biologic Response Modifier	Route of Administration	Examples of Conditions Where Drug is Used
Cyclophosphamide	X	X	X	Monthly IV pulse, daily PO	WG and SLE
Methotrexate	X	X	X	Weekly PO, SC or IM	WG and RA
Cyclosporin A		X	X	Daily PO	RA
Azathioprine		X	X	Daily PO	WG and RA
Mycophenolate mofetil		X	X	Daily PO	SLE and WG
Anakinra (anti–IL-1)			X	SC	RA
Etanercept (anti-TNF/LTa)			X	SC	RA and WG
Infliximab (anti-TNF)			X	IV	RA
Daclizumab (anti-CD25)			X	SC and IV	WG
Rituximab (anti-CD20)			X	IV	RA, SLE, and WG
Adalimumab (anti-TNF)			X	IV	RA

Abbreviations: WG, Wegener's granulomatus disease; RA, rheumatoid arthritis; SLE, systemic lupus erythematosus.

Health care facilities across the nation are faced with the need for a greater degree of sophisticated knowledge and skills for all disciplines, from nursing to pharmacy to medicine. This need must be met in an escalating staff crisis, as more of the baby boomer generation retires and the workforce shrinks at the same time that the target therapeutic population expands. Health care administrators are demonstrating resourcefulness by providing cancer internships and specialty programs to attract and retain quality staff members. Institutions that have such programs and establish high standards recruit more patients to their facility as word of the quality of care goes out not only from patients and families but also from staff.

Within the hospital setting, collaboration between health care providers is needed and must include team members from pharmacy, medicine, and nursing departments as well as quality control experts. For example, the health care institution should establish and maintain policies and standards required for safe management of patients receiving cytotoxic drugs, monoclonal antibodies, and biologic response modifiers. Representatives from key disciplines, such as medicine, nursing, and pharmacy, should review policies, standards, and procedures for any department involved with cytotoxic agents, biologic response modifiers, and monoclonal antibodies. Issues to be addressed by the institution include:

1. Maintaining a list of institutional dispensed agents
2. Establishing the process for drug-related issues including:
   a. dosage and dose modification
   b. recommended premedications
   c. patient history and allergies
   d. administration contraindications
   e. review of safety laboratory testing
   f. labeling
   g. preparing
   h. dispensing
   i. returning hazardous drugs
   j. double checking within each department the drug, dose, route, use, and schedule and intended patient
3. Documentation requirements
4. Occurrence review and follow-up actions
5. Staff (pharmacy, medicine, and nursing) education

Additionally, the process for obtaining the material safety data sheets (MSDS) for all dispensed hazardous drugs should be established. Material safety data sheets (MSDS) provide critical information about drug profiles for exposures in the event of an accidental spill of the agent. Once a spill occurs, the first priority is to take actions to protect patients, visitors, and staff. Individuals accidentally exposed should follow procedures for immediate first aid depending on the type of exposure: mucus membranes or skin. Any containment or clean-up measures require personal protective equipment such as chemotherapy gloves, non–strike-through chemotherapy gowns, masks, and safety goggles.

Individuals exposed to the spilled agent should obtain a written copy of the MSDS document, which lists potential adverse effects associated with the agent. Occurrence reports should be completed and follow-up should be conducted as indicated for care with the occupational health services or primary physician. Table 7.5 is an example of the National Institutes of Health Procedure for the Safe Handling and Disposal of Hazardous Drugs (HD). It should be noted that each institution develops procedures based on individual institutional programs. This procedure was developed by the National Institutes of Health, a research institution and elements of the standard may not apply in other centers.

An effective method and timely schedule for review of medication errors should be established. Complete reporting of any errors and investigation of causative factors contributing to errors must be explored by all relevant departments involved. Strategies for prevention of future errors

TABLE 7.5   Procedure: Safe Handling of Hazardous Drugs

National Institutes of Health (NIH)
Warren Grant Magnuson Clinical Center
Nursing Department

PROCEDURE: Safe Handling and Disposal of Hazardous Drugs (HD) including:

    I. Essential Information
    II. Administration of HD (Safe Work Practices)
        ■ Intravenous
        ■ Oral
        ■ Intravesical
        ■ Intraperitoneal
        ■ Agents given in the OR or Special Procedures
    III. Safe Handling of Trace Contamination of HD
    IV. Safe Handling of HD Spills on Hospital Mattresses (e.g., Intraperitoneal Chemotherapy)
    V. Safe Handling of HD Spills
    VI. Employee, Patient, or Visitor: Accidental Skin, Eye, or Sharp Exposure to HD

PROCEDURE: Safe Handling of Hazardous Drugs (HD)
I. Essential Information

A. Studies in cooperation with the Occupational Safety and Health Administration (OSHA) indicate potential risks for health care workers who are exposed to HDs or investigational agents with unknown risks. Potential risks of HD include: genotoxicity, carcinogenicity, teratogenicity, infertility, and organ toxicity. Because of the potential risks, it is the responsibility of all health care workers and Clinical Center personnel to comply with the safety measures recommended by OSHA and other regulatory and advisory agencies to minimize exposure to HDs. A principle of "ALARA" or keeping exposures "As Low As Reasonably Achievable" will be followed when handling HD or investigational agents where the risks are not fully known.

B. Accessing the Pharmacy Department's "Medical Information" website, NIH personnel can obtain Material Safety Data Sheets (MSDS) from the Pharmacy website. The documents may be downloaded or printed. If for some reason the website should not be available, contact the Clinical Center (CC). Pharmacy MSDS are documents, which contain information about commercially marketed HD, including recommendations for acute exposure treatments and health hazards after exposure to HD. In the event of an occupational exposure to a HD, staff, patients, and visitors have the right to obtain drug information in a timely manner. Information about the drug may be in the form of an MSDS to identify potential risks of exposure. Persons outside the NIH who wish to obtain MSDS should contact the drug product's manufacturer or distributor.

C. Patient Care Unit personnel are recommended to refer to drug information resources that are located on their units. The Pharmacy Department prepares and distributes to each patient care unit DRUG FACT SHEETS for investigational study drugs used on each patient care unit. DRUG FACT SHEETS are updated whenever protocol-related drug treatments are amended and when updated pharmaceutical data become available for investigational compounds used at the Clinical Center. DRUG FACT SHEETS include information about adverse effects associated with hazardous agents.

(Continued)

TABLE 7.5   Procedure: Safe Handling of Hazardous Drugs (Continued)

D. The Clinical Center (CC) provides protective barrier equipment and practice guidelines to decrease or prevent the risk of occupational exposure to HD. Any staff who are pregnant or lactating and staff who are trying to conceive who have concerns about exposure to HD during administration and while caring for patients receiving these agents should discuss their concerns with their immediate supervisor. For questions about the CC Safety Program relative to HDs contact the NIH CC Safety Officer.

E. HD will be prepared and properly labeled by the Pharmacy with a colored label stating:

HAZARDOUS DRUG

    Special Handling

    If medication is not administered to patient,
    return to pharmacy for proper disposal
    DO NOT DISCARD ON UNIT

F. Storage areas for HD containers and contaminated equipment, trash, or linen need to be safely secured and labeled on the patient care unit restricted to authorized personnel to prevent injury to children, patients, visitors, and staff.

G. The prepackaged chemotherapy spill kit is to be used by staff on the patient care unit (e.g., Sage ChemoSafety Spill Kit). Patients, when appropriate, are discharged with the home health spill kit (e.g., Kendall ChemoBloc Home Health Spill Kit).

II. Administration of HDs (Safe Work Practices)
A. Equipment List
Supplies for Routine Handling and Disposal of HD
    Chemotherapy spill kit (see section III B)
    2 Pairs of chemotherapy gloves (powder-free Nitrile gloves, 0.11-mm thick)
    Chemotherapy gown
    Safety goggles
    Air purifying respirator (NIOSH 95 approved)
    Spill towels (e.g., Chux pads)
    Absorbent pads (e.g., Chux pads)
    Sterile gauze
    Tape
    Covered plastic double-lined medical pathological waste (MPW) box
    Plastic lined isolation linen bag
    Sharps box
    Leak-proof plastic bags that can be sealed
    Chemotherapy waste container/bucket

                                                                    Key Points

B. STEPS
    1. Wash hands
    2. Don protective personal equipment such as gown,
        chemotherapy gloves, and safety goggles as follows:
        a. Don gown and close snaps.   a. Gowns should be disposable, constructed of low
                                                                    permeability fabric, lint free, and have a closed front

b. Gloves:

Single Gloving

If single gloving, tuck the clean glove over the cuff of the gown.

Double Gloving

If double gloves are worn, one glove is inserted under the cuff and one glove goes over the cuff.

c. Change gloves at least every hour.

d. Put on a NIOSH 95–approved respirator mask and safety goggles for administration of HD where aerosol formation, spraying, or splashing is likely (e.g., if in the room with patient receiving aerosolized pentamidine and ribavirin).

3. If at any time barriers are noted to be torn, punctured, or contaminated with HD, remove the damaged items, remove contaminated clothing, and wash contaminated skin.

4. Separate HD from other drugs by storing HD drugs in a bin (like a bath basin) or in a cabinet with a front barrier.

5. Place a plastic-backed absorbent pad under the IV system to protect the patient when connecting or disconnecting the IV site to the VAD.

6. Priming IV sets with fluid when administering HD will be accomplished with one of the following techniques:

a. Pharmacy will prime IV sets for selected HD:
■ HD delivered by ambulatory pumps
■ Small volumes of HD
■ HD not compatible with standard flush solutions.
■ There should be no need to remove air from the container of HD that the Pharmacy has prepared. Do not add fluids to a container of HD that the Pharmacy has prepared.

(or front snaps with a protective panel), and long sleeves with elastic or knit closed cuffs.

b. Double gloving is recommended by OSHA but is not mandatory in the event that double gloving interferes with an individual's technique. Double gloving is not usually required if using chemotherapy gloves (Nitrile 0.11-mm thick).

c. Gloves should have minimal or no powder. Changing gloves hourly helps to prevent accidental exposure as a result of an unnoticed torn glove.

d. NIOSH 95 respirators effectively prevent the inhalation of HD. Safety goggles effectively prevent accidental exposure to the eyes.

3. Refer to section V for exposure information.

4. HD need to be stored safely in patient care areas to avoid accidental dropping of the HD container.

5. Placing a pad under the IV system when connecting or disconnecting the IV site to a VAD helps to absorb potential leakage of HD.

6. Priming IV sets with fluid to dispel air is associated with risks of spills and formation of aerosol. To avoid these risks, OSHA recommends using a non-drug-containing compatible flush solution to prime IV sets whenever possible.

a. Because of the nature of some HD, there will be some instances when the Pharmacy will prime IV sets. Pharmacy is equipped with biosafety cabinets for this procedure. The Pharmacy Department will remove air from all containers that are to be administered with an ambulatory pump. Adding fluids to a container of HD causes a potential risk for

(Continued)

TABLE 7.5 Procedure: Safe Handling of Hazardous Drugs (Continued)

b. Secondary IV sets used for HD administration will be primed with a non–drug-containing compatible flush solution using a backflow closed-system technique.

c. Primary IV sets used for HD administration will first be primed with a non–drug-containing compatible flush solution. The bag of the flush solution can then be removed and discarded and replaced with the HD solution container.

d. Vented/universal tubing with the vent open for glass containers and closed for nonglass containers.

e. Syringes with HD should be large enough so that they are never more than three fourths full when the entire dose is present. Do not clear air from the syringe.

7. Use sterile gauze when connecting or disconnecting HD containers to IV lines, extension tubing, etc.

8. Verify that all IV tubing connection sites are secured (Luer-Lok connections are tightened by hand and taped).

9. Observe the IV system for any leakage.

10. Dispose of any IV equipment keeping the system intact (e.g., do not disconnect IV tubing from infusion bag). Discard disposable used equipment into a chemotherapy waste bucket then close the lid. When the chemotherapy waste bucket is three fourths filled, close and secure the lid and then place the chemotherapy bucket in a covered double lined MPW box.

11. Dispose of glass containers contaminated with HD along with the connected IV tubing by placing them into a chemotherapy waste bucket. Close the lid. When the chemotherapy waste bucket is three fourths filled, close and secure the lid and then place in a covered double-lined MPW box.

12. Wear double gloves and gown to clean contaminated

formation of aerosol of HD as well as for changing the chemical compound of the HD.

b. Refer to the Nursing Department procedure on medication administration: backflow technique.

c. Do not prime IV sets with HD.

d. Keep the vent closed for nonglass containers and opened for glass containers. Avoid exposure to any potential aerosol.

e. Overfilled syringes increase the risk of accidental spills. The Pharmacy will safely remove air from the syringe with HD.

7. Sterile gauze should be used around IV injection sites to contain leaks or sprays of aerosol.

8. Do not tighten connections with hemostats because it causes the plastic connectors to crack and leak.

10. Placing contaminated IV equipment into a chemotherapy waste bucket with a secure lid and then placing it into a MPW box contains the HD and decreases the risk of formation of aerosol during handling of the trash.

11. To decrease the risks of exposure for staff, HD will be dispensed in nonglass containers except in situations where glass is the only approved container for the HD.

reusable equipment. Wash equipment twice with detergent and then rinse equipment with water. Wear safety goggles and/or mask if there is a risk for splashing or aerosol generation.

13. While wearing protective equipment such as gloves and gown, dispose of linen contaminated with HD or body fluids from patients who have received HD within the last 48 hours into an isolation linen bag with a plastic liner.

14. Remove protective barrier equipment like gowns and gloves before leaving the administration area. After use, dispose of equipment into a covered double-lined MPW box and then wash hands.

15. Dispose of sharps contaminated with HD in a leak-proof and puncture-resistant container (sharps box). When the sharps box is three fourths filled, close and place into a MPW box.

16. Any unused or partially used HD should be securely clamped, capped, and sealed in a plastic bag before sending it back to the Pharmacy.

17. Provide teaching to families and significant others concerning safe handling of HD or body secretions.

18. Wear protective barriers, such as double gloves, when dealing with patient secretions if the patient has received a HD within the previous 48 hours. Avoid splashing when emptying bedpans or urinals. Avoid rinsing procedures that generate spraying and formation of aerosol.

19. Wash hands after gloves are removed.

III. Safe Handling of Trace (≤ 5 cc) Contamination of HD
   A. Essential Information
   Nursing staff are responsible for management or disposal of items contaminated with trace amounts of HD (≤ 5 cc) such as clothing, linen, and drips on environmental surfaces (e.g., beds or tables). Trace waste from HD is disposed of in the chemotherapy waste container/bucket, the container is closed and then placed into MPW box and is handled as medical pathologic waste. Any spill of HD that exceeds 5 cc is considered a spill, disposed of as chemical waste, and managed by the fire department.
   B. Equipment
   Supplies for Safe Handling of Trace Contamination of HD or Chemotherapy Spills
   Chemotherapy Drug Spill Kit containing:
   2 pairs of chemotherapy gloves (powder-free Nitrile gloves 0.11-mm thick)
   Chemotherapy gowns

12. Reusable equipment, such as IV pumps, need to be cleaned by housekeeping staff before reuse.

14. Do not reuse gloves or contaminated protective equipment. If double gloves were worn, first remove the outermost gloves, then remove gown, goggles, and mask. Remove the innermost gloves last, being careful to avoid touching skin or anything with the potentially contaminated gloves. Next, wash hands.

16. HD should be transported inside sealed plastic bags. Do not use the pneumatic tube system or Mosler automatic delivery systems.

17. Follow guidelines for teaching safe handling of HD as listed in the references.

18. Wear splash goggles whenever there is potential for aerosol formation.

19. Do not reuse gloves or contaminated personal protective

(Continued)

TABLE 7.5   Procedure: Safe Handling of Hazardous Drugs (Continued)

Safety goggles
Air purifying Respirator Mask (NIOSH 95 approved)
3 Spill towels
2 Absorbent pads
2 Chemotherapy waste bags and ties
Shoe coverings
Scooper device with scraper (use if glass is involved)
Detergent
Sharps box
1 Chemotherapy waste container/bucket
Covered double plastic-lined MPW box
Plastic lined isolation linen bag
Leak-proof plastic bags that can be sealed

C. Steps

1. Immediately contain the spill by placing disposable
   absorbent plastic-backed pad (e.g., Chux) absorbent side
   down over the spill.

2. Restrict access to the area until the cleanup is completed
   and remove nonessential person(s) from the area.

3. Notify the Fire Department for any spills of HD on
   absorbent surfaces such as carpets.

4. Don protective gear: two pairs of nonpowdered
   chemotherapy gloves, chemotherapy gown, safety
   goggles, and, if needed, shoe coverings and a NIOSH
   95–approved respirator mask.

5. Remove Chux pad and place in a chemotherapy waste
   bucket; close and secure the lid and then place in a
   double plastic lined MPW box.

6. Remove glass particles if present using a scoop device and
   scraper from the chemotherapy spill kit instead of gloved
   hands. Place glass particles in a chemotherapy waste bucket
   and then close the lid.

7. Wipe the spill area with an absorbent gauze and clean spill
   area using disposable materials and detergent solution,
   washing three times.

8. Rinse the area with clean water using dampened gauze.

Key Points

1. Do not touch spill at this point.

3. The Fire Department will manage spills involving
   absorbent surfaces like carpets.

4. A NIOSH 95–approved mask is required when airborne
   powder or aerosol is likely to be generated.

6. Using a scoop device and scraper helps to prevent
   sharps injury and exposure to HD.

9. Place contaminated materials into chemotherapy waste bucket, close and secure the lid, and then place in a covered double plastic-lined MPW box.

10. Notify your Head Nurse or Service Supervisor.

IV. Safe Handling of HD Spills on Hospital Mattresses (e.g., Intraperitoneal Chemotherapy [IPC])

A. Essential Information

1. The standard Clinical Center mattress has a factory-produced cover that is vapor permeable and impervious to fluid penetration. Unless the mattress has been punctured, the fluid will pool on the surface of the cover, which can be blotted dry, washed, and rinsed.

2. IPC therapy has a potential for spills of HD mixed with body fluids because of the connections of the system, patient wound condition (e.g., wound dehiscence), and position changes of the patient from the recumbent position to sitting or standing.

3. Preventative measures for spills during IPC should help prevent or lessen the extent of any potential spill of HD and body fluids.

B. Equipment

Supplies for Safe Handling of Trace Contamination of HD or Chemotherapy Spills
Chemotherapy Drug Spill Kit containing:
2 Pairs of chemotherapy gloves (powder-free Nitrile gloves 0.11-mm thick)
Chemotherapy gowns
Safety goggles
Air-purifying respirator mask (NIOSH 95 approved)
3 Spill towels
2 Absorbent pads
2 Chemotherapy waste bags and ties
Shoe coverings
Scooper device with scraper (use if glass is involved)
Detergent
Sharps box
1 Chemotherapy waste container/bucket
Covered double plastic lined MPW box
Plastic-lined isolation linen bag
Leak-proof plastic bags that can be sealed

C. Steps

Prior to providing care to patients at risk for a spill:

1. Prepare the environment to contain any potential spills.

2. Check and tighten connections on patient drains, collection containers.

3. Assess incision lines and wound site for integrity and risk for dehiscence.

Key Points

1. Liberally use protective barriers such as draw sheets, plastic lined draw sheets, and Chux pads on the bed prior to initiation of administration of cytotoxic agents.

2. Equipment connections are a potential source of disconnection and subsequent leakage of HD.

3. Incision lines and wound sites that are not well approximated or wounds that have dehisced may allow flow of body fluids, along with trace

(Continued)

TABLE 7.5   Procedure: Safe Handling of Hazardous Drugs (Continued)

amounts of HD, to leak onto patient gowns, bed linens, and the mattress cover.

4. The earlier the spill is recognized, the greater the potential for containment of the fluids and the opportunity to minimize the impact of the spill on the patient, environment, and others.

4. Instruct patient and family to call the nurse at the first sign of any leakage of fluids associated with the IPC.

5. Once any spill associated with IPC has occurred:
   a. Don protective equipment such as double chemotherapy gloves, gown, and splash goggles.
   b. Determine the source of the spill and attempt to stop the flow of liquids (e.g., clamp any disconnected tubing).
   c. Assist the patient in immediate care including placing absorbent pads, such as sterile gauze, or Chux, over any wet skin areas.
   d. Remove any wet linens or clothing and place in plastic-lined bags in linen bag.
   e. Follow the instructions in this procedure for the safe handling of spills in section VI.

6. With patient out of bed and with protective equipment on, inspect mattress cover for any obvious perforations.

7. For mattress covers without any obvious perforations, blot any wet areas on the mattress with absorbent pad such as Chux.

8. Wash any affected areas three times with detergent solution.

9. Rinse the affected area of the mattress cover with clean water using dampened gauze.

10. Place contaminated materials into chemotherapy waste bucket, close and secure the lid, and then place in a covered double plastic-lined MPW box.

11. Notify the Head Nurse or Service Supervisor.

12. Once the mattress cover has dried, the patient may be returned to the bed.

13. In the event of a spill of HD/body fluids onto a perforated mattress cover, complete steps 5–12.

14. Once the mattress cover has dried, notify housekeeping to remove bed for inner mattress inspection.

14. A perforated mattress cover allows contamination of the inner mattress. This complication cannot be safely managed on the patient care unit.

V. Safe Handling of HD Spills (> 5 ml)

A. Equipment (same as in section III B)

B. Steps

Key Points

1. Immediately cover the area by placing a plastic-backed absorbent pad, such as a Chux, absorbent side down, over the spill.

2. Remove nonessential person(s) from the room.

3. Isolate contaminated person(s) to minimize the spread of contamination (e.g., use a bathroom to isolate the person).

3. Remove any contaminated clothing and follow steps for skin exposure in section VI. Obtain and review the HD MSDS.

4. Close doors and notify the NIH Fire Department. Report the following:
   ■ Location of the spill
   ■ Name of HD spilled
   ■ Approximate volume of the spill
   ■ Interventions taken

4. The Fire Department will respond and clean the spill.

5. Notify the Head Nurse or Service Supervisor.

VI. Employee, Patient, or Visitor: Accidental Skin, Eye, or Sharp Exposure to HD

A. Equipment
   ■ Soap and water
   ■ Saline solution (room temperature: 1 liter of 0.9% sodium chloride injection or irrigation normal saline or tap water)
   ■ IV tubing to be used for the eye irrigation
   ■ Covered double plastic-lined MPW box
   ■ 2 Pairs of powder-free chemotherapy gloves/Nitrile gloves
   ■ Leak-proof plastic bags that can be sealed
   ■ 3–4 Plastic-backed pads (e.g., Chux)
   ■ Chemotherapy gowns
   ■ Safety goggles
   ■ Plastic-lined isolation linen bag

B. Steps

Key Points

1. For staff: Remove contaminated gown and gloves and place in leak-proof plastic bag, seal, and then place in MPW box.

   For patients and visitors: Remove contaminated clothing and place in plastic bag and seal.

1. Contaminated clothing and linen should be washed separately to avoid contamination of other clothes. They can then be washed a second time in the regular laundry.

Using Cytotoxic Agents in Nonmalignant Conditions   281

(Continued)

TABLE 7.5   Procedure: Safe Handling of Hazardous Drugs (Continued)

2. Immediately wash the affected areas:

   a. Skin areas should be washed with soap and copious amounts of water for at least 10 minutes. Do not use a scrub brush.

   b. For eye exposures, have the individual lie down, place absorbent pads under the head and chin, have a staff member assist by keeping the affected eye open, and then gently irrigate the eye for at least 15 minutes with copious amounts of water or isotonic eye wash, 0.9% sodium chloride irrigation or injection.

   c. For mucous membranes such as the mouth, instruct the individual not to swallow, and flush the mouth with copious amounts of tepid water.

3. After initial treatment measures are taken for employees, patients, or visitors, send employees to the Occupational Medical Services (OMS) for medical examination and treatment. For visitor HD emergencies requiring more than initial treatment measures, call the NIH Fire Department and the Service Supervisor. Notify the Head Nurse or Service Supervisor for all exposures to HD. Notify the primary care physician if the patient is exposed.

C. Document in Medical Record

2.

   a. Scrub brushes may tear the skin and worsen the exposure.

   b. Assistance from a second person may be needed to adequately irrigate the eyes of the affected individual. Both staff members should wear gowns, gloves, and goggles.

3. If OMS is closed, the on-call physician and the Service Supervisor will determine whether the exposure warrants an immediate visit to Suburban Hospital's Emergency Room or if the employee can postpone reporting the exposure until OMS reopens. Obtain and review the MSDS.

Source: Modified from National Institutes of Health. Warren Grant Magnuson Clinical Center.
Note: Each institution develops procedures based on individual institutional programs. This procedure was developed for a research institution and elements of the procedure may not apply in other centers.

are ideally planned using a multidisciplinary team. Setting the stage in every institution for readiness to document and report not only actual errors but also close calls is crucial in creating an atmosphere of safety and a team approach to care. Punitive or blaming strategies in institutions are counterproductive to problem solving and prevention. Staff in all departments must feel secure enough to report errors or close calls to ensure system changes that will promote patient safety. Recently, the practice of public disclosure of health facility errors has facilitated prevention measures nationwide. Mistakes occurring in one facility are possible or probable in another facility. Prevention strategies set in place after medication errors once disclosed can be shared and replicated in other institutions. This will help to reduce the incidence of morbidity and mortality for many patients.

The effectiveness of using a multidisciplinary team approach, which includes a consensus planning conference for patients, is described in a publication by Dr. Rabinowitz. The article outlines the benefits of communication and the advantages of bringing experts within disciplines together for collaborating on the treatment plan (Rabinowitz 2004). Creative use of phone conferencing and telemedicine technologies affords even small facilities the ability to successfully coordinate care in this way.

Health care centers, clinics, doctor offices, and outpatient centers will be increasingly challenged to establish comprehensive safety measures because significant resources are required to establish and maintain a safe environment. Smaller health care facilities may profit from joining with other groups or linking with larger operations as a way to collaborate and share resources. To meet educational needs, smaller health care facilities may want to send staff outside their institution to attend courses in other facilities. Sometimes, larger institutions will contract for educational programs and also make the classes available to smaller facilities. It is a common practice to have experts in larger institutions provide classes or consultations to smaller facilities or even develop consortia of hospitals to share the education of staff.

Oncology Nursing Society Guidelines and Relevance to Staff Caring for Patients with Nonmalignant Conditions

Oncology national organizations, such as the Oncology Nursing Society (ONS), have set the standards for oncology patient care at a high desirable level (Brown *et al.* 2001). These standards could serve as guidelines for multidisciplinary teams providing care to patients with nonmalignant diagnoses. The section of these guidelines on the clinical practicum is particularly helpful because it addresses course description. Each of the objectives in the ONS guidelines for education applies to staff caring for patients with nonmalignant conditions. Clinical activities and staff evaluation are also applicable, with the exception of the section on vesicants, irritants, and extravasation.

The ONS guidelines lists specific agents, such as cytotoxic agents, cytokines, and monoclonal antibodies; patterns of occurrences or complications associated with the drugs; rationale for use; monitoring parameters; and interventions. This information is presented in table formats, which make the references easy to use. Using an evidence-based practice approach, the data is referenced, which allows for rapid exploration of further information applicable to an individual patient. Information in the ONS guidelines is accurate and relevant to nursing practice whether the patients have malignancies or nonmalignant conditions because the drugs and administration strategies are often the same.

Similarities and Differences Between Drug Administration in Malignant and Nonmalignant Conditions

The review of the types of agents used for nonmalignant conditions in patients, found in Table 7.4 reveals some similarities and also some differences between the oncology and the nononcology areas. Some of the same drugs are used in patients both in cancer therapy and in treatment for rheumatic diseases. In individuals with non-Hodgkin's lymphoma who are HIV+, cyclophosphamide and other cytotoxic agents are used along with rituximab in a dose such as 375 mg/m² by intravenous (IV) infusion once weekly for 4–8 doses. In patients with RA, rituximab may used as a single agent for a flare but has been shown to be more effective in combination with methotrexate or cyclophosphamide.

For some of the chemotherapies involving cytotoxic agents, the dosages used in nonmalignant patients will be significantly lower than for oncology patients. Therefore, adverse effect profiles related to drug dosage may differ somewhat between the two groups of patients. For example, individuals with WG may be prescribed cyclophosphamide at a dose of 2 mg/kg/day orally, together with prednisone at 1 mg/kg/day. This dosage is considerably lower than the dosage used in non-Hodgkin's lymphoma. Nadirs for neutropenia may not be as profound for the rheumatic disease patient compared with the patient with a malignancy.

For some time, patients with WG have received oral cytotoxic agents such as cyclophosphamide. Clinicians working with these patients have appreciated the importance of using multiple systems for assuring understanding of drug dosage, schedule, and side effects. Patients are taught about their drug regimens with nurse and pharmacist teaching sessions. Evaluation of understanding is accomplished with verbal feedback from the patient and family. Drug log books are used for patients to document dosages, schedule, and side effects. Case managers and clinic nurses phone patients between clinic visits to help ensure accuracy and safety in drug administration. Patients are asked to bring their drug log books with them to clinic visits. The log books are reviewed, and findings are discussed with the patient. In 2000, Dr. Thomas and colleagues described the onset of use of oral chemotherapy in oncology medicine with agents such as capecitabine, cyclophosphamide, and etoposide (Thomas *et al.* 2000). As programs using oral agents increase for oncology patients, oncology clinicians may choose to incorporate some of the successful clinical teaching strategies used with the rheumatology patients into their practice.

Hypersensitivity reactions may occur with drug administration despite patient condition. Clinicians must be able to recognize the early signs and symptoms of hypersensitivity reactions and take prompt actions to discontinue the drug infusion. The physician or nurse practitioner must be contacted immediately for orders of emergency medications such as epinephrine, benadryl, and IV steroids. The experienced nurse will understand how to manipulate the IV line in such a way as to maintain IV access and patency while minimizing any additional medication from infusing into the patient.

In general, at this time, cytotoxic regimens used in the rheumatic disorders do not contain irritant or vesicant drugs. Therefore, the knowledge of management of extravasation for vesicants or irritants is not required for staff caring for patients with nonmalignant treatments.

The routes of some of the cytotoxic agents may be either oral or IV for rheumatic patients. Some patients with WG receive low-dose oral cyclophosphamide therapy long term, whereas, at other times, these patients receive pulse IV therapy of cyclophosphamide for a disease flare. Issues of safe handling of hazardous agents apply for both groups of patients. For example, an accidental spill of IV cyclophosphamide will have similar ramifications for safety regardless of patient diagnosis, hospital, or clinic area. Therefore, nursing and other institutional staff must understand and use protective personal equipment, such as gloves, gowns, goggles, and masks, as well as safe disposal practices. An example of a procedure for safe handling of hazardous drugs can be found in Table 7.5.

Clinical Competency

Individual oncology nursing staff in large hospitals or medical centers will usually administer cytotoxic agents frequently enough to maintain their competency. This may not always be the case in other centers. In some facilities, staff frequently administer cytotoxic agents and biologic response modifiers with oncology patients but rarely administer these drugs to patients with nonmalignant conditions. Because of this discrepancy of experience, the challenge will be greater for the maintenance of competency with nursing staff if their frequency of using their skills is low.

For example, oncology nurses may administer chemotherapy to more than 4–8 patients a day, 5–7 days a week. Compare this experience to a nurse working on a medical surgical unit caring for patient rheumatic disease who only has the opportunity to administer a cytotoxic agent 2–3 times a year. It is obvious that clinical knowledge and competencies are more difficult to maintain in low-frequency areas.

Patients in every health care setting have a right to receive a high standard of care. Patients expect that the health team will be knowledgeable and experienced with their therapies. How is this accomplished in settings where the staff has a low frequency of use of these powerful agents? Some of the strategies for obtaining and maintaining clinical competency for nursing staff include the following:

1. Cluster care of the patients in limited inpatient or outpatient areas with staff who will have a high frequency of experience in administering the agents. For example, one facility may decide that any patient receiving cytotoxic agents, monoclonal antibodies, or biologic response modifiers will come to the oncology area whether the patient has a malignancy or rheumatic disorder. This decision will ensure that staff will be familiar with the drugs and process for drug administration. Educational needs of the staff will need to expand to concepts related to the rheumatic diseases to ensure that staff understand the differences between patient diagnoses and drug dosages.

2. Prepare a core group of nursing staff throughout an institution for knowledge and skill acquisition. Ensure that updated policies and structure to maintain competencies with the core staff are available. Follow through with evaluation of staff competency and knowledge at prescribed intervals. Staff significant

numbers of the core group of staff on any inpatient or outpatient area of the institution where the special agents are used.

3. Provide comprehensive education and validation of competency for all staff on any area where the patient may require the agents. Establish policies about the minimum required number of drug administrations for each staff nurse each year. Periodically assign nurses requiring more drug administration experiences to a unit where the agents are given frequently. Validate knowledge and competency according to institution policy.

4. Obtain the acceptance of staff for the need to be accountable for their knowledge and competency to not only enhance their own clinical repertoire but also to ensure patient safety.

5. Obtain the support of the management team for staff education, competency, and periodic revalidation of competency. The nurse manager support is essential for staff to obtain and maintain knowledge and skills through course work and adequate scheduling to high-frequency areas for drug administration.

6. Encourage staff to challenge their assignment if they are asked to administer cytotoxic agents, monoclonal antibodies, and biologic response modifiers if they have knowledge and skill deficits. Nurses should recognize not only personal limitations of knowledge and competency but also be able to help identify any other deficiencies in the facility for the safe administration of these agents. In these instances, direct communication between the nurse and manager will help ensure a high standard of care. These efforts will not only protect patients but help ensure that the staff are in alignment with national and regional standards of care.

Educational Program

Some institutions are requiring nurses who care for patients with nonmalignant conditions but administer these specialized drug therapies to attend cancer chemotherapy education courses. Other institutions are requiring a separate course.

An example of an initial educational program for preparing nononcology nursing staff for administration of cytotoxic agents, monoclonal antibodies, and biologic response modifiers begins with a 1-day didactic program and a simulation experience for chemotherapy administration. This day is followed by a knowledge test and clinical competency validation experiences. The sequence of test taking and successful passing of the test prior to the clinical situation is important.

Presenters for the didactic program include nursing staff, clinical nurse specialists, pharmacists, physicians, and nurse practitioners. The specific drugs presented are selected based on actual agents dispensed by the institution. Food and Drug Administration (FDA)–approved therapies as well as active research protocol regimens constitute the list of agents presented in the class. Class content relevant to agents is updated as new drugs are introduced by the institution.

The following topics constitute an example of an initial didactic program that was developed at the National Institutes of Health by a nursing group led by an experienced clinical oncology nurse educator.

- Cell function and pathophysiology
- Principles of administration for cytotoxic agents, monoclonal antibodies, and biologic response modifiers
- Rationale for use of these agents in nonmalignant conditions
- Specific drugs
  - Drug classification
  - Mechanism of action
  - Dosage routes
  - Intravenous (IV) compatibilities
- Administration of drugs
  - IV therapy techniques
    - Personal protective equipment (PPE) requirements
    - Use of gauze and protective pads during spiking of IV tubing or use of syringe
    - Back flow methods using non–drug-containing flushes to purge air from IV tubing
    - Special tubing issues for certain agents
    - IV access issues
    - Techniques for IV push, piggyback, and continuous therapies
- Nursing implications, including management of complications and adverse effects
  - Initial patient nursing history and physical examination, including patient weight, height, body surface area (BSA), previous therapies and responses, and allergies
  - Common nursing assessments and interventions based on expected or untoward drug complications
  - Medical record review (progress notes; medical orders including drug, dose, and any modifications based on condition or laboratory results; drug diluent type; route; schedule; and duration of infusion), safety laboratory test results, such as pregnancy test, and treatment and research informed consents
  - Verification process for calculations of drugs and drug label
  - Teaching patients and family members about expected effects of drug therapies, potential complications, and patient and family actions for management or prevention of complications; assessment of patient and family understanding of planned therapies.
  - Drug-specific preventative therapies for common complications, including but not limited to: pretherapy hydration, monitoring intake and output, use of agents, such as mesna and antiemetics, and laboratory safety testing
  - Standards of practice, policies, and procedures for administration of cytotoxic and biologic agents; see Table 7.5 for an example of a standard of practice for administration of cytotoxic or biologic agents and a procedure for safe handling of hazardous drugs
  - Documentation requirements

- Procedures for spills of hazardous agents
  - Use of hospital spill kit and patient spill kit
  - Patient and family teaching about hazardous drugs and body fluids
- Disposal of equipment (e.g., IV tubing and residual drug)
- Institution policies and procedures
  - Emergency equipment and medications
  - Oxygen therapy
  - Suction therapy
  - Emergency medications including but not limited to:
    - Epinephrine 1:1000 units per 1 ml SC route
    - Benadryl 50 mg/ml
    - Solu Cortef IV 100 mg/2 ml
- Common interventions for adverse events occurring during administration (e.g., anaphylaxis and hypersensitivity); crash cart use
- Institutional documents
  - Policies denoting prerequisite administration competencies for cytotoxic agents, monoclonal antibodies, and biologic response modifiers
  - Procedures for management of hazardous agents
  - Standard of practice for administration of agents
  - Knowledge test
  - Clinical validation of competency (Quint-Kastner *et al.* 2000)

Formal didactic programs must be linked with a system for observation of clinical competency. Institutions may opt to use a mentor or preceptor system where the experienced competency-validated nurse demonstrates care of the patient and administration of agents to the novice. Next, the novice cares for the patient and administers the agents under the close supervision of an experienced nurse. Some staff will require more than one return demonstration of patient preparation and drug administration to validate competency.

Prerequisite courses and competency validation are required prior to course work and include:

- IV administration and vascular access class
- Basic cardiac life support
- Mock cardiac life support scenarios on clinical units

Conclusion

From this chapter, it can be determined that the administration of cancer therapies, especially the newer agents, is more than just pushing poisons. It is both an art and a science that requires didactic knowledge and technical skills. The process of chemotherapy administration involves the entire team, including the patient and the family, and covers the gamut of informed consent through prescription writing, dose calculation, assessment, and evaluation of the patient for side-effect management. It is medication administration at its very finest. The administration of cancer therapies involves every aspect of the nursing process and working with every member of the multidisciplinary team. It is a very humbling experience for every nurse who ventures to care for the cancer patient requiring this type of treatment.

The care of patients with nonmalignant conditions is complex because the therapies are high risk, and many of the patients are exceptionally vulnerable because of their illnesses. Fortunately, outstanding guidelines for clinical care of these patients are available. By using the relevant elements of the ONS guidelines and through the use of best practice strategies, patients have the opportunity to achieve disease remission. Successful clinical management is achievable through the compliance to standards of care and procedures, best practices in administration, staff education, validation of competency, multidisciplinary planning, use of evidence-based practice models, quality assurance efforts, and dedication to the patients and families. This process is difficult, but the rewards are satisfying as we observe the relief of disease in our patients.

References

American Society of Clinical Oncology (ASCO). 2004a. *Statement regarding the use of outside services to prepare or administer chemotherapy drugs.* Alexandria, VA: American Society of Clinical Oncology.

American Society of Clinical Oncology (ASCO). 2004b. Criteria for facilities and personnel for the administration of parenteral systemic antineoplastic therapy. *Journal of Clinical Oncology* 22(22):1–3.

American Society of Health-Systems Pharmacists (ASHP) Council on Professional Affairs. 2002. ASHP guidelines on preventing medication errors with antineoplastic agents. *American Journal of Health-System Pharmacy* 59(17):1648–1668.

Barton-Burke, M., Wilkes, G., and Ingwersen, K. 2001. *Cancer chemotherapy: A nursing process approach* (ed 3). Sudbury, MA: Jones & Bartlett Publishers, Inc.

Birner, A. 2003. Safe administration of oral chemotherapy. *Clinical Journal of Oncology Nursing* 7(2):158–161.

Brown, K.A., Esper, P., Kelleher, L., O'Neill, J.E.B., Polovich, M., and White, J.M. 2001. *Oncology Nursing Society chemotherapy and biotherapy: Guidelines and recommendations for practice.* Pittsburgh: Oncology Nursing Society.

Buyon, J. 2001. Systemic lupus erythematosus: B. Clinical and laboratory features. In J.H. Klippel, L.J. Crofford, J.H. Stone, and C.M. Weyand (Eds): *Primer on the rheumatic diseases* (ed 12). Atlanta: Arthritis Foundation, pp 335–346.

Connor, T., Anderson, R.W., Sessink, P.J., Broadfield, L., and Power, L.A. 1999. Surface contamination with antineoplastic agents in six cancer treatment centers in Canada and the United States. *American Journal of Health-System Pharmacy* 56(14):1427–1432.

Department of Health and Human Services (DHHS). 2004. *Antineoplastic agents: Occupational hazards in hospitals.* DHHS (NIOSH) Publication Number 2004-102. Cincinnati: NIOSH–Publications Dissemination.

Fischer, D.S., Alfano, S., Knobf, M.T., Donovan, C., and Beaulieu, N. 1996. Improving the cancer chemotherapy use process. *Journal of Clinical Oncology* 14(24):3148–3155.

Fortenbaugh, C., and Rummel, M. 2004. Chemotherapy safety. *Clinical Journal of Oncology Nursing* 8(4):424–425.

Institute of Medicine (IOM). 1999. *To Err is human: Building a Safer Health System.* Washington, DC: National Academy Press, http://www.nap.edu/books/0309068371/html.

Langhorne, M., and Barton-Burke, M. 2001. Chemotherapy administration: General principles for nursing practice.

In M. Barton-Burke, G.M. Wilkes, and K.C. Ingwersen (Eds): *Cancer chemotherapy: A nursing process approach* (ed 3). Sudbury, MA: Jones and Bartlett, pp 608–643.

Martin, S., and Larson, E. 2003. Chemotherapy-handling practices of outpatient and office-based oncology nurses. *Oncology Nursing Forum* 30(4):575–581.

National Institute for Occupational Safety and Health (NIOSH). 2004. *Preventing occupational exposure to antineoplastic and other hazardous drugs in health care settings.* DHHS (NIOSH) Publication Number 2004-165. Cincinnati: NIOSH–Publications Dissemination.

Opfer, K.B., Wirtz, D.M., and Farley, K. 1999. A chemotherapy standard order form: Preventing errors. *Oncology Nursing Forum* 26(1):123–128.

Polovich, M. (Ed.) 2003. *Safe handling of hazardous drugs.* Pittsburgh: Oncology Nursing Society.

Quint-Kastner, S., Woolery-Antil, M., and Peterson, A. 2000. *Course: Administration of cytotoxic and biologic agents for non-malignancies.* Bethesda, MD: National Institutes of Health.

Rabinowitz, B. 2004. Interdisciplinary breast cancer care: Declaring and improving the standard. *Oncology* 18(10):1263–1267.

Rogers, B.B. 1999. Preventing and detecting cancer chemotherapy drug errors. *Oncology Nursing Updates: Patient Treatment and Support* 6(1):1–12.

Schulmeister, L. 1999. Chemotherapy medication errors: Descriptions, severity, and contributing factors. *Oncology Nursing Forum* 26(6):1033–1041.

Sitzia, J., and Wood, N. 1998. Patient satisfaction with cancer chemotherapy nursing: A review of the literature. *International Journal of Nursing Studies* 35(1–2):1–12.

Spath, M.L., Rimkus, C.F., and Saenz, D.A. 1998. A chemotherapy and infusion therapy flow sheet for outpatient oncology settings. *Oncology Nursing Forum* 25(1):129–135.

Thomas, F., Cahill, A., Mortenson, L., and Schoenfeldt, M. 2000. Oral chemotherapy, cytostatic, and supportive care agents new opportunities and challenges. *Oncology*, 15(2):23–25.

Tse, H., and Shaw, M. 2004. Autoimmunity and disease. In G.B. Pier, J.B. Lyczak, and L.M. Wetzler (Eds): *Immunology, infection, and immunity.* Washington, DC: American Society for Microbiology, pp 625–648.

Wilkes, G., and Barton-Burke, M. 2005. *2005 Oncology drug handbook.* Sudbury, MA: Jones & Bartlett Publishers.

Womer, R.B., Tracy, E., Soo-Hoo, W., Bickert, B., DiTaranto, S., and Barnsteiner, J.H. 2002. Multidisciplinary systems approach to chemotherapy safety: Rebuilding processes and holding gains. *Journal of Clinical Oncology* 20(24):4705–4712.

Drug Interactions with Antineoplastic Medications

Michael Steinberg, Pharm.D., BCOP

Introduction

Drug interactions are known to occur with many common drugs through a variety of mechanisms involving all aspects of pharmacokinetics including absorption, distribution, metabolism, and elimination. Absorption is the process by which medications move away from the site of administration. For example, drugs taken orally must move from the lumen of the gastrointestinal tract into the systemic circulation. Bioavailability is the fraction of the drug dose that actually reaches the site of action. Factors that may affect absorption and bioavailability include properties of the drug, drug delivery systems, and the environment of the area where the drug is absorbed. Drugs then spread throughout the body in the distribution phase in various concentrations to different tissues depending on the drugs physicochemical characteristics and physiological factors. Plasma protein binding, hydrophobic characteristics, tissue binding, and pH could all affect distribution. Over time, the drugs may be altered by metabolic processes converting the molecules to a form that may or may not provide additional pharmacologic activity and may even be toxic in certain concentrations but are easier to eliminate from the body. These biotransformation reactions may be performed by enzymes such as the cytochrome P450 (CYP450) enzyme system. The CYP450 system is a superfamily of about 50 enzymes that metabolize many drugs and

other chemicals. The CYP450 enzymes are identified through a nomenclature that uses a number to designate each family, followed by a capitalized letter to indicate the subfamily and another number for the individual isoform of each enzyme in the subfamily. Some drugs are metabolized through other methods besides CYP450 enzymes or may not undergo any metabolic transformation prior to elimination from the body. Finally, the elimination process is the method by which the body seeks to rid itself of the original chemical entity or its metabolites (Hardman *et al.* 2001).

Some interactions are pharmacodynamic in effect and thus involve the actual activity of the drugs. Any factor that could affect the mechanism of action of the drug would alter its pharmacodynamics. For example, changes in the molecular target of the drug, the number of targets for the drug, or changes in the way the drug interacts with the target could all change the ultimate benefits or adverse effects of the drug.

With regard to drug interactions, chemotherapeutic drugs to treat cancer are no different than drugs used for other conditions. However, there are some factors that make drug interactions involving chemotherapy more important as well as less understood. For example, significant side effects, such as myelosuppression, nausea, vomiting, hepatotoxicity, nephrotoxicity, and others, can occur with use of chemotherapy and vary from patient to patient. Drug interactions can prolong the presence of chemotherapy drugs in the body, leading to a worsening of already difficult to tolerate adverse effects or increasing the risk of toxicity. Likewise, many chemotherapeutic drugs have characteristics that make them carcinogenic, mutagenic, and teratogenic. Drug interactions that reduce active levels of chemotherapy may reduce the efficacy and limit the therapeutic benefits. These effects make direct study of drug interactions unethical. Therefore, drug interactions are often described anecdotally or as theoretical possibilities based on drug characteristics. Furthermore, dose adjustments based on the potential for a drug interaction may be controversial because of the risk of either reducing the anticancer effect or increasing the adverse effects because of the unpredictability of the interaction. Therefore, even though many interactions with chemotherapy exist, caution is suggested, but changes in dosing are often not available. Given the highly variable nature of potential drug interactions, it is crucial to take into consideration each patient's clinical condition when assessing the likelihood or clinical significance of such interactions. Therefore, when assessing the potential for a drug interaction involving chemotherapy, one must consider the overall status of the patient and what result may occur with changes in therapy. The broad use of many medications by each patient increases the risk of a drug interaction. The evaluation of all drugs a patient is receiving allows for the assessment of the potential for a drug interaction. Upon identification of these interactions, steps may or may not be made to ameliorate the impact these interactions have on the effect of the patient's medications. This activity necessitates the need to determine all medications a patient is taking, both prescription and over-the-counter, each time the patient is prescribed a chemotherapy medication. It is also important to keep in mind that chemotherapy medications are available in an assortment of dosage forms and classes, such as oral and intravenous medications and targeted immunotherapy or traditional chemotherapy.

This chapter will discuss a number of interactions and their mechanisms that exist with chemotherapy medications. Although some of these interactions are manageable with alterations in administering or dosing the drugs, most interactions with chemotherapy are poorly understood, and resolutions to minimize the impact of the effects are not formally available. Therefore, in some cases, although an interaction may occur, no change in therapy is recommended.

Pharmacokinetic Interactions

Absorption (Including Drug–Food) Interactions

Absorption of most drugs taken orally occurs in the small intestine. Drug interactions that affect absorption of drugs either increase or decrease the percentage of drug that is absorbed and available for systemic action. Additionally, some interactions may change the rate at which drugs are absorbed, while the actual amount remains unchanged.

In general, the absorption of oral digoxin may be substantially decreased in patients receiving certain antineoplastic agents. Some cancer chemotherapy agents may cause transient damage to the intestinal mucosa, resulting in altered digoxin absorption. This effect has been reported in patients receiving bleomycin, carmustine, cyclophosphamide, cytarabine, doxorubicin, methotrexate, procarbazine, and vincristine (Tatro 1991), but other drugs may cause the effect as well. Thus, serum levels of digoxin, as well as the desired response, need to be monitored, and dosing regimens of digoxin may need to be adjusted accordingly. Using alternative dosage forms, such as digoxin elixir or liquid-filled capsules, may reduce the risk of this interaction because of more rapid absorption.

Likewise, phenytoin absorption may be decreased in patients receiving agents such as bleomycin, carboplatin, carmustine, cisplatin, methotrexate, and vinblastine (Tatro 1991) potentially predisposing patients to subtherapeutic levels and the risk of

TABLE 8.1 PharmacoKinetic Drug Interactions

Substrate	Affecting Agent	Result	Mechanism	Response
Digoxin	Various agents, i.e., bleomycin, carmustine, cyclophosphamide, cytarabine, doxorubicin, methotrexate, procarbazine, vincristine	Decreased digoxin absorption	Damage to intestinal mucosa	Use digoxin elixir or liquid-filled capsules; monitor serum digoxin level and effect
Phenytoin	Various agents, i.e., bleomycin, carboplatin, carmustine, cisplatin, methotrexate, vinblastine	Decreased phenytoin absorption	Damage to intestinal mucosa	Consider using parenteral phenytoin; monitor serum phenytoin level and effect
Tamoxifen, theophylline, warfarin	Aminoglutethimide	Increased metabolism of substrates	Inhibits metabolism	Avoid combinations with aminoglutethimide; monitor substrate levels or effect
Carmustine	Cimetidine	Enhanced myelosuppression	Inhibits metabolism	Avoid cimetidine use with carmustine; monitor blood counts
Mercaptopurine (MP)	Allopurinol	Increased side effects	Inhibits metabolism	Avoid allopurinol use with MP or reduce MP dose to 25–33% of original dose
Methotrexate (MTX)	NSAIDs, large doses of penicillins	Increased MTX toxicity	Alter renal tubular secretion of MTX	Avoid combination of NSAIDs and MTX
Methotrexate	Salicylates	Increased MTX toxicity	Delay renal excretion	Avoid combination of salicylates and MTX
Methotrexate	Salicylate, sulfonamides, sulfonylureas, phenytoin	Increased MTX toxicity	Displacement of MTX from plasma proteins	Avoid concomitant use of MTX with these agents

NSAIDS, nonsteroidal anti-inflammatory drugs.
Source: King, R. 1995. Drug interactions with cancer chemotherapy. *Cancer Practice* 3(1):58–59. Reprinted with permission.

seizures. In these patients, serum levels of phenytoin must be monitored, and doses should be adjusted accordingly. The use of parenteral phenytoin can avoid this potential interaction by bypassing the absorption process from the gastrointestinal tract altogether.

Because of the altered immune function of oncology patients to fight off infection, they are often at risk of potentially fatal fungal infections. Severe and prolonged neutropenia, stem-cell transplantation, and acute leukemia are risk factors for fungal infections. Because of this known risk, antifungal agents, such as itraconazole, voriconazole, amphotericin, or caspofungin, are indicated to manage oropharyngeal and esophageal candidiasis as well as serious systemic infections caused by *Aspergillus* and other fungi. Long-term use of these agents is not uncommon. The widespread use of these agents and the likelihood of drug interactions suggests that a brief discussion of these drugs is appropriate.

Itraconazole and voriconazole are available both orally and intravenously. Optimal absorption of these agents would be ideal to achieve therapeutic systemic concentrations. Itraconazole capsules require an acidic environment for optimal absorption. Concomitant use of medications that reduce the acidity of the stomach (i.e., increase pH) can reduce bioavailability and reduce the antifungal effectiveness. These medications include liquid antacids, histamine type 2 (H2) receptor blockers (e.g., cimetidine, ranitidine, nizatidine, famotidine), and proton pump inhibitors (e.g, omeprazole, lansoprazole, pantoprazole, rabeprazole).

Often, the use of antacid therapy is unavoidable. In these cases, antacid therapy should be administered at a minimum of 2 hours following itraconazole. The itraconazole capsules should also be taken with food to enhance absorption. Itraconazole is available in an oral solution, which has a greater bioavailability than the capsules when taken on an empty stomach and is not affected by antacids. Other alternatives to using oral itraconazole include the intravenous formulations of itraconazole, voriconazole, amphotericin, or caspofungin or the oral voriconazole, the absorption of which is not affected by pH.

Induction or Inhibition of Metabolism

The cytochrome P450 (CYP450) enzyme system is a group of enzymes that metabolize many medications. The active levels of these enzymes can be induced or inhibited by certain drugs, resulting in increases or decreases, respectively, in the rate of the metabolism of drugs that are affected, referred to as the substrate. If the metabolism of a drug is reduced by the inhibition of an enzyme, clearance of the drug is slowed. This can result in prolonged and/or increased levels of the drug, causing a greater effect and/or risk of adverse effects or toxicity. If the metabolism of a drug is increased because of the induction of an enzyme, the drug is cleared faster from the circulation. This can result in less drug activity and failure of therapy.

CYP450 enzyme inducers include barbiturates such as phenobarbital and other anticonvulsants such as phenytoin and carbamazepine. The H2 receptor blocker cimetidine, the antimicrobial rifampin, and azole antifungals such as ketoconazole, fluconazole, itraconazole, and voriconazole are considered enzyme inhibitors. There are many different CYP450 enzymes, and the effect each drug has on each enzyme varies significantly. Furthermore, interactions involving the CYP450 system can be unpredictable and depend on the presence of other factors that may influence metabolism and need to be taken into consideration when assessing the possibility of a drug interaction.

Aminoglutethimide

Aminoglutethimide, an aromatase inhibitor used in breast cancer, increases the activity of CYP450 3A4, which is the enzyme responsible for metabolizing most drugs. One of the drugs affected is tamoxifen, which is also used in breast cancer. This enzyme-inhibiting interaction effect has been proposed to have occurred in six women with breast cancer who received the combination of tamoxifen and aminoglutethimide for 6 weeks (Lien *et al.* 1990). These patients were observed to have a decreased area under the concentration versus time curve (AUC) because of increased enzymatic clearance of tamoxifen. The mean decrease in AUC was 73%, with a mean increase in clearance of 222%. If possible, these two agents should not be administered together because the response of breast cancer patients to tamoxifen may be compromised. Fortunately, concomitant administration of both drugs usually does not occur because aminoglutethimide is typically reserved for use as a second-line agent in women who may have already received tamoxifen in the past but are no longer receiving it.

The metabolism of warfarin can be affected by aminoglutethimide. A case report describes two breast cancer patients receiving both of these agents who experienced a reduced anticoagulant effect secondary to a significant increase in warfarin metabolism (Lonning *et al.* 1984). Because of the risks of suboptimal actions of warfarin, close monitoring of the international normalized ratio (INR) is necessary to confirm adequate anticoagulation. Doses of warfarin should then be adjusted based on the target INR of the particular indication. If aminoglutethimide therapy is discontinued during treatment with warfarin, the warfarin dose may need to be readjusted to reflect the removal of the aminoglutethimide effect.

Aminoglutethimide can increase the metabolism of other drugs as well. For instance, there is a known effect to increase metabolism of theophylline, resulting in potentially subtherapeutic serum concentrations. The availability of newer bronchodilators combined with a new generation of aromatase inhibitors for breast cancer has reduced the frequency of this interaction, and thus, it stands mainly as an example of the effects of an interaction.

Carmustine

As previously mentioned, cimetidine is an enzyme inhibitor. It has been reported to enhance the myelosuppressive effects of carmustine either by inhibiting the usual metabolism of carmustine, resulting in increased levels of the drug, or through additive effects of the two agents on the bone marrow. Concomitant administration of the drug with cimetidine should be avoided if possible to decrease the potential for greater myelosuppression, delayed neutrophil recovery, and the resulting increased risk for infection. Resolution of this interaction can be made by using an alternative H2 blocker, such as ranitidine, famotidine, or nizatidine, or a proton pump inhibitor such as pantoprazole, lansoprazole, or omeprazole. These alternatives would provide the reduced levels of stomach acid that are often necessary in cancer patients for stress or peptic ulcer prophylaxis or treatment and management of stress-related mucosal bleeding.

6-Mercaptopurine

6-Mercaptopurine (6-MP) is commonly used in the treatment of acute lymphocytic leukemia. Allopurinol is frequently used to either treat or prevent hyperuricemia associated with tumor lysis syndrome that may occur in patients with acute leukemia. Allopurinol works by inhibiting the enzyme xanthine oxidase, which is used to convert hypoxanthine to xanthine and then xanthine to uric acid. Xanthine oxidase is also responsible for the metabolism of 6-MP after oral administration. When allopurinol and oral 6-MP are used simultaneously, allopurinol inhibits the metabolism of 6-MP, resulting in large increases of active drug. This can increase the antineoplastic effects as well as the adverse effects, such as nausea, vomiting, and myelosuppression. Therefore, if the two agents must be given together, the 6-MP dose should be reduced to 25–33% of the usual dose (i.e., a 67–75% dose reduction). Because the interaction occurs upon first pass metabolism of the 6-MP directly after absorption, administration of the intravenous form of 6-MP avoids the interaction. Another practice is to discontinue the use of allopurinol when the threat of hyperuricemia from tumor lysis has resolved. This allows the 6-MP dosing to occur without the threat of the interaction.

Warfarin

Because of the anticoagulant action of warfarin, bleeding is an inherent risk of its usage. Therapy in the setting of cancer chemotherapy is no different. In fact, there are multiple drug interactions that practitioners must be aware of when a patient is receiving warfarin during treatment with some antineoplastic agents. The rhythmic use of chemotherapy over a period of many weeks to months can produce an on/off effect, with warfarin necessitating very close monitoring to safeguard against thrombotic or hemorrhagic complications.

Fluorouracil (5-FU) is one agent that has been described in many case reports to have the potential to interact with warfarin. One case report described a patient treated with low-dose warfarin (1 mg/day) for prevention of thrombosis associated with the placement of a hepatic artery catheter. Prior to starting 5-FU, to treat liver metastases from a primary lung cancer, the patient's INR was normal despite the use of drugs such as trimethoprim-sulfamethoxazole and dexamethasone. During follow-up evaluation of the patient 16 days after receiving the 5-FU, the patient's INR was 8.4. Phytonadione was given, and the INR was reduced. It was felt by the author that the 5-FU was directly responsible for the elevated INR (Brown 1999).

This case is significant because it shows that the effect can occur with even low doses of warfarin. Another case report described multisite mucous membrane bleeding and hematuria in a patient with metastatic colon cancer who was receiving chronic anticoagulation therapy and was initiated on a chemotherapy regimen with 5-FU and leucovorin (Brown 1997). 5-FU was administered as a weekly bolus for 4 weeks. This resulted in an elevated INR to 35.9, although it had been in the therapeutic range prior to starting 5-FU. To resolve the interaction, the patient was restarted on a lower dose of warfarin.

Five patients at another institution were reported to have a similar interaction between 5-FU and warfarin (Kolesar *et al.* 1999). These patients had either metastatic colon or breast cancer and were treated with 5-FU–containing regimens. 5-FU appears to have been administered as a bolus in the majority of cases. All patients had been receiving chronic anticoagulation prior to initiation of chemotherapy. An increased INR dictated warfarin dose reductions in all patients. One patient had a major bleeding event. This effect may be a result of the inhibition by 5-FU on the CYP450 enzyme CYP2C9, which is responsible for metabolizing warfarin.

5-FU has been shown to affect other drugs with narrow therapeutic indexes. For example, a case report of a patient maintained on phenytoin for a generalized seizure disorder began treatment with 5-FU for rectal cancer. After the second cycle of 5-FU, the patient was noted to have a 1-week history of unsteadiness, blurred vision, and bilateral and horizontal nystagmus during lateral gaze. Her phenytoin level at this time was measured to be 47.5µg/ml (target 10–20 µg/ml). Phenytoin is metabolized primarily by CYP2C9, with secondary metabolism by CYP2C19, and then conjugated, and the metabolites are excreted in the urine. 5-FU may inhibit CYP2C9, resulting in reduced metabolism of phenytoin and potentially increased levels (Rosemergy 2002). This represents another interaction by 5-FU on hepatic enzymes that can result in potentially supertherapeutic levels. Patients receiving 5-FU along with other drugs require close monitoring for signs of toxicity as well as therapeutic drug levels to recognize situations that require adjustments in dosage.

Capecitabine

Capecitabine is an oral prodrug of 5-FU indicated for the treatment of metastatic breast cancer. Because capecitabine and 5-FU result in the same active component, their interactions with other drugs are similar. Therefore, as expected, there have been reports of altered coagulation parameters and/or bleeding in patients receiving warfarin and capecitabine concomitantly (Xeloda [capecitabine] product information 2003). As with 5-FU, because of the increased risk of bleeding with an elevated INR, close monitoring is warranted in patients receiving warfarin and capecitabine, and a dose reduction of warfarin may be necessary.

Imatinib

Imatinib represents one of the newer, targeted therapies used in oncology. It is used to treat leukemias, such as chronic myelogenous leukemia, that involve the Philadelphia chromosome, a pathologic gene rearrangement that results in overactive tyrosine kinase activity. Imatinib is known to have increased serum levels when taken in combination with ketoconazole because of the CYP3A4-inhibitory effect of the antifungal. This effect is likely to occur with other drugs that inhibit CYP3A4 as well, just as CYP3A4 inducers could decrease imatinib plasma concentrations. Interestingly, imatinib also has CYP3A4-inhibitory effects, which have been shown to increase the area under the concentration versus time curve (AUC) of the antihyperlipidemia drug simvastatin by 3.5-fold. In vitro studies have also shown that imatinib also is a potent inhibitor of CYP2C9, 2D6, and 3A5, which increases the chances for other drug interactions (Gleevec [imatinib] product information 2004). This could increase the risk of side effects for people taking this medication.

Cyclosporine/Tacrolimus

Cyclosporine (CSA) and tacrolimus are immunosuppressant agents frequently used to prevent graft-versus-host disease (GVHD) in patients after allogeneic stem-cell transplantation. Tacrolimus and CSA are metabolized in part by CYP3A4. The azole antifungals, such as voriconazole, itraconazole, and fluconazole, can inhibit the metabolism of CSA and tacrolimus by inhibiting CYP3A4, leading to increased blood levels. Even at therapeutic doses of these immunosuppressants, toxicity can occur and may include hepatotoxicity, neurotoxicity, nephrotoxicity, and hypertension. When voriconazole is used, the tacrolimus dose is recommended to be reduced to one third of the original dose (66% dose reduction), and CSA is recommended to be reduced to

one half of the original dose (50% dose reduction) (Vfend [voriconazole] product information 2004). As for fluconazole or itraconazole use with these immunosuppressants, close monitoring or serum levels for clinical signs and symptoms of increased toxicity is warranted. Close observation of a patient for excessive tremors, increases in blood pressure, serum creatinine, or liver function tests are examples of better ways to assess increased toxicity (Diflucan [fluconazole] product information 2004; Sporanox [itraconazole] product information 2004).

Grapefruit juice is an unlikely inhibitor of CYP3A4, but it can lead to increased blood levels of CSA or tacrolimus. Patients who drink grapefruit juice regularly should be made aware of the potential interaction and monitored closely for signs of increased toxicity. This type of interaction, although highly variable, represents the significant effect foods may have on metabolism of drugs.

There are many other drugs that interact with CSA through the CYP450 system, and each needs to be assessed individually for their impact on therapy. The antiepileptics phenytoin, carbamazepine, and phenobarbital represent a group of agents that are infamous for their induction effects on hepatic CYP450 enzymes. A study by Relling et al. (2000) looked at the effect enzyme-inducing anticonvulsants could have on the treatment of patients with acute lymphoblastic leukemia with chemotherapy. The authors retrospectively looked at 716 patients treated with chemotherapy including different combinations of prednisone, vincristine, cytarabine, etoposide, teniposide, daunorubicin, asparaginase, mercaptopurine, cyclophosphamide, and methotrexate. Of these 716 patients, 40 were found to have received phenytoin, a barbiturate, or carbamazepine for at least 30 days. The patients were then analyzed for event-free survival and duration of remission. It was found that the use of an anticonvulsant resulted in a significantly worse event-free survival ($P = .0009$). The mean plasma clearances of teniposide and methotrexate were found to be significantly lower in patients who did not receive an anticonvulsant (teniposide, $P = .0001$; and methotrexate, $P = .051$). Therefore, the levels of these agents were lower in patients on the anticonvulsants. This lower chemotherapy exposure may be a result of the induction of the CYP3A4 enzyme. This may put patients at risk of a reduced effect of treatment for their leukemia. This is one of the few studies available that actually shows that chemotherapy levels can be affected by drugs taken concomitantly and that this can affect the response to chemotherapy. Another drug that has been suggested to interact with antiepileptics is paclitaxel, which can have an increased metabolism associated with enzyme induction from anticonvulsants (Baker 2001). Unfortunately, many of these and other interactions require more investigation, and formal recommendations are not available to guide decision making. Table 8.2 shows enzymes that are involved in metabolizing many chemotherapy agents. Table 8.3 lists drug interactions involving chemotherapy agents and the metabolic enzyme effectors.

The combination antibacterial quinupristin and dalfopristin can be used for the treatment of vancomycin-resistant *Enterococcus faecium* (VRE) and other complicated skin and skin structure infections. Quinupristin/dalfopristin has been demonstrated *in vitro* to significantly inhibit CYP450 metabolism of CSA (Synercid I.V. [quinupristin and dalfopristin] product information 1999). If quinupristin/dalfopristin is used concomitantly with CSA, monitoring of CSA blood levels and signs and symptoms of toxicity should be performed.

Distribution and/or Elimination Interactions

Distribution interactions typically involve the displacement of one highly protein-bound drug by another. Only the unbound, free fraction of a drug is active. Therefore, competition for the limited amount of protein binding sites by two drugs can increase the free fraction, or availability, of one drug over the other. Increased availability of the free drug most likely will lead to an increased activity as well as side effects.

Because the kidneys are major sites of drug elimination or excretion, they are involved in most elimination interactions. Normal elimination can be impaired if changes in glomerular filtration rate, tubular secretion, or urine pH occur. These changes often result from the administration of other drugs.

Paclitaxel

Paclitaxel is another commonly used chemotherapy agent that carries the risk of increasing warfarin activity. A report described a woman with ovary cancer receiving treatment with warfarin for a deep vein thrombosis for 2 months prior to receiving paclitaxel. With the first dose of paclitaxel, her INR rose to 5.2. Temporary discontinuation of the warfarin allowed the INR to drop back to the target level, at which time warfarin was restarted. A similar scenario occurred after the next five cycles of paclitaxel. Although the patient was on other medications at the time, including ranitidine, dexamethasone, and ondansetron, pharmacokinetics of paclitaxel support its culpability. Both paclitaxel and warfarin are highly plasma protein bound. The two drugs competing for binding sites could easily result in an increase in the free, active levels of warfarin. When considering the effect paclitaxel may have on CYP450 enzymes, it is seen that CYP2C8 and CYP3A4 are used for paclitaxel, but CYP2C9 and CYP1A2 metabolize warfarin. Therefore, the effect is unlikely to be a result of effects on liver enzymes (Thompson 2003).

Methotrexate

Potentially significant drug interactions of methotrexate (MTX), especially when given in high doses, occur with nonsteroidal anti-inflammatory drugs (NSAIDs) such as ibuprofen (Motrin, Advil), diclofenac (Voltaren), ketoprofen (Orudis) and, naproxen (Anaprox, Naprosyn, Alleve); penicillins such as amoxicillin, amoxicillin with clavulanic acid (Augmentin), piperacillin with tazobactam (Zosyn), and penicillin; and salicylates such as aspirin and bismuth subsalicylate (Pepto Bismol).

TABLE 8.2 CYP450 Enzymes Responsible for Chemotherapy Metabolism

CYP3A4	CYP1A1	CYP2D6	CYP2B6
Bortezomib Busulfan Cyclophosphamide Ifosfamide Thiotepa (major) Fluorouracil Docetaxel (required for activation) Vincristine Vinorelbine Etoposide (major) Teniposide (major) Irinotecan Doxorubicin Flutamide Toremifene Glucocorticoids (metabolism and induction) Imatinib	Dacarbazine (required for activation)	Bortezomib Fluorouracil Tamoxifen (required for potent active metabolite) Imatinib (minor)	Ifosfamide: enhanced activity of 2B6 can increase the production of the toxic metabolite chloroacetadehyde Thiotepa (minor)

CYP2C8	CYP1A2	CYP2E1	CYP2C9
Paclitaxel	Bortezomib Etoposide (minor) Teniposide (minor) Flutamide (major) Dacabazine (required for activation) Imatinib (minor)	Etoposide (minor) Teniposide (minor) Dacarbazine (required for activation)	Imatinib (minor) Bortezomib **CYP2C19** Imatinib (minor) Bortezomib

TABLE 8.3 Chemotherapy Drug Interactions Through the CYP450 Enzymes

Thiotepa	Inhibits CYP2B6	Increases cyclophosphamide
Doxorubicin	Inhibits CYP3A4	Increases paclitaxel
Tamoxifen	Inhibits CYP3A4	Multiple drugs
Anastrozole	Inhibits CYP1A2, 2C9, and 3A4	Multiple drugs
Fluorouracil	Inhibits CYP2C9	Increases warfarin, phenytoin
Capecitabine	Inhibits CYP2C9	Increases warfarin, phenytoin

Penicillins may interfere with the elimination of MTX by blocking its renal tubular secretion. This results in a reduction of MTX elimination, causing prolonged and increased levels. This can lead to MTX toxicity, including severe neutropenia, stomatitis, and hepatotoxicity. Several case reports have described patients receiving various doses of MTX in combination with penicillins.

These patients developed the adverse effects just described (Nierenberg and Mamelok 1983; Ronchera *et al.* 1993; Mayall *et al.* 1991).

Nonsteroidal anti-inflammatory drugs (NSAIDs) pose another threat to increasing MTX levels. The mechanism of this interaction may be a result of the decrease in renal perfusion secondary to NSAID inhibition of renal prostaglandin synthesis (McEvoy 1994). Competition with MTX for renal secretion is a second postulated mechanism (McEvoy 1994). This interaction is significant because of the potential for toxicities caused by high levels of MTX persisting over several days.

Salicylates, such as aspirin, can also inhibit the renal excretion of MTX (McEvoy 1994). This effect may last for several days. Therefore, aspirin should not be taken within 10 days of a dose of MTX to avoid the interaction.

It is also usually recommended to avoid the concomitant administration of MTX and other drugs, such as salicylates, sulfonamides (e.g., sulfamethoxazole-containing products such as Bactrim), sulfonylureas (e.g., tolbutamide, tolazamide, chlorpropamide, glyburide, glipizide), and phenytoin, that highly bind to plasma proteins. Competition for protein binding sites can lead to displacement of MTX and result in an increased amount of active MTX available. This can increase the likelihood of greater myelosuppressiona and/or gastrointestinal toxicity. The extent to which toxicity may be enhanced is difficult to predict and varies depending on the presence of other confounding factors that may also worsen expected adverse effects.

Because of the potential for drug interactions between many drugs a patient may be taking, a complete medication history, including all over-the-counter drugs, needs to be routinely conducted whenever a new medication is added. Drugs identified to have potential for a clinically significant interaction should not be given. If a potentially interacting drug cannot be discontinued because of medical need, the patient receiving this drug needs to be monitored carefully.

Pharmacodynamic Interactions

Additive Toxicity

In oncology, additive toxicities of chemotherapy combinations with similar side effect profiles can be problematic. In some cases, concomitant administration of some of these agents is unavoidable. For example, cancer chemotherapy regimens often contain more than one agent that has myelosuppression or mucositis as a dose-limiting toxicity. Because chemotherapy regimens have been designed for the antineoplastic effects of their agents when given in combination, changes in these regimens are uncommon except in individual cases when dosage modifications or discontinuation of certain agents may be done to reduce the risk of toxicity seen in a patient with previous chemotherapy cycles. Table 8.4 summarizes the pharmacodynamic interactions known to date. When alternative therapy is available, it should be pursued. Advances in supportive care for patients receiving chemotherapy does allow for administering agents with some overlapping toxicities.

Cisplatin

The toxicity profile of cisplatin includes both nephrotoxicity and ototoxicity. These adverse effects may be potentiated by the use of additional agents that also may cause nephrotoxicity and/or ototoxicity. Antimicrobials, such as gentamicin, tobramycin, amikacin, vancomycin, and amphotericin B, as well as other drugs like cyclosporine, ethacrynic acid, and furosemide should be used with caution when using cisplatin.

The severity of these additive toxicities varies among different patients. Common methods used to prevent cisplatin-induced renal impairment include vigorous prehydration, concurrent hydration, and posthydration with saline-based fluid as well as administration of a diuretic, such as mannitol, to facilitate urinary flow. Ensuring nontoxic levels of contributing agents will allow for

TABLE 8.4 Medication Pharmacodynamic Interactions and Practice Implications

Chemotherapy Agent	Interacting Drug	Result	Resolution
Cisplatin	Aminoglycosides, vancomycin, amphotericin B, cyclosporine, loop diuretics, trimethoprim/sulfamethoxazole, erythromycin	Nephrotoxicity and ototoxicity side effects may be potentiated	Avoid drug combinations that potentiate nephrotoxicity and ototoxicity; monitor for ototoxicity, tinnitus, and auditory discomfort; monitor for nephrotoxicity: BUN and serum creatinine; hydrate vigorously
L-asparaginase	Prednisone	Impaired pancreatic function resulting in decreased insulin synthesis and potential for decreased glucose tolerance resulting in hyperglycemia	Monitor blood glucose levels; sliding-scale insulin therapy may be needed
Paclitaxel	Cisplatin	More severe myelosuppression when cisplatin is followed by paclitaxel	Monitor for paclitaxel side effects such as neutropenia and peripheral neuropathy
Procarbazine	Monoamine oxidase inhibitors (MAOIs)	Serotonin syndrome that may include hypertensive crisis	Concomitant administration with products such as decongestants and sympathomimetic agents should be avoided; avoid concomitant administration with aged foods, such as wine, beer, and cheese, that contain tyramine, an amino acid with sympathomimetic activity

BUN, blood urea nitrogen.
Source: King, R. 1995. Drug interactions with cancer chemotherapy. *Cancer Practice* 3(1):58–59. Reprinted with permission.

appropriate dosage adjustments if necessary. Discontinuation of the causative agent(s) is another alternative if other therapeutic choices are available.

L-Asparaginase

Asparaginase therapy can lead to impairment of pancreatic function, which may lead to decreased insulin synthesis. Hyperglycemia can result but is usually temporary and should resolve once the effects of asparaginase have diminished, usually within several weeks. Hyperglycemia is a common adverse effect of corticosteroids like prednisone. In patients receiving both asparaginase and prednisone, the potential for increased hyperglycemic effects needs to be considered because of the decreased glucose tolerance associated with corticosteroids. Close serum glucose monitoring as well as the use of sliding-scale insulin therapy may need to be temporarily initiated for glucose control.

Trastuzumab

Trastuzumab is a monoclonal antibody directed against human epidermal growth factor receptor 2 (HER2/neu). HER2/neu is overexpressed in about 25–30% of breast cancer patients. Trastuzumab may be used as a single agent or in combination regimens to treat patients with breast cancer who have this overexpression of HER2/neu. Trastuzumab use in women may cause the development of ventricular dysfunction and congestive heart failure. In clinical trials, patients who received trastuzumab in combination with an anthracycline and cyclophosphamide experienced a higher incidence and severity of cardiac dysfunction (Herceptin [trastuzumab] product information 1999). Patients with prior use of anthracyclines and cyclophosphamide, especially the elderly or patients with preexisting cardiac dysfunction, are at higher risk of developing or worsening cardiac dysfunction. Prior radiation therapy to the chest is also considered to be a risk factor. Therefore, any patient initiated on trastuzumab needs to have a baseline cardiac assessment and continued follow-up during therapy to assess any changes that may occur in cardiac function.

Administration Sequence-Dependent Interactions

Chemotherapy regimens commonly include multiple agents that are administered in a fashion that is most convenient with regard to availability of intravenous (IV) line access. IV push medications are often given first, followed by medications that require a continuous infusion, especially if over 24 hours. Alternatively, IV push medications may be administered while another agent is infusing. Sequence of administration usually is not an issue, but there are several instances in which a specific sequence of administration of two chemotherapy agents may be more beneficial to the patient with respect to optimal antineoplastic effects and decreased severity of adverse effects.

L-Asparaginase and Methotrexate

Because MTX requires actively dividing cells for its effects, the administration of asparaginase immediately prior to or with MTX may limit the anticancer effects of MTX (McEvoy 1994). The inhibition of protein synthesis in tumor cells by asparaginase is thought to prevent the entry of these cells into the S phase of the cell cycle, which is the phase during which MTX has its maximum activity. In contrast, when asparaginase is given to leukemia patients 9–10 days prior to or shortly after MTX, the antitumor effects appear to be enhanced (McEvoy 1994). Gastrointestinal and hematologic toxicity also may be reduced in these patients (McEvoy 1994). Therefore, asparaginase therapy should be given several days before or after the administration of methotrexate.

Paclitaxel and Cisplatin

As previously established, cisplatin is a nephrotoxin. When paclitaxel is given shortly after cisplatin, more severe myelosuppression has been demonstrated (Rowinsky *et al.* 1991). The mechanism for this interaction is not clear. However, one postulation is that cisplatin slows paclitaxel clearance because of its nephrotoxic actions, resulting in an increased exposure to paclitaxel and thus worsened neutropenia. The more severe myelosuppression prolongs the period during which a patient is at risk for infection. Therefore, in chemotherapy regimens that include both drugs, such as in the treatment of ovary cancer, paclitaxel should be given before cisplatin.

Therapeutic Interactions

Therapeutic interactions are interactions that are used in a beneficial sense to enhance efficacy or reduce toxicity. The three classic interactions of this type are the use of mesna for protection against hemorrhagic cystitis induced by either ifosfamide or cyclophosphamide, leucovorin rescue following methotrexate infusions, and potentiation of fluorouracil's antineoplastic activity by leucovorin.

Ifosfamide/Cyclophosphamide and Mesna

The alkylating agents ifosfamide and cyclophosphamide have numerous metabolites in common, including acrolein, which does not possess antitumor activity but is associated with bladder damage, specifically hemorrhagic cystitis. The result of acrolein's toxic effects can range from microscopic hematuria to frank hemorrhage. The risk of hemorrhagic cystitis with cyclophosphamide has increased with the advent of high-dose infusions as part of stem-cell transplantation preparative chemotherapy regimens. The lower milligram potency of ifosfamide compared with cyclophosphamide necessitates the need for higher relative doses when used in clinical practice. This results in a higher acrolein level for ifosfamide, which carries an increased risk of hemorrhagic cystitis.

Mercaptoethane sulfonate sodium (mesna) is a compound that protects the bladder epithelium by complexing with acrolein in the bladder to form an inactive product that can be readily eliminated. Vigorous hydration with or without urinary alkalinization to ensure frequent voiding is also recommended to reduce the risk of hemorrhagic cystitis.

Methotrexate and Leucovorin

One drug interaction is commonly used to reduce toxicities, such as neutropenia, mucositis, and hepatotoxicity, that may occur with the use of methotrexate (MTX). The beneficial drug interaction of leucovorin and MTX assists in reducing MTX toxicity. Leucovorin is a form of folic acid that helps "rescue" normal cells from the cytotoxic effects of MTX. The mechanism by which MTX interferes with DNA, RNA, and protein synthesis is via inhibition of the enzyme dihydrofolate reductase, which is responsible for the production of the tetrahydrofolate cofactors required for major cellular biosynthetic reactions. After administration, leucovorin is metabolized to tetrahydrofolate, providing a source of the molecule that MTX action has prevented from being synthesized. Leucovorin administration is typically started sometime within 24–48 hours after the completion of the MTX infusion. The leucovorin is continued until the serum MTX level has dropped to a concentration of less than 3×10^{-8} M, which does not contribute to cell toxicity.

Fluorouracil and Leucovorin

In treatment of advanced colorectal carcinoma, leucovorin can be used to potentiate the antineoplastic activity of fluorouracil (5-FU). Improved response to 5-FU and prolonged survival are the goals of this therapeutic drug interaction. Leucovorin is a form of folic acid that helps to stabilize the complex formed between 5-FU and the enzyme it inhibits, thymidylate synthetase. The more stable complex of 5-FU and thymidylate synthetase results in enhanced activity of 5-FU to interfere with DNA synthesis. The enhanced activity of 5-FU can also result in a potentiation of its adverse effects. Gastrointestinal toxicity in the form of diarrhea, nausea, stomatitis, and vomiting is most likely to be more pronounced. The myelosuppression commonly associated with 5-FU may also be enhanced. Because of the risk of increased toxicity, patients must be monitored to identify those effects that are dose limiting and avoid any potential fatalities.

Miscellaneous
Procarbazine

Procarbazine has been shown to possess the ability to inhibit monoamine oxidase activity. Monoamine oxidase (MAO) is an enzyme responsible for the degradation of neurotransmitters as well as other sympathomimetic agents such as pseudoephedrine. Accumulation of sympathomimetic agents has the potential to cause hypertensive crisis. Products containing this ingredient, such as decongestants, should be avoided in patients receiving procarbazine. Likewise, drugs that increase the levels of serotonin, such as the family of serotonin selective reuptake inhibitors that includes fluoxetine (Prozac), sertraline (Zoloft), paroxetine (Paxil), citalopram (Celexa), escitalopram (Lexapro), and others, should also be avoided. The use of these drugs in combination with an MAO inhibitor can lead to high levels of serotonin, resulting in serotonin syndrome.

Tyramine, an amino acid contained in certain foods, also has sympathomimetic activity that can be enhanced by the concurrent ingestion of procarbazine. Most of these foods are foods that are aged, such as wine, beer, and cheese, and should be avoided in patients receiving procarbazine.

In addition, procarbazine has been reported to have some disulfiram-like activity (McEvoy 1994). Disulfiram (Antabuse) is an alcohol deterrent used in the management of alcohol dependence. When alcohol or alcohol-containing products are ingested after someone has taken disulfiram, a feeling of nausea is triggered. Thus, the simultaneous ingestion of alcohol, including that found in many medicinal preparations such as cough and cold products, should be avoided to prevent severe gastrointestinal toxicity.

Finally, procarbazine crosses the blood-brain barrier and distributes into the cerebrospinal fluid. Thus, it has the potential to cause central nervous system (CNS) effects such as sedation. The administration of other CNS depressants with procarbazine should be avoided or given with caution to prevent additive CNS toxicity. These agents include narcotic analgesics, antihistamines, phenothiazines, benzodiazepines, and barbiturates, among others.

Alternative Therapy

Cancer patients increasingly are considering alternative therapies to maintain their health or treat conditions, including cancer and adverse effects of chemotherapy. The risk of negative drug interactions between chemotherapy and alternative medicine choices, like high-dose vitamins, antioxidants, and other herbal preparations, necessitates the questioning of patients about their use of nontraditional products. Garlic, gingko, ginseng, St. John's wort, milk thistle, echinacea, and coenzyme Q_{10} are some commonly used alternative therapies, but there are many others. Traditional health care professionals may even want to communicate with their patients' herbalists and nutritionists in deciding on the best approach to providing optimal therapy. Although more information is being made available on alternative therapies, there remains a paucity of data regarding potential interactions.

Conclusion

Drug interactions with cancer chemotherapy often can be very difficult to assess. Use of multiple drugs, varying levels of an interaction, and the frequent inability to distinguish which drug is responsible for a certain toxicity compound the issue. Some of the common interactions that occur in oncology have been discussed. As more information becomes known about the pharmacokinetics and pharmacodynamics of all drugs, more interactions will be found, and known interactions will be better understood. Because of the clinical differences a particular drug interaction will cause in different individuals, all patients need to be provided with the same level of caution regarding interactions. Available literature should be used as a guide in identifying potential drug interactions.

Finally, although many interactions have been discussed here, other interactions exist. This further emphasizes the need for practitioners to carefully inspect each patient's medication list and evaluate drug interactions using up-to-date texts.

TABLE 8.5   CYP450 Enzyme Drug Interactions Involving Chemotherapy Agents

CYP450 Enzyme	Inhibitor	Inducer	Substrate
1A2	Anastrozole Cimetidine Ciprofloxacin Citalopram Enoxacin Erythromycin Fluvoxamine Grapefruit juice Mexiletine Mibefradil Mirtazapine Norfloxacin Propranolol Ritonavir Sildenafil Tacrine Ticlopidine	Charbroiled food Cigarette smoke Omeprazole Phenobarbital Primidone Rifampin	Ondansetron Tamoxifen
2A6	Ketoconazole Methoxsalen Miconazole Pilocarpine Ritonavir		Tamoxifen
2B6		Phenobarbital Phenytoin Primidone	Cyclophosphamide Ifosfamide Tamoxifen
2C8-10	Amiodarone (2C9) Anastrozole (2C8/9) Chloramphenicol (2C9) Cimetidine (2C9) Diclofenac (2C9) Disulfiram (2C9) Fluconazole (2C9) Fluoxetine (2C9) Flurbiprofen (2C9) Fluvastatin (2C9) Fluvoxamine (2C9) Ketoprofen (2C9) Metronidazole (2C9) Omeprazole (2C8) Phenylbutazone (2C9) Ritonavir (2C9) Sertaline Sildenafil (2C9) Sulfonamides (2C9) Sulfadiazine (2C9) Sulfamethizole (2C9) Sulfamethoxazole (2C9) Sulfinpyrazone (2C9)	Carbamazepine (2C9) Ethanol (2C9) Phenytoin (2C9) Primidone (2C8) Rifampin (2C9)	Paclitaxel (2C8)

(Continued)

TABLE 8.5   (Continued)

	Ticlopidine (2C9) Trimethoprim (2C9) Troglitazone (2C9) Zafirlukast (2C9)		
2D6	Amiodarone Chloroquine Cimetidine Citalopram Codeine Delavirdine Doxorubicin Fluoxetine Fluphenazine Fluvoxamine Haloperidol Lomustine Methadone Mibefradil Mirtazepine Nefazodone Paroxetine Perphenazine Primaquine Propafenone Propranolol Quinidine Ranitidine Ritonavir Sertraline Sildenafil Thioridazine Ticlopidine Venlafaxine Vinblastine Vinorelbine Yohimbine		Dolasetron Ondansetron Tamoxifen
2E1	Disulfiram Ritonavir Sildenafil	Ethanol Isoniazid	Ondansetron Tamoxifen
3A4	Amprenavir Anastrozole Cimetidine Clarithromycin Clotrimazole Danazol Delavirdine Diltiazem Erythromycin Fluconazole	Carbamazepine Dexamethasone Efavirenz Macrolide antibiotics Phenobarbital Phenylbutazine Phenytoin Prednisone Primidone Rifabutin	Busulfan Dolasetron Doxorubicin Etoposide Granisetron Ifosfamide Imatinib Ondansetron Paclitaxel Tamoxifen

(Continued)

TABLE 8.5   (Continued)

	Fluozetine	Rifampin	Teniposide
	Fluvoxamine	Sulfinpyrazone	Tretinoin
	Grapefruit juice		Vinblastine
	Indinavir		Vincristine
	Itraconazole		
	Ketoconazole		
	Mibefradil		
	Miconazole		
	Mirtazapine		
	Nefazodone		
	Nelfinavir		
	Norfloxacin		
	Paroxetiner		
	Propranolol		
	Quinine		
	Quinidine		
	Ranitidine		
	Ritonavir		
	Saquinavir		
	Sertraline		
	Sildenafil		
	Troglitazone		
	Troleandomycin		
	Zafirlukast		
3A5-7	Clotrimazole	Phenobarbital	Vinblastine
	Ketoconazole	Phenytoin	Vincristine
	Metronidazole	Primidone	
	Miconazole	Rifampin	
	Troleandomycin		

Source: Tatro, D.S. 2005. *Drug interaction facts*. St.Louis: Wolters Kluwer Health, Inc.; and Gleevec (imatinib) product information. Hanover, NJ: Novartis Pharmaceuticals Corporation, 2004.

TABLE 8.6 Drug Interactions with Chemotherapy*

	Bisphosphonate	Bleomycin	Busulfan	Capecitabine	Carboplatin	Carmustine	Cisplatin	Cyclophosphamide	Cytarabine	Daunorubicin	Dolasetron	Doxorubicin	Etoposide	Fluorouracil	Gemcitabine	Ifosfamide	Imatinib	Interferon alfa	Irinotecan	Mercaptopurine	Methotrexate	Mitoxantrone	Ondansetron	Tamoxifen	Trastuzumab	Vinblastine	Vincristine
Allopurinol								X												X							
Aminophylline																		X									
Amiodarone																					X						
Amobarbital												X															
Amoxicillin																					X						
Ampicillin																					X						
Aspirin																					X						
Atovaquone													X														
Atracurium																				X							
Azathioprine																					X						
Bismuth subsalicylate																					X						
Bumetanide							X																				
Butalbital												X															
Carbamazepine																	X									X	X
Chloramphenicol								X																			
Chloroquine																					X						
Chlorthiazide								X				X									X						
Chlorthalidone								X				X															
Choline magnesium salicylate																					X						
Cimetidine						X								X													
Ciprofloxacin								X	X	X		X										X					X
Cisplatin																						X					
Cloxacillin																					X						
Cyclophosphamide																					X	X					
Cyclosporine													X														
Diclofenac	X																				X						
Digoxin		X				X		X	X			X															X
Dicloxacillin																					X						
Doxycycline																					X						
Erythromycin																	X									X	
Ethacrynic acid						X																					
Etodolac	X																				X						
Fenoprofen	X																				X						
Fluconazole																	X									X	X
Flurbiprofen	X																				X						
Fosphenytoin														X					X								
Furosemide								X																			

306   CHAPTER 8: Drug Interactions with Antineoplastic Medications

TABLE 8.6   (Continued)

	Bisphosphonate	Bleomycin	Busulfan	Capecitabine	Carboplatin	Carmustine	Cisplatin	Cyclophosphamide	Cytarabine	Daunorubicin	Dolasetron	Doxorubicin	Etoposide	Fluorouracil	Gemcitabine	Ifosfamide	Imatinib	Interferon alfa	Irinotecan	Mercaptopurine	Methotrexate	Mitoxantrone	Ondansetron	Tamoxifen	Trastuzumab	Vinblastine	Vincristine
Grapefruit juice													X														
Haloperidol																					X						
Hydro-chlorthiazide								X						X							X						
Ibuprofen	X																				X						
Indapamide								X						X							X						
Indomethacin	X																				X						
Itraconazole			X														X									X	X
Ketoconazole																	X									X	X
Ketoprofen	X																				X						
Ketorolac	X																				X						
Levofloxacin								X	X	X		X										X					X
Lomefloxacin								X	X			X										X					X
Magnesium salicylate																					X						
Meclofenamate	X																										
Mefenamic acid	X																				X						
Meloxicam	X																										
Mesalamine																				X							
Methicillin																					X						
Methotrexate								X												X	X						
Metolazone								X						X							X						
Mezlocillin																					X						
Nabumetone	X																				X						
Naproxen	X																				X						
Nifedipine																											X
Norfloxacin								X	X	X		X										X					X
Ofloxacin								X	X	X		X										X					X
Olsalazine																				X							
Omeprazole																					X						
Ondansetron					X		X																				
Oxaprozin	X																										
Pancuronium																				X							
Pantoprazole																					X						
Penicillin																					X						
Pentobarbital												X															
Phenobarbital												X				X											
Phenytoin		X		X	X	X								X			X	X			X					X	
Piperacillin																					X						
Piroxicam	X																				X						

(Continued)

TABLE 8.6 (Continued)

	Bisphosphonate	Bleomycin	Busulfan	Capecitabine	Carboplatin	Carmustine	Cisplatin	Cyclophosphamide	Cytarabine	Daunorubicin	Dolasetron	Doxorubicin	Etoposide	Fluorouracil	Gemcitabine	Ifosfamide	Imatinib	Interferon alfa	Irinotecan	Mercaptopurine	Methotrexate	Mitoxantrone	Ondansetron	Tamoxifen	Trastuzumab	Vinblastine	Vincristine
Potassium acetate																					X						
Potassium citrate																					X						
Prednisone								X																			
Primidone												X															
Probenecid																					X						
Procarbazine																					X						
Rifabutin																								X	X		
Rifampin																	X							X	X		
Salsalate																					X						
Sodium acetate																					X						
Sodium bicarbonate																					X						
Sodium citrate																					X						
Sodium lactate																					X						
Sodium salicylate																					X						
Sparfloxacin								X	X	X		X											X				X
St. John's wort																		X	X								
Succinylcholine								X																			
Sulfadiazine								X													X						
Sulfamethizole								X													X						
Sulfamethoxazole								X													X						
Sulfasalazine																				X	X						
Sulfasoxazole																					X						
Sulindac	X																				X						
Tetracycline																					X						
Theophylline																	X										
Ticarcillin																					X						
Tolmetin	X																				X						
Trimethoprim																					X						
Trimethoprim-sulfamethoxazole																					X						
Trovofloxacin								X	X	X		X											X				X

TABLE 8.6   (Continued)

	Bisphosphonate	Bleomycin	Busulfan	Capecitabine	Carboplatin	Carmustine	Cisplatin	Cyclophosphamide	Cytarabine	Daunorubicin	Dolasetron	Doxorubicin	Etoposide	Fluorouracil	Gemcitabine	Ifosfamide	Imatinib	Interferon alfa	Irinotecan	Mercaptopurine	Methotrexate	Mitoxantrone	Ondansetron	Tamoxifen	Trastuzumab	Vinblastine	Vincristine
Tubocurarine																				X							
Vancomycin																					X						
Vecuronium																				X							
Warfarin				X	X		X						X	X	X	X	X			X				X	X		
Ziprasidone								X																			

*This table represents the existence of the potential for an interaction involving the listed drugs but in no way suggests any therapeutic decision based on an interaction that may occur. Specific product information should be consulted regarding concomitant use of multiple drugs.

X denotes potential for interaction

Source: Tatro, D.S. 2005. *Drug interaction facts*. St. Louis: Wolters Kluwer Health, Inc.; and Gleevec (imatinib) product information. Hanover, NJ: Novartis Pharmaceuticals Corporation, 2004.

References

Baker, A.F., *et al.* 2001. Drug interactions with the taxanes: Clinical implications. *Cancer Treatment Reviews* 27(4):221–233.

Balis, F.M. 1986. Pharmacokinetic drug interactions of commonly used anticancer drugs. *Clinical Pharmacokinetics* 11(3):223–235.

Balmer, C., and Valley, A.W. 1994. Basic principles of cancer treatment and cancer chemotherapy. In J.T. DiPiro, R.L. Talbert, P.E. Hayes, *et al.* (Eds): *Pharmacotherapy: A pathophysiologic approach* (ed 6). Norwalk, CT: Appleton and Lange.

Bosanquet, A.G., and Gilby, E.D. 1984. Comparison of the fed and fasting states on the absorption of melphalan in multiple myeloma. *Cancer Chemotherapy and Pharmacology* 12(3):183–186.

Brown, M.C. 1997. Multisite mucous membrane bleeding due to a possible interaction between warfarin and 5-fluorouracil. *Pharmacotherapy* 17(3):631–633.

Brown, M.C. 1999. An adverse interaction between warfarin and 5-fluorouracil: A case report and review of the literature. *Chemotherapy* 45(5):392–395.

Diflucan (fluconazole) product information. 2004. New York: Pfizer, Inc.

Dorr, R.T., and von Hoff, D.D. 1994. *Cancer chemotherapy handbook* (ed 2). Norwalk, CT: Appleton and Lange.

Finley, R.S. 1992. Drug interactions in the oncology patient. *Seminars in Oncology Nursing* 8(2):95–101.

Gleevec (imatinib) product information. 2004 Hanover, NJ: Novartis Pharmaceuticals Corporation.

Gunnarsson, P.O., Davidsson, T., Andersson, S.B., *et al.* 1990. Impairment of estramustine phosphate absorption by concurrent intake of milk and food. *European Journal of Clinical Pharmacology* 38(2):189–193.

Hansten, P.D., and Horn, J.R. 1994. *Drug interactions & updates*. Vancouver, WA: Applied Therapeutics.

Hardman, J.E., Limbird, L.E., (Eds) and Goodman Gilman, A. 2001. *Goodman and Gilman's pharmacological basis of therapeutics* (ed 10). New York: McGraw Hill.

Herceptin (trastuzumab) product information. 1999 San Francisco: Genentech, Inc.

Ignoffo, R.J. 1989. Drug interactions with antineoplastic agents. *Highlights on Antineoplastic Drugs* 7(1):2–7.

Inman, W., and Kubota, K. 1992. Tachycardia during cisapride treatment. *BMJ* 305(6860):1019.

Janetzky, K., and Morreale, A.P. 1997. Probable interaction between warfarin and ginseng. *Am J Health-Syst Pharm* 54(6):692–693.

King, R. 1995. Drug interactions with cancer chemotherapy. *Cancer Practice* 3(1):58–59.

Klepser, T.B., and Klepser, M.E. 1999. Unsafe and potentially safe herbal therapies. *American Journal of Health-System Pharmacy* 56:125–138.

Kolesar, J.M., Johnson, C.L., Freeberg, B.L., *et al.* 1999. Warfarin-5-FU interaction—A consecutive case series. *Pharmacotherapy* 19(12):1445–1449.

Lien, E.A., Anker. G., Lonning, P.E., *et al.* 1990. Decreased serum concentrations of tamoxifen and its metabolites induced by aminoglutethimide. *Cancer Research* 50(18):5851–5857.

Lonning, P.E., Kvinnsland, S., and Bakke, O.M. 1984. Effect of aminoglutethimide on antipyrine, theophylline, and digitoxin disposition in breast cancer. *Clinical Pharmacology Therapy* 36(6):796–802.

Lonning, P.E., Kvinnsland, S., and Jahren, G. 1984. Aminoglutethimide and warfarin: A new important drug interaction. *Cancer Chemotherapy and Pharmacology* 12(1):10–12.

Mayall, B., Poggi, G., Parkin, J.D. 1991. Neutropenia due to low-dose methotrexate therapy for psoriasis and rheumatoid arthritis may be fatal. *Medical Journal of Australia* 155:480–484.

McEvoy, G.K. (Ed). 1994. *AHFS drug information 94.* Bethesda, MD: American Society of Health-System Pharmacists.

Michalets, E.L. 1998. Update: Clinically significant cytochrome P-450 drug interactions. *Pharmacotherapy* 18(1):84–112.

Nierenberg, D.W., and Mamelok, R.D. 1983. Toxic reaction to methotrexate in a patient receiving penicillin and furosemide: A possible interaction. *Archives of Dermatology* 119:449–450.

Reece, P.A., Kotasek, D., Morris, R.G., *et al.* 1986. The effect of food on oral melphalan absorption. *Cancer Chemotherapy and Pharmacology* 16(2):194–197.

Relling, M.V., Pui, C.H., Sandlund, J.T., *et al.* 2000. Adverse effects of anticonvulsants on efficacy of chemotherapy for acute lymphoblastic leukaemia. *Lancet* 356(9226):285–290.

Ronchera, C.L., Hernandez, T., Peris, J.E., *et al.* 1993. Pharmacokinetic interaction between high-dose methotrexate and amoxycillin. *Therapeutic Drug Monitoring* 15:375–379.

Rosemergy, I., *et al.* 2002. Phenytoin toxicity as a result of 5-fluorouracil administration. *New Zealand Medical Journal* 115(1159):124–125.

Rowinsky, E.K., Gilbert, M.R., McGuire, W.P., *et al.* 1991. Sequences of taxol and cisplatin: A phase I and pharmacologic study. *Journal of Clinical Oncology* 9(9):1692–1703.

Sporanox (itraconazole) product information. 2004. Titusville, NJ: Janssen Pharmaceutica Products, L.P.

Stevens, D.A. 1999. Itraconazole in cyclodextrin solution. *Pharmacotherapy* 19(5):603–611.

Synercid I.V. (quinupristin and dalfopristin) product information. 1999. Collegeville, PA: Rhone-Poulenc Rorer Pharmaceuticals, Inc.

Tatro, D.S. 1991. *Drug interaction facts.* St. Louis: Facts and Comparisons.

Tatro, D.S. 2005. *Drug interaction facts.* St. Louis: Wolters Kluwer Health, Inc.

Thompson, M.E. 2003. Interaction between paclitaxel and warfarin. *Annals of Oncology* 14(3):500.

Velcade (bortezomib) product information. 2004. Cambridge, MA: Millennium Pharmaceuticals, Inc.

Vfend (voriconazole) product information. 2004. New York: Pfizer, Inc.

Xeloda (capecitabine) product information. 2003. Nutey, NJ: Roche Laboratories, Inc.

Standardized Nursing Care Plans

TABLE A1.1 Plan of Care for Patients Receiving Biotherapy

Nursing Diagnosis (Potential/Actual)	Expected Outcomes	Assessment	Nursing Interventions
I. *Altered comfort related to:* A. Chills	I. A. 1. Pt/significant other demonstrates self-care behaviors for management of chills 2. Pt reports acceptable control of chills	I. A. 1. Assess severity and duration of chills and document 2. Monitor vital signs frequently and report changes to physician	I. A. 1. Keep pt warm 2. Avoid icy fluids 3. Medicate with meperidine 25–50 mg IVPB, as ordered 4. Instruct pt/significant other in self-management of chills
B. Fever 101°–104°F (38.4°–40.0°C)	B. 1. Pt/significant other demonstrates self-care behaviors for management of fever 2. Pt reports acceptable control of temperature 3. Pt reports temperatures uncontrolled with medication of unrelated to normal pattern	B. 1. Monitor temperature every 1–4 hrs 2. Report to physician fevers > 104°F despite antipyretics or other control measures	B. 1. Encourage po fluids 2. Medicate with antipyretic as ordered 3. For temps > 103°F despite antipyretic, consider tepid sponge bath or shower; ice packs to temperature-control areas; hypothermia blanket, if indicated 4. Instruct pt/significant other to monitor temperature 5. As therapy continues, teach family to monitor temperature pattern in response to medication; report unusual spikes to health care team 6. Instruct pt/significant other in self-management of fever 7. Instruct pt/significant other to report to physician if fever does not resolve after therapeutic measures
C. Pruritus	C. 1. Pt/significant other identifies/demonstrates	C. 1. Assess pruritus onset/duration and characteristics,	C. 1. Water-based lotion and/or cream to affected area prn

measures to control pruritus
2. Pt reports acceptable control of pruritus

factors that relieve/aggravate the condition, treatment used previously

2. Use colloidal oatmeal baths in bathwater (tepid water instead of hot)
3. Consider use of room humidifier
4. Administer medications as ordered; may need aggressive, around-the-clock administration
5. Encourage use of distraction (relaxation techniques, reading, needlework, etc.)
6. Teach signs/symptoms of skin changes to report
7. Discuss measures to promote skin hydration
8. Teach measures to prevent further skin irritation
9. Teach relaxation techniques as necessary
10. Teach pt to substitute rub, pressure, or vibration for scratching (e.g., rub arms with lotion)

II. Pain related to myalgias, arthralgias, headaches

II. A. Pt/significant other demonstrates self-care behaviors for the management of myalgias and headaches
B. Pt reports acceptable control of pain

II. A. Assess need for analgesia
B. Assess characteristics of pain
C. Assess adequacy of pain control

II. A. Acetaminophen 650 mg po q 3–4 hs as ordered
B. Apply moist heat to aching areas
C. Instruct pt/significant other in self-management of myalgias and headaches

III. Diarrhea related to treatment with biologic agents

III. A. Pt/significant other identifies measures to correct or control diarrhea
B. Pt reports acceptable control of diarrhea

III. A. Abdominal assessment every 8 hs and prn
B. Monitor intake and output every 8 hs
C. Monitor stools for frequency, volume,

III. A. Administer IV fluid as ordered
B. Encourage adequate po fluid intake
C. Administer medications that control diarrhea as ordered
D. Encourage hygiene measures. May consider use of sitz bath and/or barrier creams

(Continued)

TABLE A1.1   Plan of Care for Patients Receiving Biotherapy (Continued)

Nursing Diagnosis (Potential/Actual)	Expected Outcomes	Assessment	Nursing Interventions
		and consistency and document	E. Teach complications of diarrhea (e.g., fluid electrolyte imbalance, skin breakdown) and prevention measures
		D. Assess for complications of diarrhea (e.g., dehydration)	F. Teach signs and symptoms to report
		E. Assess perineal/perianal region for skin status	
IV. Altered nutritional status (less than body requirements) related to anorexia, mucositis, nausea, vomiting	IV. A. Pt maintains adequate nutritional status B. Pt/significant other verbalizes understanding of nutritional needs C. Pt/significant other demonstrates measures to increase nutritional uptake	IV. A. Weigh pt regularly and record B. Initiate a calorie count if indicated to assess intake	IV. A. Provide appetizing foods consistent with pt preference B. Provide high-calorie, low-bulk foods C. Use nutritional supplements D. Refer to dietitian for consultation E. Try small, frequent meals F. Try cool foods if pt is sensitive to food odors G. Give antiemetics as ordered; in some cases, around-the-clock administration might be necessary H. Discuss with health care team the need for tube feedings, or hyperalimentation (IVH), if nutritional status becomes severely compromised I. Instruct pt/significant other in measures to provide adequate nutrition
V. Altered oral mucous membranes related to treatment with biologic agents	V. A. Pt recognizes and reports changes in mucous membranes B. Pt demonstrates oral hygiene protocol	V. A. Perform oral exam to include palate, gingiva, dorsum of tongue, undersurface of tongue, floor of	V. A. Encourage pt to perform oral hygiene after meals and at bedtime B. Begin use of salt and soda mouth rinses every 2 hs and prn

mouth, buccal mucosa, oral pharynx, and inner surface of lips

B. Assess normal oral hygiene routine

C. Provide lubricant for lips

D. Encourage use of soft toothbrush

E. Consider oral irrigations prn to hydrate mouth and for comfort

F. Avoid use of agents that further dry the oral mucosa

G. Explain rationale for prophylactic oral hygiene protocol

H. Teach proper oral hygiene protocol

I. Teach signs/symptoms to report to nurse/physician

VI. Fatigue related to treatment with biologic agents

VI.
A. Pt maintains independence in activities of daily living and/or uses measures to prevent further immobility

B. Pt verbalizes understanding of cause of fatigue

VI.
A. Assess effect of fatigue on activities of daily living

B. Assess usual pattern of sleep and rest

C. Assess for signs and symptoms associated with fatigue

D. Assess for cofactors that may influence fatigue (e.g., anemia, poor nutritional intake, pain)

VI.
A. Encourage pt to arrange most strenuous activities according to peak energy level

B. Encourage pt to seek assistance with activities of daily living as necessary

C. Encourage pt to maintain mobility
1. Ambulatory pt: mild exercise (e.g., walking as tolerated)
2. Bedridden pt: turn every 2 hs; active/passive range of motion

D. Encourage pt to take short naps as required to increase energy level

E. Treat cofactors that may contribute to fatigue as appropriate

F. Teach pt/significant other about fatigue as an expected side effect of biotherapy and self-management strategies to prevent sequelae

---

VII. Altered skin integrity related to treatment with biologic agents

VII.
A. Pt/significant other verbalizes understanding of factors that may cause alteration in skin integrity

VII.
A. Observe skin daily for any breaks, discoloration, redness

B. Observe injection sites for changes

VII.
A. Turn bedfast pt every 2 hs

B. Rotate injection sites for IM/SQ agents

C. Apply moist heat to any inflamed areas

(Continued)

TABLE A1.1 Plan of Care for Patients Receiving Biotherapy (Continued)

Nursing Diagnosis (Potential/Actual)	Expected Outcomes	Assessment	Nursing Interventions
	B. Skin integrity is maintained C. Pt/significant other demonstrates behaviors to maintain skin integrity	(e.g., inflammatory reactions) C. Observe IV sites for phlebitis	D. Apply water-based lotion and/or cream to entire body 2–3 times a day for dry desquamation E. Consider use of room humidifier for dryness F. Instruct pt/significant other in individual measures for maintenance of skin integrity G. Instruct pt/significant other in causative factors
VIII. Altered tissue perfusion related to treatment with biologic agents	VIII. A. Pt maintains adequate blood pressure	VIII. A. Assess orthostatic vital signs every 1–4 hs, daily weights, intake and output every 8 hs B. Assess respiratory and cardiovascular system every 8 hs or clinic visit for increased heart rate, decreased blood pressure, complaints of dizziness, complaints of shortness of breath, rales C. Assess for fluid shifts as evidenced by peripheral edema, ascites rales, weight gain, decreased urine output	VIII. A. Administer IV fluids, colloids, and vasopressors as ordered B. Institute comfort measures as necessary C. Institute safety concerns: ambulate with assistance, rise from lying to sitting position slowly D. Encourage po fluid intake E. Teach pt/significant other about expected side effects of biotherapy and temporary nature of side effects F. Teach pt/significant other to monitor for side effects while at home (daily weight, temperature tid, etc.) and notify physician of any changes or problems G. Teach pt/significant other to recognize these signs and symptoms: peripheral edema, shortness of breath, decreased

Nursing Diagnosis	Patient Outcomes	Nursing Assessment	Nursing Interventions
			urinary output, weight gain ≥ 5 pounds H. Teach pt to rise from lying position slowly
IX. Potential for injury related to allergic reaction	IX. A. Pt immediately reports signs and symptoms of anaphylaxis	IX. A. Prior to administration, review prior allergic episodes to include agent thought to be responsible, description of the episode (reaction to agent) B. During administration, assess for shortness of breath/wheezing, sneezing/coughing, local or generalized urticaria and/or erythema/itching, hypotension, tachycardia cyanosis unconsciousness, emesis and/or diarrhea	IX. A. Administer test dose if ordered B. Ensure that emergency equipment is available C. Ensure that emergency drugs (epinephrine, diphenhydramine, hydrocortisone) are available when administering MABs D. Teach pt to report pain or tightness in chest; dyspnea; inability to speak; generalized itching; symptoms of uneasiness, agitation, warmth, dizziness; desire to urinate or defecate
X. Altered thought processes related to treatment with biologic agents (e.g., confusion slowed mentation, somnolence)	X. A. Pt/significant other verbalizes understanding of factors that may cause alteration in thought processes B. Pt/significant other recognizes changes in thinking or behavior C. Pt maintains reality orientation	X. A. Assess mental status prior to therapy B. Assess mental status on each shift or clinic visit and when indicated C. Assess amount of premedication and/or analgesics pt is receiving	X. A. Orient to time and place if necessary B. Allow verbalization of feelings C. Refer to mental health professional if indicated D. Report changes in mental status to physician E. Initiate safety measures if indicated F. Provide memory prompts for orientation (e.g., clocks, calendar, family photos)

(Continued)

TABLE A1.1 Plan of Care for Patients Receiving Biotherapy (Continued)

Nursing Diagnosis (Potential/Actual)	Expected Outcomes	Assessment	Nursing Interventions
			G. Instruct pt/significant other how biologic therapy may cause alteration in thought process H. Inform pt/significant other that this side effect is temporary
XI. Altered coping related to changes in disease status and/or new therapy	XI. A. Pt recognizes potential/actual stressors and facilitates own coping strategies	XI. A. Assess pt's perception of stressors and beliefs about the causes B. Assess pt's past use of coping strategies C. Evaluate pt's ability to solve problems	XI. A. Encourage pts to verbalize thoughts and feelings about changes in disease status and new therapy B. Identify available resources for support and encourage participation (e.g., American Cancer Society, support groups, chaplain) C. Teach relaxation techniques D. Teach problem-solving techniques
XII. Knowledge deficit related to medication self-administration	XII. A. Pt/significant other demonstrates self-administration of agent if indicated	XII. A. Assess ability of pt/significant other to be responsible for self-administration	XII. A. Utilize teaching aids (e.g., written materials, videotape, injection models) B. Instruct pt/significant other in reconstitution of agent C. Instruct pt/significant other in IM/SQ injection technique
XIII. Knowledge deficit related to treatment with biologic therapy	XIII. A. Pt/significant other verbalizes expected side effects of agent, reportable signs and symptoms, and treatment plan	XIII. A. Assess knowledge of side effects B. Assess understanding of therapeutic plan	XIII. A. Instruct pt/significant other of expected side effects and reportable signs and symptoms B. Instruct pt/significant other regarding required laboratory and diagnostic tests C. Instruct pt/significant other on therapeutic plan

Source: Barton-Burke, M., Wilkes, G.M., and Ingwersen, K. 2001. *Cancer chemotherapy: A nursing process approach* (ed 3). Sudbury, MA: Jones and Bartlett Publishers, pp. 63–67.

TABLE A1.2 Standardized Nursing Care Plan for the Patient Experiencing Bone Marrow Depression

Nursing Diagnosis	Expected Outcomes	Nursing Interventions

I. A. *Potential for altered health maintenance*	I. A. Pt will manage self-care as evidenced by verbal recall or return demonstration of instructions for self-assessment of oral temperature; examination of skin and mucous membranes; signs and symptoms of infection and bleeding; measures to avoid exposure to infection; measures to avoid injury and bleeding; and when and how to notify the health care provider	I. A. 1. Assess baseline knowledge, learning style, and level of anxiety of pt and significant other
		2. Develop and implement teaching plan
		  a. Purpose and goal of chemotherapy
		  b. Specific drugs
		    1) mechanism of action
		    2) potential side effects, including bone marrow suppression as appropriate
		  c. Self-care measures
		    1) assessment and care of skin, oral mucosa to prevent infection, trauma
		    2) assessment of temperature BID, or if feels as if fever, and instructions to call health care provider if temperature is over 101°F (38.5°C)
		    3) signs and symptoms of infection (fever, sore throat, cough, painful urination)
		    4) signs and symptoms of bleeding (nose or gum bleeding, capillary or large "black and blues")
		    5) measures to minimize exposure to infection and trauma as described in NCI booklet *Chemotherapy and You: A Guide to Self-Help*
		  d. Provide written information to reinforce teaching, such as the booklet above, free from the NCI

B. *Potential for non-compliance with self-care activities*	B. Pt and significant other will comply with pre-scribed measures 90% of the time	B. 1. Reinforce teaching prior to treatment as nurse does prechemo assessment and prior to pt leaving clinic or hospital after treatment administration 2. Evaluate compliance through telephone call to pt following treatment or discharge or visiting nurse home visit 3. If pt or significant other is having difficulty with managing self-care activities, consider visiting nurse referral or hospitalization if pt is neutropenic or thrombocytopenic and unable to safely care for self

(Continued)

TABLE A1.2   Standardized Nursing Care Plan for the Patient Experiencing Bone Marrow Depression (Continued)

Nursing Diagnosis	Expected Outcomes	Nursing Interventions
C. *Knowledge deficit related to purpose and self-administration techniques of cytokine growth factors, which may be given to prevent complications of febrile neutropenia, anemia, or bleeding*	C. Pt and significant other will verbally describe and demonstrate technique for administration of growth factors if ordered	C. 1. Provide teaching regarding side effects and administration techniques using video, pt education booklets, and demonstration/return demonstration 2. If unable to manage administration, contact community nursing agencies 3. Pt/family teaching materials available through the pharmaceutical companies that make cytokine growth factors
II. *Potential for altered nutrition: less than body requirements*	II. A. Pt will maintain within 5% of pretreatment weight B. Recovery from nadir approximates expected time based on specific chemotherapy agents	II. A. Assess food preferences B. Encourage foods high in proteins, calories, iron, and folic acid C. Discourage excessive alcohol intake D. Review dietary instructions with pt and person responsible for preparing food E. Review teaching material with pt and family from NCI booklet *Eating Hints*, a free publication, for pts receiving chemotherapy.

III. *Potential for injury: infection and bleeding related to bone marrow depression*	III. A. Pt will remain free of infection, bleeding, and tissue hypoxia	III. A. Assessment of potential for injury related to bone marrow depression
		1. Expected nadir from specific agents administered, nadir from prior treatment cycle if appropriate
		2. Major life stressors and coping ability
		3. Sexual history and self-care habits re: hygiene
		4. Sleep pattern
		5. Elimination pattern
		6. Nutritional pattern
		7. History and physical exam
		  a. Symptoms of infection: fever, pain (swallowing, with elimination, etc.), erythema, presence of exudates
		  b. Symptoms of bleeding: dizziness, presence of blood in excretia

c. Symptoms of anemia: fatigue, dyspnea on exertion, angina
d. Skin, mucous membranes: are they intact, color, evidence of petechiae or ecchymoses, exudates
e. Breath sounds, pulmonary exam
f. CNS exam
g. Laboratory data: complete blood count, WBC differential, absolute neutrophil count

B. Institute neutropenic precautions for absolute neutrophil count < 500/mm^3
1. Protect pt from exposure to microorganisms
   a. Provide private room if possible
   b. Place sign on door requiring *all* persons who enter to wash their hands meticulously prior to entering the room, that persons with colds or infections should not enter, and that no flowers, fresh fruits, or vegetables should be brought into the room
   c. Place card in nursing cardex instructing that *no* intramuscular injections, rectal temperatures, or medications should be administered PR
   d. Plan scrupulous hygiene with pt for oral care, daily bath, and meticulous perineal hygiene
   e. Inspect all intravenous sites and change dressings using aseptic technique; sites should be changed every 96 hours or earlier if there is any indication of phlebitis
   f. Avoid invasive procedures, such as urinary catheterization if possible
   g. Wash hands meticulously prior to entering room and between each physical contact with the pt; monitor that all other persons wash their hands prior to entering; ensure that the nurse caring for the pt does not care for any other pt who is infected

B. Pt will experience minimal complications of bone marrow suppression as evidenced by return to normal temperature and neutrophil count and absence of major bleeding

(Continued)

TABLE A1.2   Standardized Nursing Care Plan for the Patient Experiencing Bone Marrow Depression (Continued)

Nursing Diagnosis	Expected Outcomes	Nursing Interventions
		2. Continually assess for presence of infection
		a. Monitor vital signs every 4 hours or more frequently if temperature is elevated
		b. Monitor absolute neutrophil count
		c. Inspect potential sites of infection: mouth, pharynx, rectum, wounds, intravenous sites, and others, remembering that usual signs of infection, such as pus and erythema, may be absent
		d. Monitor for changes in character, color, and amount of excretia (sputum, urine, stool)
		e. Report signs and symptoms of infection to physician and obtain cultures, administer antipyretics and antibiotics as ordered
		3. Instruct pt in stress-reducing activities to promote relaxation and satisfactory sleep/rest patterns
		C. Institute platelet precautions for pt with platelet count less than 50,000/mm³
		1. Protect pt from trauma and potential bleeding
		a. Place sign in nursing cardex that no IM or rectal medications should be administered, no aspirin or prostaglandin inhibiting medications should be administered, and no rectal temperatures should be taken
		b. Minimize number of venipunctures and apply pressure to site at least 5 minutes until bleeding stops
		c. Avoid invasive procedures, such as deep endotracheal suctioning, enemas, douches
		d. Teach pt to brush teeth with soft brush or sponge applicator to prevent trauma to gums; avoid flossing
		e. Provide safe environment, padding side rails when in use and removing clutter and obstructing furniture from room

f. Prevent constipation by administering stool softeners as ordered, and encourage fluid intake of 3 liters per day

2. Continually monitor for signs and symptoms of bleeding
   a. Minor bleeding, such as petechiae, ecchymoses, epistaxis; occult blood in stool, urine, emesis
   b. Major bleeding, such as hematemesis, melena, heavy vaginal bleeding; changes in orthostatic vital signs > 10 mmHg in blood pressure or increase in heart rate > 100 beats per minute; changes in neuro vital signs
   c. Monitor platelet count, hematocrit daily
   d. Notify MD re: signs and symptoms of bleeding, and transfuse platelets as ordered

IV. *Potential for altered tissue perfusion related to anemia*

IV. A. Pt will be without signs and symptoms of severe anemia

IV. A. Assess signs and symptoms of anemia
   1. Hematocrit: mild (31–37%), moderate (25–30%), or severe (< 25%)
   2. Presence of symptoms of mild anemia (paleness, fatigue, slight dyspnea, palpitation, sweating on exertion); moderate anemia (increased severity of symptoms of mild anemia); and severe anemia (headache, dizziness, irritability, angina, dyspnea at rest, compensatory tachycardia, and tachypnea)

B. Encourage pt to change positions gradually, slowly moving from lying to sitting position and sitting to standing position. Encourage slow, deep breathing during position changes

C. Reassure pt that fatigue is related to anemia and hopefully will improve with transfusion

D. Replace red blood cells as ordered, expecting that the 1 unit of RBCs will increase the hematocrit; washed or leukocyte-poor red blood cells are used to prevent antibody formation if the pt is planning to go for a bone marrow transplantation

E. Assess activity tolerance and need for oxygen for activity or at rest

F. Review foods that are high in iron and folic acid and encourage pt to include these in the diet

(Continued)

TABLE A1.2 Standardized Nursing Care Plan for the Patient Experiencing Bone Marrow Depression (Continued)

Nursing Diagnosis	Expected Outcomes	Nursing Interventions
V. *Potential for constipation*	V. A. Pt will move bowels at least once every day	V. A. Provide pt education about the goal and means of preventing constipation, such as stool softeners, oral fluids to 3 quarts per day, high-fiber diet, adequate exercise B. Discuss a bowel regime with physician to promote soft, regular bowel movements, especially if the pt is receiving narcotic analgesia

VI. *Potential for activity intolerance related to fatigue of anemia, malaise*	VI. A. Pt will maintain minimal activity	VI. A. Teach pt to increase rest and sleep periods and to alternate rest and activity periods
		B. Encourage pt to incorporate foods high in iron in diet, such as liver, eggs, lean meat, green leafy vegetables, carrots, and raisins
		C. Assess need for homemaker, home health aide, and visiting nurse at home
		D. Assess for psychological manifestations of fatigue:
		  1) depression
		  2) anxiety
		  3) loss of independence
		  4) decreased level of concentration
		  5) difficulty making decisions
		E. Teach pt to prioritize activities deciding what pt must do and those that can be delegated
		F. Teach pt to eat several small meals a day, and select high-energy foods, such as potatoes, rice, pasta
		G. If pt able, teach pt to start and maintain an exercise program, starting slowly
		  1) gradually increase activity
		  2) low-impact exercises, such as stretching, muscle strengthening
		  3) cardiovascular exercises

Source: Barton-Burke, M., Wilkes, G.M., and Ingwersen K. 2001. *Cancer chemotherapy: A nursing process approach* (ed 3). Sudbury, MA: Jones and Bartlett Publishers, pp. 104–108.

TABLE A1.3 Standardized Nursing Care Plan for the Patient Experiencing Neuropathy

Nursing Diagnosis	Expected Outcomes	Nursing Interventions

I. *Potential for injury related to* → *sensitivity to temperature, gait disturbance,* → *proprioception*	I. A. Pt will be without injury
	B. Pt will report changes in tactile and proprioceptive function
	C. Pt will develop safe measures to compensate for losses
		I. A. Assess integrity of *tactile* and *proprioceptive* functions
		   1. Sensory perception to light touch, pinprick, vibration, temperature; vision, color vision
		   2. Pt's ability to tolerate light touch, cool water, presence of numbness and tingling, presence of painful sensations
		   3. Proprioception testing of station, gait, deep tendon reflexes, muscle weakness or atrophy, and balance
		   4. Pt's ability to sense placement of body parts, ability to write, evidence of muscle weakness
		  B. Discuss alterations in sensation, proprioception, and impact on ability to do activities of daily living (ADLs)
		  C. Discuss alternative strategies to prevent injury
		   1. Instruct pt in safety measures and use of visual cues
		   2. Encourage pt to take time to complete activities, focus attention to task
		   3. Use potholder when cooking
		   4. Use gloves when washing dishes, gardening
		   5. Inspect skin for cuts, abrasions, burns daily, especially arms, legs, toes, fingers
		  D. Refer as appropriate for occupational or physical therapy, diagnostic testing using EMG
		  E. If pt presents with S/S of peripheral neuropathy, hold chemotherapy and discuss with physician

II. *Potential for impaired self-care related to tactile and proprioception dysfunction*	II. A. Pt will identify activities of self-care that are difficult
	B. Pt will identify strategies to meet needs
		II. A. Assess pt's ability to perform ADLs such as eating, hygiene, dressing, walking, and handwriting
		  B. Discuss and develop strategies to meet self-care needs
		   1. Referral to occupational therapy for splint, etc.
		   2. Involve family members in care planning
		   3. Community resource referral as appropriate (homemaker, home health aide, visiting nurse)

III. *Potential for alteration in comfort related to painful paresthesias*	III. A. Pt will have decreased pain	III. A. Assess comfort level and presence of severe tingling or prickling sensation, cramping or burning B. Assess intensity, quality, and frequency of discomfort

(Continued)

TABLE A1.3   Standardized Nursing Care Plan for the Patient Experiencing Neuropathy (Continued)

Nursing Diagnosis	Expected Outcomes	Nursing Interventions
		C. Identify precipitating factors, such as warm or cold stimulation, and develop realistic plan to avoid precipitating factors
		D. Consider adjunctive analgesics with neurologic action for dysaesthetic pain: gabapentin (Neurontin), amitriptyline HCl (Elavil), phenytoin sodium (Dilantin)
		E. Consider nonpharmacologic intervention: teach pt guided imagery, progressive muscle relaxation, massage, etc.
IV. Impaired mobility related to decreased proprioception, muscle dysfunction	IV. A. Pt will ambulate safely	IV. A. Assess pt's level of activity, muscle strength, and mobility level prior to chemotherapy, then prior to each treatment, and at each visit once therapy is completed
		B. Encourage pt to use visual cues to determine position of body parts
		C. Teach measures to prevent injury
		D. Refer for physical, occupational therapy, and assistive devices as needed
V. Potential for sexual dysfunction related to altered tactile sensation, muscle weakness, changes in role	V. A. Pt and significant other will identify alterations in sexual expression	V. A. Discuss with pt the impact of treatment-related dysfunction on sexuality, social role, and self-esteem
	B. Pt and significant other will identify alternative methods of sexual expression	B. Discuss appropriate alternative means of sexual expression
		C. Refer for specific sexual counseling if diminished ability to have erection
		D. Observe for changes in needs related to affection and emotional support
VI. Potential for role change with changes and alterations in self-esteem and self-concept related to sensory/perceptual dysfunction, changes in social function, changes in ability to perform occupational role	VI. A. Pt and family will demonstrate positive coping strategies	VI. A. Assess impact of sensory/perceptual dysfunction on social and work roles: ability to meet role expectations of self and family
		B. Discuss modifications in job and role, as appropriate and available
		C. Refer pt to OT/PT to see if appliances available to foster rehabilitation (braces, etc.)
		D. Encourage independence and provide positive reinforcement for accomplishments
		E. Support pt as he or she grieves loss(es); assess need for support groups or counseling

VII. Potential for alteration in nutrition: less than body requirements related to taste distortions, anorexia, hypersensitivity to foods	VII. A. Pt will eat balanced diet from four food groups B. Pt will attain ideal body weight following completion of treatment	F. Support pt and family by providing information to help explain these behavioral responses to treatment-related dysfunction VII. A. Assess dietary preferences, changes in food tolerances B. Teach pt to select high-calorie, high-protein foods C. Suggest dietary modifications based on taste changes (e.g., Crazy Jane Salt and spices if foods are tasteless) D. Perform periodic weights prior to each treatment cycle E. Evaluate pt's ability to do fine-motor movement to feed self, cook F. Refer to nutritionist or dietitian as needed G. Monitor laboratory values, especially magnesium and calcium, on cisplatin therapy
VIII. Potential for constipation related to autonomic neuropathy (vinca alkaloids)	VIII. A. Pt will move bowels at least every other day	VIII. A. Assess normal elimination pattern B. Encourage pt to drink at least 3 liters of fluid/day C. Encourage daily exercise D. Teach pt to include bulky, high-fiber foods in diet E. Teach pt to self-administer stool softeners and laxatives as needed

IX. Knowledge deficit related to self-care measures related to neuropathic changes	IX. A. Pt will identify risk of development of neuropathy
	B. Pt will identify signs and symptoms to report to health care provider
		IX. A. Teach pt re: potential side effect(s) of neuropathy
		1. Constipation
		2. Numbness/tingling in hands/feets
		3. Motor weakness
		  a. Gait changes (e.g., foot drop)
		  b. Loss of fine-motor movement (buttoning shirt, picking up dime)
		4. Inability of males to have erection
		5. Difficulty urinating
		B. Teach pt to report the occurrence of signs and symptoms of neuropathies

Source: Barton-Burke, M., Wilkes G.M., and Ingwersen, K. 2001. *Cancer chemotherapy: A nursing process approach* (ed 3). Sudbury, MA: Jones and Bartlett Publisher, pp. 173–175.

TABLE A1.4 Standardized Nursing Care Plan for Patient Experiencing Stomatitis

Nursing Diagnosis	Expected Outcomes	Nursing Interventions

I. Potential for altered oral mucous membranes	I. A. Oral mucosa will remain pink, moist, intact, without debris	I. A. Assess oral mucosa (baseline)
		1. Assess history of alcohol use, smoking
		2. Assess history of dental problems, oral hygiene practices, and prior or concurrent radiation to head or neck
		3. Perform oral exam
		  a. Lips
		  b. Upper inner lip and gums
		  c. Tongue (dorsum, lateral borders, ventral surface)
		  d. Inner cheeks (buccal mucosa)
		  e. Hard and soft palate
		  f. Floor of mouth
		  g. Oral pharynx
		4. Assess amount, consistency of saliva
		5. Assess condition of teeth
		B. Assess nutritional status
		C. Initiate and discuss dental referral as needed prior to therapy
		D. Instruct in oral hygiene self-care measures (see IV. Potential for knowledge deficit)

II. Altered oral mucous membranes, Grade I (generalized erythema) Grade II (small ulceration or white patches)	II. A. Oral mucosa will be pink, moist, intact, and painless within 5–7 days	II. A. Assess oral mucosa q shift or at each clinic visit; document size and location of abnormality and intervention B. Assess comfort and ability to eat, drink C. Institute oral hygiene q 2 hrs during day and q 6 hrs during night 1. Warm normal saline rinses *unless* crusts, debris, thick mucus or saliva; then use sodium bicarbonate (1 tsp in 8 oz water) q 4 hrs alternating with warm saline rinses q 4 hrs 2. (Warm) sterile normal saline rinses if WBC < 1000/mm^3 3. Reserve hydrogen peroxide (1:4 strength) for *resistant*, thick secretions or white patches (*candida*) and resistant debris, and rinse afterward with water

III. Altered oral mucous membranes, Grade III (confluent ulcerations with white patches > 25% or unable to drink liquids) Grade IV (hemorrhagic ulcerations and/or unable to drink liquids and eat solid food)

III. A. Oral mucosa will heal within 10–14 days, and white patches (*candida*) are absent

IV. Potential for knowledge deficit, re: risk for stomatitis and self-care management

IV. A. Pt verbally repeats steps of self-assessment
B. Pt demonstrates self-care techniques (mouth rinse, brushing, flossing)

D. Encourage flossing qd and brushing with soft-bristled brush pc and hs unless plt < 40,000/mm³ or WBC < 1500/mm³
E. Encourage pt to remove dentures during oral hygiene rinsing and if irritating mucosa
F. Encourage pt to moisten lips with medicated lip ointment, water-soluble lubricating jelly, or lanolin
G. Encourage pt to avoid citrus fruits and juices, spicy foods, hot foods, and to eat bland, cool foods
H. Discuss use of antifungal therapy if candidiasis present

III. A. Assess oral mucosa q 4 hrs for evidence of infection, response to therapy
B. Assess ability to eat, drink, communicate
C. Assess level of comfort, discomfort
D. Culture ulcerated areas that appear infected
E. Cleanse mouth q 2 hrs while awake, q 4 hrs during night
   1. Alternate warm saline mouth rinse with antifungal or antibacterial oral suspension q 2 hrs
   2. Use sodium bicarbonate solution for thick secretions, debris: if ineffective in removing debris, use 1:4 hydrogen peroxide followed by water or saline rinse
F. Suggest soft sponge-tipped applicator to cleanse teeth, mouth pc and hs
G. Apply lip lubricant q 2 hrs

IV. A. Instruct pt in stomatitis as potential side effect of chemotherapy as appropriate
B. Instruct pt in daily oral exam
   1. Use of mirror and self-exam
   2. Signs and symptoms to report (burning, redness, blisters, ulcers; difficulty swallowing; swelling of lips, tongue; pain)
C. Instruct pt in oral care
   1. Remove dentures; wash and rinse mouth; and then replace
   2. Floss daily with unwaxed dental floss
   3. Brush with soft toothbrush and nonabrasive toothpaste pc and hs
   4. Rinse with water, saline, dilute sodium bicarbonate solution, or mouthwash without alcohol

(Continued)

TABLE A1.4 Standardized Nursing Care Plan for Patient Experiencing Stomatitis (Continued)

Nursing Diagnosis	Expected Outcomes	Nursing Interventions

		5. Avoid oral irritants (tobacco, alcohol, poorly fitting dentures, mouthwashes containing alcohol)
		D. Instruct pt in self-care q 2 hrs if actual stomatitis occurs
		  1. Cleansing solution of warm normal saline or sodium bicarbonate solution unless resistant thick secretions, debris; then can use 1:4 hydrogen peroxide with water rinse following
		  2. Medication application as indicated
		  3. High-calorie, high-protein, cool, bland foods
		  4. Small, frequent feedings; fluids to 3 liters/day

V. *Pain related to stomatitis*	V. A. Pt states relief from oral pain	V. A. Use mild analgesic q 2 hrs, timing 15 mins ac; gargles must be swished 2 min
		  1. Viscous zylocaine 2% gargles, 10–15 cc swish/spit q 3 hrs, duration 20 mins (max 120 mg/24 hrs; Brager and Yasko 1984)
		  2. Orabase emollient for local relief
		  3. 1:1:1 viscous zylocaine:diphenhydramine HCl (12.5 mg/ml):Kaopectate swish and swallow q 2–4 hrs
		  4. Benzocaine 20%—apply directly or swish and spit (duration 20 mins)
		  5. Dyclonine HCl (Dyclone) 0.5% 15 mins ac: 5–10 cc swish for 2mins, gargle and spit, onset 10 mins, duration 1 hr
		B. Parenteral analgesics may be necessary, including morphine infusion

VI. *Impaired verbal communication related to pain, increased or thickened saliva*	VI. A. Pt will communicate needs effectively	VI. A. Assess pt's ability to communicate B. If secretion is thick, copious, instruct pt in tonsil-tip suctioning technique C. Develop satisfactory communication tool if pt unable to talk (i.e., magic slate, writing message) D. Respond promptly to pt call light
VII. *Potential for altered nutrition: less than body requirements*	VII. A. Pt will regain baseline weight within 5%	VII. A. Premedicate with analgesics 15 mins ac B. Encourage high-calorie, high-protein, small, frequent feedings with cool, bland liquid or pureed foods; also, creative popsicles, custards

related to pain of mucositis

VIII. *Potential for infection*

IX. *Potential for altered tissue perfusion related to hemorrhage*

X. *Xerostomia (uncommon)*

VIII. A. Pt will be free of infection
B. Infection will be detected early and treated

IX. A. Pt will be without oral bleeding
B. Bleeding will be detected early and terminated

X. A. Pt will have moist mucosa with thin secretions

C. If inability to eat persists, discuss with MD need for enteral, parenteral nutrition
D. Encourage popsicles, ice creams as desired
E. Discourage citrus juices, fruits, hot and spicy foods, rough or hard foods

VIII. A. Assess oral mucosa q 4–8 hrs for s/s infection—culture any suspicious sites
B. Monitor vs, T q 4 hrs; if outpatient, teach pt to monitor temperature at least BID
C. Encourage pt to cleanse oral mucosa prior to administration of antibiotic or antifungal medication—keep NPO for 15–30 mins p̄ medication administration
D. Consider administration of antifungal or antibiotic as frozen popsicle if extreme pain, as this can decrease discomfort
E. Administer systemic antibiotics if ordered

IX. A. Assess for s/s bleeding in gingiva, mucosa
B. Remove dentures, partial plates
C. If *bleeding*, monitor platelet count, hematocrit
  1. Transfuse platelets as ordered
  2. Topical thrombin, aminocaproic acid, or microfibrillar collagen may be ordered (Peterson 1984)
  3. Leave clots undisturbed—discontinue mechanical oral care
D. Use sponge-tipped applicator rather than toothbrush if platelets $< 50,000/mm^3$ to minimize trauma to gingiva, mucosa
E. Encourage liquid, cool or cold, high-calorie, high-protein supplements as tolerated; pt should be NPO if bleeding

X. A. Encourage frequent mouth moisturizing with ice chips, artificial saliva (containing carboxymethyl cellulose)
B. Oral hygiene pc and hs
C. Encourage fluids as tolerated, offering fluids every 1–2 hrs
D. Discourage mucosal irritants (smoking, alcohol)

(Continued)

TABLE A1.4 Standardized Nursing Care Plan for Patient Experiencing Stomatitis (Continued)

Nursing Diagnosis	Expected Outcomes	Nursing Interventions
		E. Encourage soft, moist foods with sauces
		F. Encourage use of sugarless candy or gum to stimulate saliva production
		G. Increase air moisture as needed by humidifier or vaporizer
		H. Oral assessment q day, as xerostomia may precede stomatitis (erythema)
		I. Pilocarpine as ordered

Source: Barton-Burke, M., Wilkes G.M., and Ingwersen, K. 2001. *Cancer chemotherapy: A nursing process approach* (ed 3). Sudbury, MA: Jones and Bartlett Publishers, pp. 119–122.

TABLE A1.5 Standardized Nursing Care Plan for Patient Experiencing Diarrhea

Nursing Diagnosis	Expected Outcomes	Nursing Interventions
I. *Potential for altered nutrition: less than body requirements*	I. A. Pt will maintain baseline weight within 5% B. Serum electrolytes will be within normal limits	I. A. Assess pt's usual weight, dietary preferences, and usual pattern of bowel elimination B. Monitor intake/output, daily weight, calorie count as appropriate C. Encourage high-calorie, high-protein, low-residue diet in small, frequent meals (cottage cheese, cream cheese, yogurt, broth, fish, poultry, custard, cooked cereals, peeled apples, macaroni, cooked vegetables) D. If diarrhea is severe, recommend liquid diet E. Discourage foods that stimulate peristalsis (bran, whole-grain bread, fried food, fruit juices, raw vegetables, nuts, rich pastry, caffeine-containing foods and drinks) F. Encourage foods high in potassium as appropriate (bananas, baked potatoes, asparagus tips); monitor serum potassium, other electrolytes
II. *Potential for fluid volume deficit*	II. A. Pt's skin will have normal turgor B. Mucous membranes will be moist	II. A. Encourage 3 liters of fluid/day, especially bouillon, Gatorade B. If nutritional supplements are needed, recommend lactose-free or low-osmolality products C. Monitor intake/output

III. *Diarrhea*
 A. Mild/moderate (4–6 stools/day above baseline)
 B. Severe (> 6 stools/day above baseline)
	III. A. Pt will have normal baseline elimination pattern	III. A. Assess bowel sounds and abdomen for rigidity
		 B. Assess frequency, consistency, and volume of stooling and document, have pt maintain diary if an outpatient
		 C. Administer antidiarrheal medication as ordered; assess response to therapy; assess need for antispasmodics, antianxiety (anxiolytic) medications
		 D. Instruct pt in self-care measures
		   1. Self-administration of medications
		   2. Low-residue diet, fluids to 3 liters/day
		   3. Perianal skin care
		   4. Alternate rest/activity periods
		 E. Discuss interruption of chemotherapy with physician

(Continued)

TABLE A1.5 Standardized Nursing Care Plan for Patient Experiencing Diarrhea (Continued)

Nursing Diagnosis	Expected Outcomes	Nursing Interventions
IV. Potential for impaired mucosal and skin integrity, perianal skin, related to diarrhea	IV. A. Skin and perianal mucosa will remain intact	IV. A. Assess perineal, perianal skin, and mucous membranes for integrity and for s/s irritation B. Recommend sitz baths $\bar{P}$ each stool, if diarrhea severe C. Provide skin cleansing with water and mild soap $\bar{P}$ each stool, and application of skin barrier as needed, if pt unable to perform care; otherwise instruct pt in self-care D. Apply topical anesthetic as needed E. Use absorbent pads under pt to prevent maceration of skin
V. Potential for pain	V. A. Pt will verbalize decreased pain	V. A. Give symptomatic treatment to minimize or alleviate pain
VI. Potential for fatigue	VI. A. Pt will verbalize decreased fatigue	VI. A. Assess energy level and help pt to plan activities when energy level is maximal B. Assess for changes in lifestyle necessitated by diarrhea C. Encourage pt to alternate rest and activity periods D. Provide care that pt is unable to perform; encourage pt to involve family if pt is at home; consider/refer community agencies as needed (for homemaker, home health aide) if diarrhea is severe and resistant to treatment E. Assist pt in determining activity priorities and measures to conserve energy
VII. Potential for activity intolerance	VII. A. Pt will participate in activities important to him or her	VII. A. Activities will be consistent with pt's level of well-being

Source: Barton-Burke M., Wilkes G.M. and Ingwersen K. 2001. *Cancer chemotherapy: A nursing process approach* (ed 3). Sudbury, MA: Jones and Bartlett Publishers pp. 125–126.

TABLE A1.6   Standardized Nursing Care Plan for Patient Experiencing Alopecia

Nursing Diagnosis	Defining Characteristics	Expected Outcomes	Nursing Interventions
I. *Potential body image disturbances related to alopecia*	I. A. Chemotherapy agents attack rapidly dividing normal as well as abnormal cells. The cells and tissues responsible for hair growth have a high mitotic rate and are sensitive to the effects of chemotherapy. The potential depends on the activity of the drug in specific phases of replication. The drugs most commonly implicated in causing alopecia because they affect the S phase of the cell cycle are bleomycin hydroxyurea cisplatin ifosfamide cyclophos- melphalan phamide methotrexate dactinomycin mitomycin-C daunorubicin paclitaxel docetaxel topotecan doxorubicin vinbastine etoposide vincristine 5-fluorouracil vinorelbine B. Doxorubicin causes alopecia in greater than 80% of pts treated, usually within 21 days. Alopecia caused from cyclophosphamide depends on dose (occurs more frequently with higher doses). Alopecia from methotrexate is also dose related. With 5-fluorouracil, thinning	I. A. Pt, significant other, or family member will verbalize an understanding of factors that cause alopecia (chemotherapy, radiation therapy) B. Pt will discuss impact of alopecia on his or her lifestyle C. Pt will demonstrate knowledge of appropriate measures to minimize alopecia	I. A. Assess pt for being at risk for developing alopecia B. Instruct pt about hair loss, temporary or permanent, and the effects of chemotherapy on hair follicles C. Instruct pt on the potential for regrowth and for the potential change in color and texture D. Assess the impact of alopecia on pt E. Encourage verbalization of feelings F. Encourage pt to cut long hair short so as to minimize the shock of alopecia G. Discuss various measures to take during hair loss: wigs, scarves, hats, turban, use of makeup to highlight other features, baseball caps, cowboy hats H. Encourage support groups with people experiencing alopecia I. Encourage pt to help maintain personal identity by wearing own clothes in hospital and retaining social contacts J. Instruct pt on proper scalp care 1. Use baby shampoo or mild soap 2. Use soft brush to minimize pulling at hair

(Continued)

TABLE A1.6 Standardized Nursing Care Plan for Patient Experiencing Alopecia (Continued)

Nursing Diagnosis	Defining Characteristics	Expected Outcomes	Nursing Interventions
	of eyebrows and loss of eyebrows may be observed in addition to loss of scalp hair. Range of alopecia may be from thinning of hair to a total body hair loss. C. Regrowth depends on schedule of treatments and doses administered. Usually regrowth begins 2–3 months after cessation of therapy. D. Whole-brain radiation (5000–7000 rads) usually results in permanent alopecia as a result of permanent damage to hair follicles. Radiation to lower levels of brain may not cause permanent alopecia.		3. Use mineral oil or Vitamin A&D ointment to reduce itching 4. Always use a sunscreen when exposed to sun (SPF 15 or higher) K. If pt loses eyelashes or eyebrows instruct pt to use methods for protecting eyes (eyeglasses, hats with wide brim)

Source: Barton-Burke M., Wilkes GM., Ingwersen K. 2001. *Cancer chemotherapy: A nursing process approach* (ed 3). Sudbury, MA: Jones and Bartlett Publishers pp. 129.

TABLE A1.7 Standardized Nursing Care Plan for the Patient Experiencing Sexual Dysfunction

Nursing Diagnosis	Defining Characteristics	Expected Outcomes	Nursing Interventions
I. *Sexual dysfunction related to disease process, treatment, or infertility*	I. A. Cancer pts often experience some sexual alteration as a result of physical or psychological insults by the disease process, diagnosis, side effects of chemotherapy, surgical intervention, or radiation B. Some chemotherapy causes sexual infertility: chlorambucil cyclophosphamide doxorubicin cytarabine procarbazine vinblastine C. Dimensions altered by cancer therapy may affect behavior used to express sexual identity	I. A. Pt will demonstrate knowledge of factors that may potentially affect sexuality B. Pt will verbalize the potential impact of diagnosis on sexual activity C. Pt will maintain satisfying sex role and sexual self-image D. Pt will identify strategies used to minimize sexual dysfunction E. Pt or significant other will identify other measures used for sexual expression	I. A. Establish a trusting relationship with the pt B. Assess pt's knowledge regarding the effects of the disease and treatment on sexuality C. Provide a comfortable, relaxed environment in which to discuss with pt the effects of disease and treatment on sexuality D. Allow pt and significant other to verbalize perceptions of how disease and treatment will affect sexual function and sexuality E. Discuss strategies to minimize sexual dysfunction 1. Alternative forms of sexual expression 2. Alternative positions to decrease pain and prevent injury 3. Encourage sexual activity when energy levels are highest (in morning, after naps) 4. Help pt to recognize sexual feelings and urges 5. Include sexual partner in counseling and teaching 6. Explain effects of drugs and treatment on fertility 7. Refer for further counseling, if necessary F. Discuss options regarding alternative methods of family planning 1. Foster parenthood 2. Adoption 3. Provide information on sperm banking

Source: Barton-Burke M., Wilkes G.M., and Ingwersen, K. 2001. *Cancer chemotherapy: A nursing process approach* (ed 3). Sudbury, MA: Jones and Bartlett Publishers, pp. 131.

TABLE A1.8   Standardized Nursing Care Plan for Patient Experiencing Nausea and Vomiting

Nursing Diagnosis	Expected Outcomes	Nursing Interventions
I. *Potential for altered nutrition, less than body requirements*	I. A. Pt will maintain weight within 5% of baseline B. Pt will be without nausea and vomiting and, if it occurs, it is minimal	I. A. Administer antiemetics prior to chemotherapy, and then regularly through expected duration of nausea and vomiting (depending on specific chemotherapeutic agent) 　1. Evaluate past effectiveness of antiemetic regime 　2. Evaluate need for continuing antiemetics 12–24 hrs after treatment 　3. Attempt to prevent nausea and vomiting during first treatment cycle to prevent anticipatory nausea and vomiting B. Administer chemotherapy at night or late afternoon if possible C. Experiment with eating patterns: suggest pt avoid eating prior to, during, and immediately after initial treatment to assess tolerance; discourage heavy, greasy, fatty, sweet, and spicy foods D. Encourage small, frequent, bland meals on day of therapy (if tolerates eating day of therapy) and increase fluid intake to 3 quarts/day E. Encourage pt to suck hard candy during therapy F. Provide environment that is clean, quiet, subdued, without odors G. Encourage weekly weighings; if pt unable to stabilize weight, refer to dietitian for intensive counseling, together with person responsible for doing the cooking H. Teach pt self-care measures 　1. Self-administration of antiemetics, including indications, dose, schedule, and potential side effects 　2. Dietary counseling encouraging bland, cool foods, cottage cheese, toast, if experiencing nausea and vomiting

II. *Potential for comfort alteration related to nausea and vomiting*

III. *Potential powerlessness*

---

3. Encourage favorite high-calorie, high-protein, small, frequent feedings as tolerated; encourage fluids to 3 quarts/day, including chicken soup, Gatorade, sherbet, ginger ale

4. Give pt copy of *Eating Hints* (NCI free publication), with ideas such as whole milk plus 1–2 T powdered milk in eggnogs, snacks to increase protein, calorie intake

II. A. Pt will verbalize decreased anxiety and increased physical comfort

    A. Encourage pt to verbalize feelings re: prior treatments, if any, and significance of treatment to the pt

    B. Provide emotional support

    C. Consider anxiety-reducing drugs in antiemetic regimen, such as lorazepam

    D. Minimize time pt is in waiting room or chemotherapy room

    E. Provide distraction using VCR/TV or radio as pt desires; for some pts, having a chaplain read the Psalms during therapy can be quite therapeutic

    F. Teach pt progressive muscle relaxation exercises and help pt to imagine peaceful past experiences; encourage fresh air

    G. Keep emesis basin within reach, provide cloth for face and hands if pt vomits

    H. Assist pt with mouth care after emesis

    I. Telephone pt, if treated as an outpt, the evening of or the day after chemotherapy administration to assess tolerance and comfort

III. A. Pt will have control over self-care activities

    A. Pt and family teaching re: potential side effects and self-care measures; offer pt and family *Chemotherapy and Use: A Self-Help Guide* (free NCI publication)

    B. Encourage pt to live as normal a lifestyle as possible, going out and engaging in usual activities; often doing something "nice" for oneself *after* treatment helps to minimize the distress and increase control

    C. Involve pt and family in appropriate decisions in treatment

(Continued)

TABLE A1.8 Standardized Nursing Care Plan for Patient Experiencing Nausea and Vomiting (Continued)

Nursing Diagnosis	Expected Outcomes	Nursing Interventions
IV. Potential for knowledge deficit of self-care measures	IV. A. Pt will verbally repeat self-care measures and schedule for carrying them out	IV. A. Instruct pt and family member in self-care measures 1. Self-administration of antiemetics postchemotherapy 2. Drink 3 quarts fluids per day, especially chicken soup, etc. 3. Bland, cool, frequent, high-calorie, high-protein foods as tolerated 4. Call health care provider for persistent nausea and vomiting > 3 times/day, inability to keep fluids down B. Use a positive approach in teaching re: the potential side effect of nausea and vomiting, stressing efforts to prevent nausea and vomiting from occurring C. If nausea and vomiting occur, reassure pt that there are other antiemetic regimens that can be used to control, and hopefully prevent, it for the next cycle
V. Potential for injury related to nausea and vomiting (esophageal tears, bleeding)	V. A. Pt will be free from injury B. Injury, if it occurs, will be detected early	V. A. Reinforce teaching to call clinic or health care provider if persistent nausea and vomiting occur, as well as if pain, bleeding, or any other abnormality occurs B. If pt is taking steroids as part of chemotherapy or antiemetic regimen, teach pt to take pills with food

Source: Barton-Burke M., Wilkes G.M., and Ingwersen K. 2001. *Cancer chemotherapy: A nursing process approach* (ed 3) Sudbury, MA: Jones and Bartlett Publishers, pp. 140–142.

TABLE A1.9 Chemotherapeutic Agents Associated with Cardiac Toxicities

Drug	Dosage	Cardiac Toxicity	Occurrence	Comments
Aminoglutethimide	250 mg po qid	Hypotension, tachycardia	10%	Can occur at any time during treatment.
Amsacrine (AMSA)	100 mg/m² IV qd × 3 or 75–150 mg/m² IV qd × 5	Ventricular fibrillation Cardiomyopathy	5%	Risk is increased by accumulative dose of greater than 900 mg/m² or greater than 200 mg/m² of AMSA in 48 hrs. Increased incidence with previous anthracycline exposure. Cardiac toxicity is enhanced by preexisting hypokalemia.
Cisplatin	Unknown	Cardiac ischemia	Rare	
Cisplatin-based combination therapy	Unknown	Arterial occlusion events, MI, CVA	Rare	Reports of myocardial infarction (MI), cerebrovascular accident (CVA) after treatment with cisplatin, velban, bleomycin, etoposide.
Cyclophosphamide	120–270 mg/kg × 1–4 days	Hemorrhagic myocardial necrosis	Rare	Occurs with induced myelosuppression for bone marrow transplantation. Potentiates anthracycline-induced cardiomyopathy.
Dactinomycin	0.25 mg/m² × 5 days	Cardiomyopathy	Rare	Seen with previous anthracycline exposure.
Daunorubicin	400–550 mg/m² (lifetime dose)	Transient EKG changes Cardiomyopathy	0–41% 1.5%	Increased risk with concomitant cyclophosphamide or previous chest irradiation. Young children and the elderly are most susceptible.
Diethylstilbestrol (DES)	5 mg q d	Thromboembolic myocardial infarction	CVA, frequent	Risk decreased by decreasing dose to 1 mg qd.
Doxorubicin	450–550 mg/m² (lifetime dose)	Transient EKG changes Cardiomyopathy	2.2% 1–5%	Same as for daunorubicin.
Doxydoxorubicin (DXDX; synthetic anthracycline)	25–30 mg/m²	CHF (cumulative dose-related cardiotoxicity with 250 mg/m²)	Rare	Radionuclide ejected fraction performed after pt receives 150 mg/m² cumulative dose. Repeat at each dose of 250 mg/m².
4'-Epidoxorubicin (anthracycline analogue)	100mg/m² q 3 wks or 60 mg/m² dl, 8 q 28 days; 900mg/m² (lifetime dose)	Transient EKG changes, ventricular extrasystole CHF	1%	Spectrum of activity is similar to doxorubicin. Incidence of CHF is 1.6% when cumulative when doses of 700 mg/m² are given.

(Continued)

TABLE A1.9 Chemotherapeutic Agents Associated with Cardiac Toxicities (Continued)

Drug	Dosage	Cardiac Toxicity	Occurrence	Comments
Estramustine	600 mg/m² po in 3 divided doses	Hypertension, angina, myocardial infarction, arrhythmias, pulmonary emboli	10–15%	Increased risk with history of cardiovascular disease.
Estrogens	5 mg qd	CHF with ischemic heart disease, thromboembolic CVA	39%	Increased risk with history of cardiovascular disease.
Etoposide (VP-16)	Unknown	Myocardial infarction	Rare	May be worsened with prior mediastinal XRT and preexisting coronary artery disease.
Fluorouracil	12–15 mg/kg q wk; 1000 mg/m² qd 1–4 days as continuous infusion	Angina 3–18 hrs after drug administered; or during high-dose continuous infusion	Rare	Not necessarily with preexisting cardiovascular disease. Can recur with subsequent doses. Cardiac enzymes are normal.
Mithramycin	25–50 mg/kg IV qod × 3–8 days	Cardiomyopathy	Rare	Exacerbates subclinical anthracycline-induced cardiotoxicity.
Mitomycin	15 mg/m² q 6–8 wks	Cardiomyopathy	Rare	Increased risk with previous chest irradiation or anthracycline exposure. Synergistic with anthracyclines.
Mitoxantrone	a. 12–14 mg/m² q 3 wks	a. Transient EKG changes	a. 28%	Increased risk of cardiomyopathy with previous anthracycline exposure, chest irradiation, or cardiovascular disease. CHF has occurred in pts who have not received prior anthracycline therapy.
	b. 100 mg/m² lifetime dose with prior exposure to anthracyclines	b. Decreased ejection fraction	b. 44%	
	c. 160 mg/m² lifetime dose without prior exposure to anthracyclines	c. CHF	c. 2.1–12.5%	

| | | 29% | Asymptomatic bradycardia may occur during or up to 8 hrs after paclitaxel infusion; one fatal myocardial infarction has been reported. |

Paclitaxel	135 mg/m² or higher	Asymptomatic bradycardia; rarely may progress to heart block Rarely, chest pain, brief ventricular tachycardia or supraventricular tachycardia	29%	Asymptomatic bradycardia may occur during or up to 8 hrs after paclitaxel infusion; one fatal myocardial infarction has been reported.
Vincristine and vinblastine	Unknown	Myocardial infarction	Rare	Phenomena not well described.

Source: Barton-Burke M., Wilkes G.M. and Ingwersen K. 2001. *Cancer chemotherapy: A nursing process approach* (ed 3). Sudbury, MA: Jones and Bartlett Publishers, pp. 152–153.

TABLE A1.10 Standardized Nursing Care Plan for Patient Experiencing Extravasation

Nursing Diagnosis	Diagnosis Characteristics	Expected Outcomes	Nursing Interventions
I. *Potential alteration in skin integrity related to extravasation*	I. Vesicant drugs may cause erythema, burning, tissue necrosis, tissue sloughing	I. Extravasation, if it occurs, will be detected early with early intervention	I. Careful technique is used during venipuncture. A. Select venipuncture site away from underlying tendons and blood vessels. B. Secure IV so that catheter/needle site is visible at all times. C. Administer vesicant through freely flowing IV, constantly monitoring IV site and pt response. Nurse should be thoroughly familiar with institutional policy and procedure for administration of a vesicant agent. D. If vesicant drug is administered as a continuous infusion, drug must be given through a patent central line.
II. *Potential pain at site of extravasation*	II. Vesicant drugs include A. Commercial agents 1. dactinomycin 2. daunorubicin 3. doxorubicin 4. mitomycin C 5. mechlorethamine 6. vinblastine 7. vincristine 8. vinorelbine 9. idarubicin 10. vindesine 11. epirubicin 12. esorubicin 13. cisplatin 14. mitoxantrone 15. paclitaxel	II. Skin and underlying tissue damage will be minimized	II. If extravasation is suspected: A. Stop drug administration. B. Aspirate any residual drug and blood from IV tubing, IV catheter/needle, and IV site if possible. C. Instill antidote if one exists through needle if able to remove remaining drug in previous step. If standing orders are not available, notify MD and obtain order. D. Remove needle. E. Inject antidote into area of apparent infiltration if antidote is recommended, using 25-gauge needle into subcutaneous tissue.

B. Investigational agents
   1. amsacrine
   2. maytansine
   3. bisantrene
   4. pyrazofurin
   5. adozelesin
   6. anti-B4-blocked ricin

F. Apply topical cream if recommended.
G. Cover lightly with occlusive sterile
   dressing.
H. Apply warm or cold applications
   as prescribed.
I. Elevate arm.
J. Assess site regularly for pain,
   progression of erythema,
   induration, and for evidence
   of necrosis:
   1. If outpatient, arrange to assess
      site or teach pt to and to notify
      provider if condition worsens.
      Arrange next visit for
      assessment of site depending
      on drug, amount infiltrated,
      extent of potential injury, and
      pt variables.
   2. Discuss with MD the need for
      plastic surgery consult if
      erythema, induration, pain, or
      tissue breakdown occurs.
K. When in doubt about whether drug is
   infiltrating, treat as an infiltration.
L. Document precise, concise
   information in patient's chart.
   1. Date, time
   2. Insertion site, needle size, and
      type
   3. Drug administration technique,
      drug sequence, and approximate
      amount of drug extravasated
   4. Appearance of site, patient's
      subjective response
   5. Nursing interventions performed
      to manage extravasation, and
      notification of MD
   6. Photo documentation if possible

(*Continued*)

TABLE A1.10   Standardized Nursing Care Plan for Patient Experiencing Extravasation (Continued)

Nursing Diagnosis	Diagnosis Characteristics	Expected Outcomes	Nursing Interventions
III. *Potential loss of function of extremity related to extravasation*			7. Follow-up plan 8. Nurse's signature 9. Institutional policy and procedure for documentation should be adhered to
IV. *Potential infection related to skin breakdown*			

Source: Langhorne M. and Barton-Burke M. 2001. *Chemotherapy general principles for nursing practice administration.* In Barton-Burke, M., Wilkes G.M., and Ingwersen, K. (Eds). *Cancer chemotherapy: A nursing process approach* (ed 3). Sudbury, MA: Jones and Bartlett. Reprinted with permission.

TABLE A1.11 Standardized Nursing Care Plan for Patient Experiencing Hypersensitivity or Anaphylaxis

Nursing Diagnosis	Defining Characteristics	Expected Outcomes	Nursing Interventions

I. *Potential for injury related to hypersensitivity or anaphylaxis*	I. A. Allergic or hypersensitivity reactions to chemotherapy vary from simple allergic reactions to life-threatening ones
	B. The reactions are the result of a foreign substance being introduced into the body, with resultant antibody formation
	C. The reactions may worsen with subsequent exposure to the foreign substance (chemotherapeutic agent)
		I. A. Allergic reactions (hypersensitivity and anaphylaxis), if they occur, will be detected early
		B. Airway will remain patent
		C. BP will remain within 20 mmHg of baseline
		D. Future allergic responses will be prevented
			I. A. Review standing orders for management of allergic reactions (hypersensitivity and anaphylaxis) per institutional policy and procedure
			B. Identify location of anaphylaxis kit; the kit should contain:
			  1. epinephrine 1:1000
			  2. hydrocortisone sodium succinate (SoluCortef)
			  3. diphenhydramine HCl (Benadryl)
			  4. aminophylline
			  5. similar emergency drugs
			C. Prior to drug administration, obtain baseline vital signs and record mental status
			D. Observe for following s/s, usually occurring within the first 15 mins of infusion
			  1. *Subjective*
			   a. nausea
			   b. generalized itching
			   c. crampy abdominal pain
			   d. chest tightness
			   e. anxiety
			   f. agitation
			   g. sense of impending doom
			   h. wheeziness/shortness of breath
			   i. desire to urinate/defecate
			   j. dizziness
			   k. chills
			  2. *Objective*
			   a. flushed appearance (angioedema of the face, neck, eyelids, hands, feet)
			   b. localized or generalized urticaria

(Continued)

TABLE A1.11   Standardized Nursing Care Plan for Patient Experiencing Hypersensitivity or Anaphylaxis (Continued)

Nursing Diagnosis	Defining Characteristics	Expected Outcomes	Nursing Interventions
			c. respiratory distress and wheezing
			d. hypotension
			e. cyanosis
			E. ONS recommendations for generalized allergic response
			1. Stop infusion and notify MD
			2. Obtain orders for infusion of NS to maintain vascular volume and titrate infusion rate to maintain adequate BP (i.e., within 20 mmHg of baseline systolic BP)
			3. Place pt in supine position to promote perfusion of visceral organs
			4. Monitor vital signs q 2 mins until stable, then q 5 mins for 30 mins, then q 15 mins
			5. Provide emotional reassurance to pt and family
			6. Maintain patent airway and have equipment ready for CPR if needed
			7. Medications per MD order and institutional policy and procedure
			F. Document incident
			G. Discuss with MD desensitization versus drug discontinuance for further dose

Source: Langhorne, M., and Barton-Burke M. 2001. *Chemotherapy administration: General principles for nursing practice.* In Barton-Burke, M., Wilkes, G.M., and Ingwersen K. (Eds): *Cancer chemotherapy: A nursing process approach* (ed 3). Sudbury, MA: Jones and Bartlett.

TABLE A1.12 Management of Hypersensitivity and Anaphylactic Reactions

1. Review the pt's allergy history.
2. Consider prophylactic medications with hydrocortisone or an antihistamine in atopic/allergic individuals (this requires a physician's order).
3. Pt and family education: Assess the pt's readiness to learn. Inform pt of the potential of an allergic reaction and report any unusual symptoms such as:
   a. Uneasiness or agitation
   b. Abdominal cramping
   c. Itching
   d. Chest tightness
   e. Lightheadedness or dizziness
   f. Chills
4. Ensure emergency equipment and medications are readily available.
5. Obtain baseline vital signs and note pt's mental status.
6. As appropriate, perform a scratch test, intradermal skin test, or test dose before administering the full dosage (this requires a physician's order). If there is no reaction, the remaining dose can be administered. If an allergic response is suspected, discontinue the test dose (unless it has been completed), maintain the intravenous line, and notify the physician.
7. For a localized allergic response:
   a. Evaluate symptoms; observe for urticaria, wheals, localized erythema.
   b. Administer diphenhydramine or hydrocortisone as per physician's order.
   c. Monitor vital signs every 15 minutes for 1 hour.
   d. Continue subsequent dosing or desensitization program according to a physician's order.
   e. If a "flare" reaction appears along the vein with doxorubicin (Adriamycin) or daunorubicin flush the line with saline.
      (1) Ensure that extravasation has not occurred.
      (2) Administer hydrocortisone 25–50 mg intravenously with a physician's order followed by a normal saline flush.

This may be adequate to resolve the "flare" reaction.
      (3) After the "flare" reaction has resolved, continue slow infusion of the drug.
      (4) Monitor for repeated "flare" episodes. It is preferable to change the intravenous site if possible.
8. For a generalized allergic response, anaphylaxis may be suspected if the following signs or symptoms occur (usually within the first 15 minutes of the start of the infusion or injection):
   a. Subjective signs and symptoms
      (1) Generalized itching
      (2) Chest tightness
      (3) Difficulty speaking
      (4) Agitation
      (5) Uneasiness
      (6) Dizziness
      (7) Nausea
      (8) Crampy abdominal pain
      (9) Anxiety
      (10) Sense of impending doom
      (11) Desire to urinate or defecate
      (12) Chills
   b. Objective signs
      (1) Flushed appearance (edema of face, hands, or feet)
      (2) Localized or generalized urticaria
      (3) Respiratory distress with or without wheezing
      (4) Hypotension
      (5) Cyanosis
9. For a generalized allergic response:
   a. Stop the infusion immediately and notify the physician.
   b. Maintain the intravenous line with appropriate solution to expand the vascular space, e.g., normal saline.
   c. If not contraindicated, ensure maximum rate of infusion if the pt is hypotensive.
   d. Position the pt to promote perfusion of the vital organs; the supine position is preferred.
   e. Monitor vital signs every 2 minutes until stable, then every 5 minutes for 30 minutes, then every 15 minutes as ordered.

(Continued)

TABLE A1.12 Management of Hypersensitivity and Anaphylactic Reactions (Continued)

f. Reassure the pt and the family.	10. Document the incident in the medical record according to institution policy and procedures.
g. Maintain the airway and anticipate the need for cardiopulmonary resuscitation.	
h. All medications must be administered with a physician's order.	11. Physician-guided desensitization may be necessary for subsequent dosing.

Source: Langhorne M. and Barton-Burke M. 2001. Chemotherapy general principles for nursing practice administration. In Barton-Burke, M., Wilkes, G.M., and Ingwersen K. (Eds). 1996. *Cancer chemotherapy: A nursing process approach* (ed 3). Sudbury, MA: Jones and Bartlett. Reprinted with permission.

Antibiotics, antitumor. *See* Antitumor antibiotics

Antibody-dependent cell-mediated cytotoxicity (ADCC), 209–210

Anti-EGFR antibodies, 19

Antigen-presenting cells (APCs), 118, 164, 218

Antigens, 118

Antimetabolites. *See also specific antimetabolites*
  common, 31
  cytotoxic activity, 31
  mechanism of action, 5, 31
  toxicities, 31

Antineoplastic drugs. *See* Chemotherapy drugs

Antisense strand, 7

Antitumor antibiotics. *See also specific antitumor antibiotics*
  common, 32
  cytotoxic activity, 31–32
  mechanisms of action, 6, 31–32
  toxicities, 32

Apaf-1 (apoptotic protease activation factor), 13–14

APC germline mutation, 189, 191

APCs (antigen-presenting cells), 118, 164, 218

Apoptosis
  extrinsic pathway, 206
  final stage of, 187, 192*t*
  growth factor absence and, 26
  intracellular malignant flaws, as targets for molecular targeted therapy, 206–207
  intrinsic pathway, 206
  process of, 13–15, 26
  p53 tumor suppressor gene and, 187, 191*t*
  purpose of, 15, 206

Apoptotic bodies, 14, 206

Apoptotic protease activation factor (Apaf-1), 13–14

Arabinosyl cytosine (cytarabine; Ara-C), 62–63, 142

Aranesp (darbepoetin alfa), 152*t*, 158

Arimidex (anastrozole), 44–45

Aromasin (exemestane), 79–80

Arrhythmias, interleukin-2-induced, 127

Arsenic trioxide (Trisenox), 45–47

Asparaginase (Elspar), 48

Asparagine, 33

Aspergillus pneumonia, 245

Autologous activated lymphocytes (AAL), 171–172

Autologous hematopoietic stem-cell transplantation
  definition of, 215, 216*t*
  indications/rationale for, 217, 218*t*
  pretransplantation phase, 219, 220, 220*f*, 222*f*
  transplantation phase, preparatory regimens, 223–224, 223*t*

Autolymphocyte therapy (ALT), 171–172

Avastin (bevacizumab), 199, 200*t*

Azacitidine (Vidaza), 200*t*, 213

5-Azacytidine (azacytidine; 5AZ), 49

B

Base pairs, 182–183, 184*f*

Bases, 182–183

Basophils, 149

Bax, 206

B-cell leukemias
  mutations in, 193
  targeted therapy for, 207

B-cell lymphomas, targeted therapy for, 207

BCG, 118, 143

BCL-2 gene, 192–193, 206

Bcl-2 protein, 206–207

BCL-2 proto-oncogene, 192, 206

BCNU (carmustine), 55–56

Bcr-abl tyrosine kinase, 192

Beta-globin, 6, 7

Bevacizumab (Avastin), 199, 200*t*

Bexxar (tositumomab), 203*t*

bFGF, 204*f*, 205*f*

Bicalutamide (Casodex), 50

BiCNU (carmustine), 55–56

Biochemical approach, 34

Bioinformatics, 181

Biologic therapy (biotherapy), 117–172
  definition of, 117
  experimental, 160–172

Cell adhesion molecules (CAMs), 10, 15
Cell cycle
  activity of chemotherapeutic drugs and,
    26–27, 26*f*
  cyclins and, 25–26, 26*f*
  "master brakes" of, 184
  stages, 24, 24*f*, 25*f*, 190*f*
    G_0 or resting phase, 10–11, 24, 24*f*, 25*f*, 184
    G_1 or first growth phase or gap, 10–11, 11*f*,
      24, 24*f*, 25*f*, 184
    G_2 or second growth period or gap, 12–13,
      24*f*, 25, 25*f*, 185
    S phase, 12, 24, 24*f*, 25*f*
    M phase. *See* Mitosis
Cell cycle-nonspecific agents, 27
Cell cycle phase-specific agents, 27
Cell cycle-specific agents, 27
Cell cycle time, 27
Cell kill hypothesis, 28
Cell-mediated immunity, 118
Cells, cancer. *See* Cancer cells
Cells, normal
  apoptosis. *See* Apoptosis
  appearance of, 10
  cell cycle. *See* Cell cycle
  contact inhibition, 10
  function of, 10
  growth, abnormal. *See* Neoplasia
  growth/division, normal. *See* Mitosis
  growth of, 193*f*
  nucleus, DNA in. *See* DNA
  ploidy, 10
  tissue adherence, 10
Cellular vaccines, 168*t*–169*t*
Centrioles, 13
Centromeres, 3
Cerubidine (daunorubicin; daunomycin),
  67–68, 341*t*
Cetuximab (Erbitux), 201*t*
Chemokines, as immunoadjuvants for cancer
  vaccines, 161, 164
Chemotherapy drugs. *See also specific*
  chemotherapy drugs
  administration, 255–256, 259–260
    check list for, 261*t*–262*t*

extravasation injuries, measuring/
  documenting, 269*f*
infrastructure for, 256–257
multidisciplinary team and, 256
nurse preparation for, 260
nursing guidelines for, 260*t*
standard practice of care for intravenous
  chemotherapy and biotherapy,
  263*t*–267*t*
systemic, 256
worksheet, 268*t*
advent of, 23–24
cell cycle activity of, 26–27, 26*f*
cell kill hypothesis and, 28
cell kinetics and, 27–29, 28*f*
classification of, 29, 30*f*, 31–34, 260, 262
cumulative doses, 258
cytostatic vs. cytotoxic, 28–29
definition of, 28
intravenous, standard practice of care for,
  263*t*–267*t*
for nonmalignant conditions.
  See Nonmalignant conditions,
  chemotherapy
orders for, 257
preparation of, 262
single-agent therapy *vs.* combination therapy,
  34–36, 35*f*
targeting of DNA processes, 5–6
vs. cytostatic agents, 28–29
Chemotherapy-induced cell death, intrinsic
  pathway, 206
Chimerism, 218
Chlorambucil (Leukeran), 56
Chlorotrianisene (Tace), 77–78
Chromatids, 3
Chromosomes
  of cancer cells, 15–16
  complement of, 186*f*
  reference points, 187*f*
  structure of, 3, 4*f*, 182, 185*f*
Chronic myelogenous (myeloid) leukemia
  (CML)
  interferon-α therapy, 140, 141*t*, 142
  molecular targets for, 192